THE BEST OF

MEDICAL HUMOR

THE BEST OF
MEDICAL HUMOR

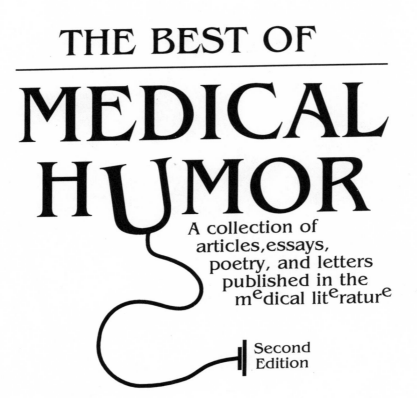

A collection of
articles, essays,
poetry, and letters
published in the
medical literature

Second
Edition

COMPILED AND EDITED BY
HOWARD J. BENNETT, M.D.
ASSOCIATE CLINICAL PROFESSOR OF HEALTH CARE SCIENCES AND PEDIATRICS
THE GEORGE WASHINGTON UNIVERSITY SCHOOL OF MEDICINE AND HEALTH SCIENCES
WASHINGTON, D.C.

HANLEY & BELFUS, INC.
PHILADELPHIA

Publisher   HANLEY & BELFUS
            210 S. 13th Street
            Philadelphia, PA 19107
            Phone: 800-962-1892
                   215-546-7293
            Fax: 215-790-9330

United States sales and distribution:

            MOSBY-YEAR BOOK, INC.
            11830 Westline Industrial Drive
            St. Louis, MO 63146

Library of Congress Cataloging-in-Publication Data

The best of medical humor : a collection of articles, essays, poetry, and letters published in the medical
    literature / compiled and edited by Howard J. Bennett. — 2nd ed.
        p.   cm.
    Includes bibliographical references.
    ISBN 1-56053-200-9 (alk. paper)
    I. Bennett, Howard J.
    [DNLM: 1. Medicine—Humor.   2. Wit and Humor.   WZ 305 B5613 1997]
PN6231.M4B47   1997
817'.54080356—cd21
DNLM/DLC
for Library of Congress
                                                                        96-37053
                                                                        CIP

The Best of Medical Humor, Second Edition   ISBN 1-56053-200-9

Last digit is the print number: 9 8 7 6 5 4 3 2 1

For Molly and Ryan

CONTENTS

MEDICAL SCHOOL

INTERNSHIP & RESIDENCY

ACADEMIA

MEDICAL LANGUAGE

WRITING & PUBLISHING

CONTENTS

POETRY

CONTENTS

CASE REPORTS

MEDICAL RESEARCH

CONTENTS

THE DOCTOR AT WORK

KEEPING UP WITH MEDICINE

INFORMED CONSENT & OTHER COMPLICATIONS OF HEALTH CARE

CONTENTS

SURGEONS & OTHER SPECIALISTS

MENTAL HEALTH HUMOR

ODDS & ENDS

CONTENTS

APPENDIX

ACKNOWLEDGMENTS

I would like to thank the following people, all of whom gave of their time to help me put this book together.

Richard Riegelman, M.D. who made a number of helpful suggestions and whose optimism convinced me that my efforts would qualify as "scholarly activity."

Mary Ryan, Karyn Pomerantz, and other staff members at George Washington University, who did all of my on-line searches.

George Paul, who helped me obtain many of the old books and articles I needed to review.

Cassandra Allen and other staff members at the National Library of Medicine, who made certain aspects of my re-search much easier than they otherwise might have been.

Marguerite Fallucco, who found material in the archives of the American Medical Association which was not available in any other library.

Judith Ratner, MD, for helping me decide whether to include certain articles when, after the twentieth reading, nothing seemed funny to me anymore.

Bill Lamsback, my editor at Hanley & Belfus, for his good ideas and for letting me play a role in all aspects of the book's production.

And finally, to all of the authors who have written medical humor over the years. Without their efforts, a book of this kind would never have been possible.

INTRODUCTION TO THE SECOND EDITION

When medical authors write an introduction to their second edition, they begin by telling the reader how much has changed since the first edition was published. What with all the new treatments and diagnostic tests, etc., a revision was absolutely necessary. So, of course, you must be wondering what's new in the field of medical humor. Are there new techniques available for recognizing a bad pun? Has it been shown that jokes reduce pimping on rounds? Will *The New England Journal of Medicine* begin publishing a weekly humor column in lieu of its boring CPCs? The answers to these questions are No, No, and Are you crazy?

So why, you might ask, did I decide to bring out a new edition of this book? My wife would say it's because I needed something to do after my children go to sleep at night. My editor would say it's because the first edition was so well received by the medical community. But the real reason is that I secretly wished to meet Dave Barry, and this is the best way to get his attention so he'll ask me to work with him on his next book. It's the one that will blow the socks off the publishing world. It's the one that will make fun of doctors and health care in ways unimaginable. It's the one that will win him his second Pulitzer Prize. Dave, are you out there?

I approached this edition pretty much like I did the first. After going "on-line" a number of times, I descended into the stacks at the National Library of Medicine. Looking through dusty old journals is a lot of fun, especially when I remembered to take along my albuterol inhaler. I not only ran into a fair number of amusing titles (Salmonella Excretion in Joy-Riding Pigs[1]), but I occasionally turned up a nugget of humor that's been buried for decades (see p. 58). Although I spent most of my time digging through the last ten years, I continued my ongoing search through the early 20th and late 19th century.

One of my most interesting finds is a poem that was published in *Guys Hospital Gazette* in 1909. William Osler was a major force in medicine at that time and the poem was meant as an affectionate roast of his book, *The Principles and Practice of Medicine*. The poem runs to fourteen stanzas, and contains 29 references to the sixth edition of Osler's classic text. Sir William had obviously impressed the English, as the following stanzas attest:

The Student's Guide to Osler[2]

Some people are keen upon Taylor
When studying medicine's wiles,
While others will steal a few moments with Wheeler
Both excellent books in their styles.
But give me the textbook of Osler
(Or don't, for I've bought it by now!)
And set *con amore* the laurel of glory
On William of Baltimore's brow.

It isn't so much that it's brainy,
Although it's undoubtedly that,
I'm not eulogistic because each statistic
Comes out so impressively pat.
It's all for the sake of the stories
He tells with a vigor so rare;
No poisonous bloater has dogged Minnesota
But goes to posterity there.

As before, after I filled a couple of boxes with material, I selected those pieces I liked best. Part of this process included a reevaluation of the first edition. Consequently, the astute reader will notice that a number of pieces were dropped this time around. I also edited some of the longer articles and did a little window dressing on a few others. All in all, about 50% of the material is new. I have also included an index to make it easier to find topics of interest.

One final comment. Anyone who looks at the contents will notice a disproportionate number of pieces written by me. There are two possible explanations for this. The first has to do with the way doctors write. Since doctors usually write light pieces as a break from the serious work they publish, most of them turn out humor infrequently. Given that I have an enzyme deficiency which prevents me from doing legitimate research, all I do is the lighter stuff. Therefore, it's not that I think my material is funnier than other people's, it's just that there's a lot more of it.

The second possibility is that I suffer from a rare condition known as *witzelsucht* (vit'sel-zookt). This is a mental state characterized by the making of poor jokes and puns of which the teller himself is intensely amused. (Check Stedman's Medical Dictionary, this really exists.)

If the first explanation is true, wish me luck (I come up for promotion next year). If the latter is true, wish my family luck (they have to live with me). Either way, I hope you enjoy the book.

Howard J. Bennett

References

1. Williams LP, Newell KW: Salmonella excretion in joy-riding pigs. Am J Public Health 1970;60:926–929.

2. Brockhouse S: The student's guide to Osler. Guy's Hosp Gazette 1909;23:420.

WHAT'S NEW IN THE SECOND EDITION

Since people don't read anthologies from cover to cover, I thought it would help if I summarized the major changes in this edition.

1. There are new references in the appendix and at the end of each chapter.

2. There is a new cartoon at the beginning of each chapter and a lot more filler throughout the book.

3. There is a new chapter called *Keeping Up With Medicine.*

4. There is an index to make it easier to find material of interest. In addition, the contents are referenced according to the journal in which they were first published. This was done to help readers figure out the type of material a journal is most likely to publish.

5. There is an article in the appendix for people who might be interested in writing medical humor.

6. Sixteen pieces were dropped from the first edition and 46 pieces are new.

A NOTE ON THE CITATIONS USED IN THE BOOK

Most of the references in the book are listed in the standard way. In some cases, however, you will notice the letter "A" before a page number. This indicates that the material was published in the journal's advertising pages. Since advertisements are not always preserved when a library binds its journals, you might have difficulty tracking down these references. If anyone is interested in one of these renegade articles but cannot find it, please drop me a note and I will send you a copy from my files.

INTRODUCTION TO THE FIRST EDITION

I got the idea for this book approximately four years ago. It was a Monday afternoon, and I was sitting in my office after a reasonably productive encounter with my filing system. Having never been schooled in efficient paper management, I usually approach this task like a child eating spinach: there are new piles every few minutes, but nothing disappears. On this particular day, however, things went smoothly. I placed a number of articles from my temporary into my permanent files and then refilled the temporary file with articles that had been blocking sunlight from the southeast corner of my desk.

It was during this last maneuver that I ran into Nancy Caroline and Harold Schwartz's article: "Chicken Soup Rebound and Relapse of Pneumonia: Report of a Case" (see p. 122). I had recently copied the article for one of my medical students and, as usual, had tossed it on my desk instead of placing it back in its folder. I reread the article, now probably for the tenth time, and laughed almost as hard as the first time I had seen it. It was and still is a marvelous parody on the case report.

After I put the article back in its folder, I began wondering how many times I had copied it for students and residents. Although it was always well received, to the best of my knowledge no one ever told me they had seen the article before. Was this really true? Was its possible that Mrs. Caroline and I were the only ones handing out copies of her daughter's article? And if that was true, what about other articles that had been published over the years? Was it possible that all medical humor was destined to obscurity?

To test my hypothesis, I set up a prospective study that same day. I administered a verbal questionnaire to the junior medical students in my clinic (with a 100% response rate) and found out that none of them had heard of Dr. Caroline's paper. A second study with our attendings revealed that 20% knew of the article, but only one could quote any of the references by heart (Bennett, unpublished disappointment). In both groups, however, over 99% said a collection of medical humor would liven up a doctor's otherwise drab and sagging bookshelves. It was at this point that I decided to search the literature to find out if such a project was feasible.

A book is a large undertaking, however, even one that collects previously published material. Therefore, I needed to consider a number of questions before I began:

1. How would I go about researching such an unusual topic? If I did a computer search using words like *humor* and *laughter,* would articles on the vitreous humor and gelastic seizures be cited? (Yes, on both accounts.)

2. Had a fair amount of humor been published in the past or would the manuscript end up being the thinnest volume ever submitted for publication?

3. Would the book encourage more editors to see the value of humor and, as a result, increase the space allotted for such writing? Might such a change in editorial policy jeopardize the future of medical research?

4. Is it possible the book would have a profound effect on the sense of humor of our profession as a whole? If that occurred, would it eliminate stereotypes that have developed over the centuries, thereby leaving nothing to parody from now on?

5. Would the book qualify for Category I CME credit?

6. Is it possible the book would influence the style of medical practice such that doctors might begin charging patients for dispensing humor in the office? Would insurance companies provide appropriate reimbursement for services rendered? And finally, would standards of practice develop such that doctors might open themselves up to possible litigation?

LAWYER: Why do you want to sue Dr. Bennett?
PATIENT: His jokes make me sick.

As you can see, this was tricky stuff. Nevertheless, the idea seemed like a good one, so I went ahead despite the possible consequences for the future.

The research itself turned out to be a lot of fun. I began by searching the "Wit & Humor" heading of *Index Medicus* and then moved on to additional data bases in allied health and nursing, medical history, and others. Despite my attempts at an organized approach, the indexing of medical humor has been uneven; consequently, much of my time was spent paging through non-indexed journals, tracking down references, and following up other leads. After 12 months, I was convinced there was enough quality material to put the collection together. In addition, I was surprised by the diversity of humor that had been published over the years.

Medical humor has appeared in a wide range of journals, from those of international reputation, to smaller specialty journals, to "throwaways." The humor itself has varied from jokes, cartoons, and anecdotes to articles, essays, and poetry. Those areas targeted for humor have varied as well, including medical school and residency, research, medical language, academia, writing and publishing, and clinical practice. Although the authors have primarily been physicians, medical humor has also been written by nurses, PhDs, and occasionally even by lay people.

As the collection grew, I began to notice certain trends in the publication of medical humor. While some journals published humor frequently, others avoided the area completely. Not surprisingly, the more prestigious journals published humor less often and usually accepted material of shorter length. For example, I am only aware of three such publications in *Chest* and while *The New England Journal of Medicine* has published a large number of poems and short pieces, these have generally been restricted to its correspondence section. Longer does not necessarily mean better, however, as some of the funniest pieces I discovered were published in *The New England Journal of Medicine.*

The most conspicuous absence, however, was in the area of mental health. Although my literature search turned up a bevy of articles on the use of humor in psychotherapy, I only uncovered a handful of humorous articles in psychiatric journals. To remedy this situation, I have stretched my definition of the term "medical literature" by including articles published in *The Journal of Irreproducible Results* and *The Journal of Polymorphous Perversity* (see Appendix). While these are not medical journals per se, they are geared to a professional audience and therefore I decided to bend the rules a little to balance the collection.

The type of humor published has also varied between journals. Cartoons, anecdotes, and articles dealing with clinical practice have appeared most commonly in journals like *Medical Economics*. On the other hand, the bulk of what I call "academic humor" has been published in the major journals and ones geared to students and residents. This trend obviously reflects editorial policy and the perceived interests of the readers.

Humorous medical poetry was the most difficult material to find because it is not well indexed and, as a general rule, turned up irregularly in journals. The one exception to this rule is a column called "The Medical Muse," which was published in *Postgraduate Medicine* from 1951 to 1972. The column appeared in almost every issue over a 20-year period and covered a wide range of topics. Interestingly, the poems were all written by the same person, a professor of English literature named Richard Armour.

Although poor indexing limited my ability to search the literature before 1960, it appears as though time has been an important factor in the publication of medical humor. For example, I found more sexist material in the 1950s and 1960s than recently, which undoubtedly reflects changes in our society as a whole. Also, many journals have changed their focus over the last two decades with regard to what and how much medical humor they publish.

The journal that has shown the greatest change over time is *JAMA*. Except for an occasional letter or essay with a light or satiric touch, *JAMA* has not published much humor in the last 20 years. In the past, things were different. Between 1903 and 1968, the journal ran four separate columns that featured cartoons, jokes, anecdotes, poetry, and satire. The names of these columns were: "Tonics & Sedatives" (1903–1962), "The Bright Side" (1954–1961), "Smile a While" (1961–1968), and "Satire" (1960–1968). While the last two columns featured medical humor almost exclusively, "Tonics & Sedatives" and "The Bright Side" also presented humor with a more general appeal. Unfortunately, these columns (like many others) were published in the journal's advertising pages. As a result, they have not been preserved in most libraries because advertisements are usually discarded in the process of binding journals. In addition to the four columns just mentioned, from 1964 to 1973 *JAMA* published a special issue each April that was called "The Book Number." Although the regular format was included, the issue featured articles on nontechnical aspects of medicine such as medical history, the illnesses of famous people, and that loosely defined area, "Literature and Medicine." Mixed in with these articles was a small sampling of medical humor and satire.

By the time I finished my research, I surpassed my initial expectations and had reviewed over 800 articles and many more short pieces. I next set about the task of wielding this material into shape. Although I enjoy cartoons and anecdotes, I decided to exclude these from the book. Not only would it be difficult to adequately search for the best in this genre, but collections of this type have been done before. The one exception I made was to include some pearls by Gary Larson, lest we forget that the medical literature is not the only source of humor poked in our direction.

In terms of style, the main issue I considered was that of humor versus satire. Although what distinguishes these two approaches can become blurred at times, satire more often relies on sarcasm to make its point. I was more interested in humor because of its general appeal and because it is more appropriate for a collection of this sort. In those instances where I did include satire, it was because the authors made their point so deftly and with such charm that they fit in with the rest of the book. Finally, because some humor is best left in the classroom, I made a conscious effort to exclude material that was overtly sexist or offensive in character.

In the final analysis, each selection had to fulfill two requirements. First, it had to say something about medicine, its clients, or its practitioners. And second, it had to make me laugh. Sometimes it was a deep, bellowing laugh like the ones reserved for Mark Twain or Woody Allen. At other times, it was the smile of recognition or a gentle laugh like the ones evoked by E. B. White or Garrison Keiller. Although I rejected a lot of older material, a number of authors have shown how durable an article can be if it is well done. One of the oldest pieces in the book is a letter published in 1884 by none other than William Osler himself—under the pseudonym Egerton Yorrick Davis. Finally, it was not uncommon to find two articles on the same subject and, in such cases, I usually chose the best one. In some instances I kept both because each one addressed the issue from a different point of view.

The book is divided into chapters to provide a framework for the variety of humor published over the years. Some chapters are shorter than others, which reflects the amount of material published in those areas and is not due to any bias on my part. For each selection, the author's name is presented with the title and a full citation is listed on the opening page. Selections that were published in a journal's advertising pages are designated with a capital "A" before the page number (e.g., A148). These references reveal a little bit about the history of medical humor by documenting which journals published what type of material. They also serve as a kind of road map for prospective authors concerning where their material might be accepted for publication. Each chapter concludes with a section called "Additional Readings" that provides annotated references for material not included in the book. Most of these references are for articles that were not quite funny enough to be selected but will be of interest to certain readers. The rest are for books that deal with the subject area of the chapter. The final section of the book is an appendix that contains information on additional books and journals of interest and a list of serious articles on the subject area of "Humor and Medicine."

Some people will undoubtedly read the book and notice the absence of their favorite article. As mentioned before, the research was difficult at times, and it is possible that I overlooked some publications. To any offended readers (or authors) I herewith apologize for my oversight. Please send me your neglected material so I can review it for the next edition.

Having now briefly discussed the history of medical humor and how the book was developed, it seems prudent to ask two final questions: What is the point of putting this collection together, and what are its goals?

First, in this age of increasingly sophisticated health care, it is important for physicians to be able to laugh at themselves and to retain a degree of humility about their profession. Contrary to popular opinion, doctors do have a sense of humor, and many editors have devoted valuable space in their journals to show this. Also, by providing a humorous look at the imperfections and oddities in medicine, the book reveals a human side of the profession that often gets lost in its technical writings.

Second, the book not only preserves the best articles in this area but also facilitates the use of humor in health care and teaching by pulling them together in one source. As an author of medical humor, I have received many letters telling me that my articles have been used in teaching rounds and case conferences, in journal clubs, and even to help relax prospective residency applicants. In my own practice, I use medical humor in lectures, to encourage the discussion of clinical issues, and to balance the serious material trainees and staff are required to read. Humor can teach, albeit from a different point of view than we are generally used to.

Third, although the book's primary goal is not to teach people to be funny, it may encourage health care workers to see the value of humor in day-to-day practice. Although few studies document the importance of humor in medicine, it is intuitive that such a connection exists.

"Whatever its origins, humor is enjoyable. We delight in those people who can laugh at the incongruities in themselves or in the world around them."

from "Humor and the Surgeon" by R. Dale Liechty, MD
Archives of Surgery 1987; 122:519

By sharing a moment of humorous insight, one can reduce the emotional distance between physician and patient and, in so doing, improve communication and mutual understanding. There are those, of course, who would argue that humor has no place in medicine (or in medical writing). To these individuals I would just say that all humor requires timing and must be used in appropriate circumstances. Like any other intervention, the beneficial effects should be weighted against the risks.

"In the undefined Good Old Days, a quality known as bedside manner was held to be important to the success of the physician. Then, the good doctor was knowing, sensitive, and above all, good-humored . . . Humor, like love is indefinable and yet is found to be important for establishing good relationships with patients, particularly the old and the young."

from "The Sense of Humor—Art & Science" Editorial,
JAMA 1970; 212:1697

So sit back and enjoy the book. Most of us will see ourselves in its pages and hopefully will get a good laugh at who we are and what we do to earn our living every day.

Howard J. Bennett

MEDICAL
SCHOOL

As long as there are medical students, there will never be a shortage of medical school humorists. Between the jokes, the stories, and the impersonations, no one is safe from their irreverent eyes. And if that isn't enough, each spring medical students put on their annual follies where they dance, sing, and perform their way into our hearts (or should that be through our hearts?). In one memorable skit from a few years ago, the students at George Washington did a take-off on *The Wizard of Oz*. In their version, however, there was a psychiatrist in search of a heart, an internist in search of courage, and a surgeon in search of a brain. Needless to say, it brought the house down.

Despite all of the creativity that goes into these events, medical students rarely publish humor. Perhaps this is because they are still test takers instead of paper-writers. Or because the medicinal value of humor is best when performed live instead of through hammering it out on a page. Either way, most of the articles in this chapter were written by physicians. The one exception is the article by Anne Eva Ricks which she published as a fourth year student. This was obviously a telling sign, however, as Dr. Ricks went on to write the successful *Official M.D. Handbook* (see Appendix).

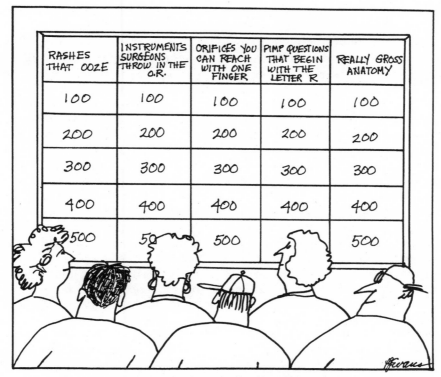

RASHES THAT OOZE	INSTRUMENTS SURGEONS THROW IN THE O.R.	ORIFICES YOU CAN REACH WITH ONE FINGER	PIMP QUESTIONS THAT BEGIN WITH THE LETTER R	REALLY GROSS ANATOMY
100	100	100	100	100
200	200	200	200	200
300	300	300	300	300
400	400	400	400	400
500	500	500		500

Jeopardy for Medical Students

THE MEDICAL SCHOOL INTERVIEW*

Eric A. Ravitz, D.O.

"Why do you want to become a physician, young man?"

"I really want to help people. Ever since I was a child, I can remember wanting to be a doctor. Watching *Ben Casey* and *Dr. Kildare* on television confirmed my desires, and no other occupation has ever entered my mind. . . . Well, yes, as a matter of fact, I have applied to dental and podiatry schools and graduate programs in anthropology, genetics, and business administration."

"Would you settle in a rural, underserved area?"

"Oh, yes, definitely. I've always wanted to help people in need in locations where no one else wants to work. I think the lack of medical support, facilities, and colleagues with whom to exchange views would be especially challenging, and as far as my family goes, well, there was life before shopping malls. Besides, I look forward to the invigorating experience of being on call 24 hours a day, seven days a week. My family won't need me."

*Reprinted with permission from Postgraduate Medicine, © 1985; 78(2):100–102.

"Why did you apply to this school?"

"Don't let my December suntan fool you. Since I was a child, I've dreamed about coming to medical school in the northern Midwest. I've always been fascinated by frigid cold and blowing snow, and I'm anxious to learn what such weather feels like and how the hearty, salt-of-the-earth midwesterner survives. I want to be a part of that culture. I figure that instead of jogging on the beach and plunging into the ocean afterward, I can cross-country ski to school for exercise. By the way, your school has a wonderful reputation in southern California. I understand that the local airline has three nonstop flights daily to Los Angeles. . . ."

And so it goes, another medical school interview successfully completed, another candidate accurately chosen. But what about some of the more pointed questions that might be asked during the interview?

"Do you like girls?"

"Well, ah, yes. I mean no. I mean yes, of course!" (I really blew it now. This trick question was intended to evoke "Hell no, medicine is my one and only love. I live, eat, and breathe medicine. I have no time for girls.")

"Do you like Oklahoma?"

"You bet, sir. Ever since I was a child, I've thought of no other place in which to live and practice medicine. Give me that good red dust any time. I just love Oklahomans too. My granddaddy traveled through Oklahoma one time. . . ."

"No, son, I meant the Sooners football team."

"Ah, well actually I have been following USC and UCLA for many years. Don't you just love John McKay? . . . I guess I could learn to love the Sooners."

"I have a letter of recommendation here that says you are intelligent and athletic and that you make a good appearance," the interviewer says with a chuckle. "Is that true?"

"Well, I would like to think my reference knows what he is talking about. He is a distinguished, well-known, best-selling novelist."

"Oh really? If he doesn't write for *Sports Illustrated* or the *Wall Street Journal*, I've never heard of him."

Would an interview accomplish more if it went as follows?

"So, while you were out of school you worked as a singing waiter at Luigi's Pizzeria on Fisherman's Wharf. How does that help qualify you to be a physician?"

"Well, sir, I met a lot of people and discovered that I'm a people person. I enjoy people, even with their complaints. (Luigi's pizza wasn't the best.) It was a challenge to put a smile on a customer's face. I think I want to be a gastroenterologist."

"Do you have any interests or talents?"

"I paint."

"Oh, what? Houses?"

"No sir, oils and watercolors. I've sold some of my work at a hometown gallery, too. As a matter of fact, since I don't have kids, I carry pictures of my paintings in my wallet. Would you like to see them?"

"Sure, son, let's have a look. Hmm, very good. Quite creative. I see that you like Picasso and Matisse. Do you think you can be this creative in your work as a physician?"

"If you folks on the committee are creative enough to give me the chance, I'll sure try."

A nurse called a resident at 3 AM. "Come quick," she said. "Your patient, Mrs. Parks, just swallowed a thermometer."

The resident hung up the phone and put on his jacket, but before he could get out the door the nurse called back.

"Never mind," she said. "I found another one."

HOW TO SURVIVE
A CASE PRESENTATION*

Howard J. Bennett, M.D.

Since the dawn of modern medical education, nearly two thousand years ago, students[1] of medicine have been faced with the delicate and unenviable task of collecting clinical information and presenting it to their attendings. History records that the first case presentation occurred in the year 174 AD when a 12-year-old intern roused Galen at 2:00 AM with the report of a slothful innkeeper who was choking on the jawbone of an ass. Galen correctly diagnosed an acute phlegmatic incarceration based on the history alone (hence the sanctity of the medical history) and dispatched the lad with the appropriate treatment.[2] Practitioners soon began priding themselves on their ability to arrive at diagnoses by reason alone, without the need of patients.[3] As the knowledge of disease and pathophysiology grew, so did the number of questions one could ask about a patient's case. As noted by Pimph (the **h** is silent) in his treatise on the case presentation, "Whether or not my questions have anything to do with the patient's disease is irrelevant."[4] Pimph's doctrine was quickly adopted by most prestigious medical schools, and the era of rounding on patients was soon at hand.[5]

Thus began the long history of having to contend with finding an appropriate response to the inquiries of overzealous, egotistical, and shortsighted professors. Being pimped, as it came to be called, was a dreaded fear of all medical students, compelling them to stay up nights studying instead of attending to the needs of their spouses. An example of the far-reaching implications of this difficult lifestyle can be found in a famous case of adultery that was widely publicized in the nineteenth century.[6] It was inevitable, however, that this system would eventually break down, and reports began to appear in the medical literature of omissions and frank fabrications in the presentation of clinical information.[7] These practices went unchecked for years until the publication of Quibble's monumental study on the psychology of case presentations

and the institutional hierarchy established therein (Table 1).[8] As a result of Quibble's work, pimping became less fashionable, although it is still rumored to be practiced somewhere in New England.

Managing Case Presentations

Managing a case presentation involves more than just reciting clinical information to your attending. It is an acquired skill, much like salivating to the dinner bell, that is passed on from generation to generation. In order to fully master the case presentation, you must first understand its structure. Fortunately, this topic has recently been reviewed, with particular attention to a new approach developed by Peeve.[9] As noted in Figure 1, Peeve's approach stands head and shoulders above the old system. Once the organization of the case presentation is understood, it is only a matter of experience to master its complexities. All students of medicine,

Table 1—Quibble's Classification of Case Presentors

The Medical Student:	Presents too much information, only half of which is relevant, and does not know what any of it means.
The Intern:	Obtains most of the information and probably knows what some of it means, but falls asleep presenting it.
The Resident:	Presents all of the information and knows what most of it means, but prefers arguing about the night call schedule.
The Chief Resident:	Obtains all of the information and knows what all of it means, but is too busy making out schedules to present it.
The Research Professor:	Has forgotten what a case presentation is, but will find a reference on it and get back to you.
The Clinical Professor:	Could obtain all of the information if he wanted to, but prefers to have others do it for him. Yes, he knows what all of it means too.
The Chief of Medicine:	Does not have time for case presentations. He is too busy editing the definitive text on differential diagnosis.

*Reprinted with permission from Chest, © 1985; 88:292–294.

Figure 1.   The Organization of Case Presentations*

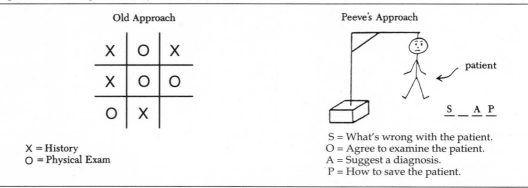

Old Approach

Peeve's Approach

X = History
O = Physical Exam

← patient

S _ _ A P

S = What's wrong with the patient.
O = Agree to examine the patient.
A = Suggest a diagnosis.
P = How to save the patient.

*Note how the O can be used in either approach, but will only solve the clinical problem using the Peeve system.

however, will occasionally find themselves in a situation where they neglected to obtain all the pertinent information about a case. The key to surviving a case presentation is knowing what to do when you have left something out.

According to Taube, the solution lies with a technique originally used in the field of education (personal communication, 1979).[10] In order to validate Taube's hypothesis, I have spent the last few years collecting information on well over four million case presentations. An initial review of the material suggested that many faltering presentations were, in fact, salvaged by the use of the clinical excuse (Bennett, unpublished doodling). In order to determine which excuses work best, the data was subjected to a detailed computer analysis using high bias tape. The results of this investigation are presented in Table 2.

Table 2—The Utilization of the Clinical Excuse to Save Your Academic Behind—and Future

Clinical Situation	Type of Information Missing from Case	Suggested Response	% Success	Alternative Response	% Success
In bed with your spouse	The case is beside the point; it's your libido that's missing	Initiate Foreplay.	72	Suggest a vacation.	100
Grand rounds	Anything (You're in big trouble)	Faint!	14	Set off your code beeper.	18
Everything else	History of the present illness	The patient argued that all history, by definition, is in the past.	58	The patient only speaks English.	74
	Past medical history	The patient said he has aphasia.	82	The patient said to get his old chart. (He might as well have aphasia.)	79
	Family history	The patient is adopted.	47	The patient suspects a history of anthrax.	88
	Physical exam	The findings are equivocal; you'll check again after vacation.	38	The area in question is either missing or congenitally absent you're not sure which.	53
	Lab data	The test is only run on the 5th Tuesday of the month.	59	The patient exsanguinated while waiting for the phlebotomy team.	37
	Consultant's report	Rounds went overtime; the patient was transferred to their service.	61	Your pet turtle ate it.	99

Conclusion

The various applications of the clinical excuse have been described in detail. When used as directed, these pearls will prevent undue embarrassment if a case presentation begins to crash. One can also expect a complete remission in the event of pimping, sneering, eye rolling, frowning, nitpicking, or should the urge to fawn or grovel arise. In closing, the reader is reminded of a well known verse by the late Ogden Cash:

> In the world of patients and places,
> There's no room for those who botch cases.

References and Notes

1. Used here in the generic sense, *ie*, a student is someone who knows less than anyone else around him, inanimate objects not included.

2. Galen: The use of an abdominal thrust to relieve acute phlegmatic incarceration: a case report. J Anachronisms 174 AD 20:188.

3. At least without having to see them. I think they still had to pay a consultant's fee or something.

4. Pimph DI: Bearing down on students for the perfect case presentation: a by-product of early toilet training. J Med Dogma 1646; 4:516.

5. Originally described by Grille (a student of Pimph's) as the "Age of Rounds." Grille was instrumental in the development of morning rounds, attending rounds, sign-out rounds and, of course, ground round.

6. Shyster B, Goose M: Goldilocks and three milkmen: a study of legal infidelity. Time Magazine, April 4, 1878.

7. Fallopian T: A third trimester pregnancy misdiagnosed as ascites due to the misrepresentation of a patient's sex by an intern. Arch Uterus 1896; 9:326.

8. Quibble D: Who follows the chief into the bathroom? A time-motion study of hospital rounds. Pedestal 1924; 44:128.

9. Peeve L: Three cheers for a new approach to the case presentation. CPC Annals 1976; 16:123.

10. Taube overheard a third grader tell his teacher that he did not have his English homework because his parakeet had eaten it the night before.

How many attendings does it take to change a light bulb?
    None—that's what medical students are for.

How many medical students does it take to change a light bulb?
    Three—one to hold the bulb, one to read the manual, and one to call the attending when it won't come out.

THE BEST OF GW FOLLIES

As noted in the introduction to this chapter, medical students rarely publish humor. What they produce instead is musical comedy—and lots of it. Every spring medical students across the country sing, joke, and cavort on stage as they make fun of their professors, medicine, and the process of becoming a physician. When I first got the idea to research these productions, I had no idea where to begin. Fortunately, the students at George Washington University have been videotaping their shows for the past 15 years. While I enjoyed the skits and monologues, this material does not translate well to the printed page. On the other hand, spoofs of popular songs do nicely in this medium. I reviewed over a hundred songs and selected those that were not only funny, but would also read well for people who did not know the original tune. In some cases I could not make out all of the lyrics and had to fill in the gaps as best I could. Finally, for anyone who wants a serious look at the value of medical school follies, see the articles by Daniel Segal and Anne Burson-Tolpin in the appendix.—H.B.

During my research, I found two classes that did takeoffs from *A Funny Thing Happened on the Way to the Forum*. The next song is a compilation of these two spoofs. It makes a great overture to the songs that follow.

Medicine Tonight

(To be sung to the tune of "A Comedy Tonight" from
A Funny Thing Happened on the Way to the Forum)

Something that's bleeding,
Something excreting,
Something for everyone,
It's medicine tonight!

IVs are clotting,
Patients are spotting,
Something for everyone,
It's medicine tonight!

Forget the books,
Forget the wards,
Who gives a lick
If we pass the boards!

Old situations,
New complications,
Nothing pretentious or polite.
Medicine tomorrow,
Comedy tonight!

Something contagious,
Something outrageous.
Something for everyone,
A comedy tonight!

Fourth years are sleeping,
Beepers are beeping,
Something for everyone,
A comedy tonight!

Cancel the scut,
We've had enough,
Let the attendings
Do their own stuff!

Something convulsive,
Something repulsive,
Something for everyone,
A comedy tonight!

Four years are through,
What can we do?
You know we'd love
To practice on you!

Something familiar,
Something peculiar,
These things and more you'll see tonight.
Medicine tomorrow,
Comedy tonight!

The next song was performed by a first year class. It begins with a skit in gross anatomy lab. The students are sitting around, cracking jokes about their professors and the consequences of smelling like formalin all the time. After they leave the stage, the lights dim and four "cadavers" get up and start singing.

Cadaver's Song

(To be sung to the tune of "The Jet Song"
from *West Side Story*)

When you're a stiff,
You're a stiff all the way
From your first night in here
To your last smelly day.

When you're a stiff,
If your guts hit the pan
You got students around
You're a cadaverous man.

You're never a whole,
You're always disconnected.
You're home with your own
When lab time is expected,
You're unprotected.

Then you are cut
With a capital K
Which you'll never forget
Till they cart you away.
When you're a stiff,
You stay a stiff!

When you're a stiff,
You're the low cat in town,
You're the gangrenous kid
With a formalin crown.

When you're a stiff,
You've lost all of your spring.
Little boy, you're a man.
Little man, you're a thing.

The stiff's are in gear,
Our abdomens are drippin'.
The knives will stay clear,
Cause every first year student's
A lousy chicken.

Here come the stiffs
Like a bat out of hell.
Someone cuts our insides,
Someone don't feel so well.

Here come the stiffs,
Freshman class step aside.
Better go underground,
Better run, better hide.

We're drawin' the line,
So keep your noses hidden.
We're hangin' a sign,
Says "Visitors Forbidden"
And we ain't kiddin'!

Here come the stiffs—Yeah!
And we're gonna rule
Every last freshman kid
In the whole crummy school.
In the whole crummy
Scalpel lovin' school!

The best part of second year is the class in physical diagnosis. After spending a year and a half in lectures, students finally get a chance to examine patients. The work is still overwhelming, of course, but at least it's a step closer to "real" medicine. The next song was performed by a group of students who just finished presenting cases to their preceptor.

My Favorite Things

(To be sung to the tune of "My Favorite Things"
from *The Sound of Music*)

Crackles and rhonchi and sibilant wheezes,
Downgoing toes in a patient who seizes,
E. multiforme with concentric rings,
These are a few of my favorite things.

Mitral valve prolapse and EKG squiggles,
Looking for pulses in babies who wiggle,
Tapping on tendons that never quite swing,
These are a few of my favorite things.

Lymph nodes in Hodgkin's and strep pharyngitis,
Tabes dorsalis and pyelonephritis,
Palpating livers from winter till spring,
These are a few of my favorite things.

When the day breaks, when my head aches, when I'm
    feeling sad,
I simply remember my favorite things, and then I don't
    feel so bad.

Rose spots with typhoid and neurofibromas,
Papilledema and cystic hygromas,
Choanal polyps that hang by a string,
These are a few of my favorite things.

FUO workups and patients with scabies,
Dipsticking urines and testing for rabies,
Talking with patients who think they are king,
These are a few of my favorite things.

Cotton-wool patches and histoplasmosis,
Sublingual masses and deep vein thrombosis,
Rectal exams that make anyone sing,
These are a few of my favorite things.

When the dean calls, when the ax falls, when I'm feeling
    sad,
I simply remember my favorite things, and then I don't
    feel so bad.

The next song was performed by a group of students during morning rounds. They are just about finished when their attending asks one final pimp question: "Okay, people. We just saw a patient with air/fluid levels in his head, chest, and abdomen. What's your diagnosis?" Two of the students are stumped, but the third one smiles and begins to sing.

Third Year Rounds

(To be sung to the tune of
"Supercalifragilisticexpialidocious" from *Mary Poppins*)

Because I was afraid to speak
When I began third year.
My intern gave my nose a tweak
And kicked me in the rear.
But then one day I learned a word
That saved my aching nose.
The biggest word you ever heard
And this is how it goes.

Oh! Naso-toxic-psycho-genic-recto-pneuma-tosis,
You could say the sound of it is really quite atrocious.
If you say it loud enough you'll always sound precocious.
Naso-toxic-psycho-genic-recto-pneuma-tosis.
Um diddle diddle diddle, um diddle aye!
Um diddle diddle diddle, um diddle aye!

I used to be afraid to go
And join my team on rounds.
I never knew the terms to use,
They'd always shoot me down.
But now I love it every day,
The critics all have softened.
When there is something you can say,
Say it loud and often.

Oh! Naso-toxic-psycho-genic-recto-pneuma-tosis,
You could say the sound of it is really quite atrocious.
If you say it loud enough you'll always sound precocious,
Naso-toxic-psycho-genic-recto-pneuma-tosis.
Um diddle diddle diddle, um diddle aye!
Um diddle diddle diddle, um diddle aye!

The beauty of this special word
Which always saves my butt,
Is no one's asked me what it means
Cause they don't have the guts.
If they knew I was bluffing
There would be a strangulation.
Because my diagnosis is
A pure confabulation.

Doing an acting internship is the hardest part of fourth year. And, as any AI knows, the nurses can make the difference between a pleasant and a miserable experience. The next song was performed by two acting interns who finally got a chance to rest during a rough night on-call.

The AI Blues

(To be sung to the tune of
Bob Dylan's "Rainy Day Women #12&35")

Well, they'll call you when the temp is 99,
And they'll call you when he's got no vital
    signs.
They'll call you just to give some Tylenol,
Oh, they'll call you just for anything at all.
Well you know it wouldn't be that bad at all,
If I didn't have to take call.

Well, they'll call you when you're walking
    out the door,
And tell you that your patient's on the floor.
They'll call you when you're crawling into
    bed,

And tell you that they think your patient's
    dead.
Well, I'd like to throw this beeper at the wall,
But that's what happens when you take call.

They'll call you when your patient didn't
    pee,
And tell you that he needs a new IV.
The patient's family thinks that I'm a creep,
But all I want to do is get some sleep.
Well, you know it's gonna happen to us all,
Cause everybody must take call.

Anyone who watches television is aware of those late night commercials that advertise collections of rock 'n roll oldies. Since medical students usually stay up late, it's not surprising that a number of shows included spoofs of these commercials. Here are some of the "hits" available on *Med School Rock*.

- *What Kind of Stool Am I?* (The Shigellas)
- *With Every Other Beat of My Heart* (The Arrhythmics)
- *Bruit, Bruit* (Sam Scott & The Aneurysms)
- *Bleeder of the Pack* (The Gel Foams)
- *Where Did Our Glove Go?* (The Rectals)
- *I Could Have Scrubbed All Night* (The Retractors)
- *50 Ways to Leave Your Med School* (The M CATs)
- *I Want to Hold Your Gland* (T_4 & the RIA Band)
- *Waking Up Is Hard to Do* (The Scut Monkeys)
- *I Am a Crock* (Simon & Carbuncle)

The next song addresses two hurdles that all medical students face. The first is deciding what they want to be when they "grow up." The second is *matching* in the program of their choice. It was performed by a fourth year student.

Residency World

(To be sung to the tune of
Sam Cook's "Wonderful World")

Don't know much about surgery.
Don't know much pathology.
Don't know why I must read these books.
Don't know much about the boards I took.
But I do know what I like.
And I know that if I match in psych.
What a wonderful world this would be.

Don't know much about neurology.
Don't know much gynecology.
Don't know much about the ICU.
Those EKGs they just make me blue.
But I do know there's little call.
There's no rectals and no bloods at all.
What a wonderful world this would be.

Now I don't claim to be an AOA student.
Cause it's not really me.
But maybe by being a psych student baby,
I can get my med degree.

Don't know much about nephrology.
Don't know much dermatology.
Don't know much about the peds I'm in,
And I'll never pull off medicine.
But I do know what I like.
And I know that if I match in psych.
What a wonderful world this would be.

See p. 111 for an entry that looks suspiciously like a follies song.—H.B.

PASSING THROUGH THIRD YEAR*

A Guide for Wary Travelers

Anne Eva Ricks

Starting third year is like going to a foreign country. You don't speak the language, you don't understand the customs, and the natives are not necessarily friendly. As in any foreign land, you must first master the vocabulary. Neither Robbins nor Bailey nor even the venerable Goodman and Gilman will help you. When substantiating a statement, you quote "the literature" or "the green journal," not "the magazines" or "you know, that little green handbook." Under no circumstances do you state, "I don't know where I read it." The more adventurous may state *"New England Journal*, March 24, 1972," but this is advisable in only two circumstances; one, if it really *is NEJM*, March 24, 1972, or two, if you *know* no one has any interest in looking it up. When a topic comes up, you can always say, "I think the [major journal of that specialty] has an article on that," because it usually does and because everyone will be impressed that you are actually reading the journals. If anyone wants more details on it, rather than elaborating, which of course you cannot do (because at most you have read the table of contents), tell him or her that you will bring in the reference tomorrow. And if you can't find the reference, don't worry, no one will likely remember by the next day.

When presenting, the format and the vocabulary are critical. Findings are "pertinent" or they are "noncontributory." Believe me, faces light up when you say the review of systems, occupational history, and past medical history are noncontributory; everyone is rushed and likes to feel confident that you understand what is and isn't important. Of course, your backside is fried if it *is* contributory.

Dress and props are important and should be tailored to the particular specialty. Appropriate props for any medical student include a white coat with at least seven pockets crammed to the top with pens, calculator, index cards, lunch money, stethoscope, ophthalmoscope, reflex hammer, tuning forks, safety pin, *The Washington Manual*, a handbook for the rotation you are on, and a notebook for pearls. Trucking around with the largest textbook put out for that field (anything over 20 lbs.) will intimidate your fellow students, and carrying the latest journal will intimidate your interns (who haven't had time to read anything since they were medical students). Of course, you will use at home whatever concise little handbook is current at the time.

On medicine, wearing almost anything from L. L. Bean but the hiking boots is appropriate; Oxford cloth shirt, knit tie, striped belt, and khaki pants are the uniform. The tie is optional for women. A bow tie is indicated only if: (1) you are either incredibly brilliant and a little strange, or (2) you are the attending who is frequently referred to as "Dr. Smith, the father of his field." Otherwise, you are putting out a lightning rod.

On surgery, scrubs are always appropriate, unless you have an alert infectious disease department. To dress up, you may put on regular trousers or perhaps a white coat. An optional touch, one to assure everyone that you are not really a medicine intern dressing up in wolf's clothing, is surgical shoe covers with something indescribably foul on them (this can be fallout from the O.R. or just lunch fragments from the VA cafeteria). Track shoes and Job stockings are definite signs that you are a gunner.

On pediatrics, the more outlandish your outfit the better. Colors which test pupillary constriction are popular, especially in combinations. Paraphernalia on your coat is absolutely *de rigueur*; koala bears hugging your stethoscope, buttons promoting fund raising or condemning smoking, and whatever symbols

*Reprinted with permission from The New Physician, © 1982; 31(8):16–19. Copyright by American Student Medical Association. Edited from the original.

of upcoming holidays that are wearable (skeletons, Easter bunnies, flags) are basics.

On ob/gyn, you can wear anything you want, but avoid being seen carrying *Ms. Magazine.* A Brooks Brothers suit and a copy of the *Wall Street Journal* (with your broker's phone number scribbled on front) is perfect camouflage for ENT. On anesthesia, adopting a foreign accent might help and *Field and Stream* will assure them that you are "just one of the guys."

Now that you know the language and some of the colorful native costumes, a few cardinal rules to insure your survival are in order.

Remain conscious at all times. Because remaining conscious at all times is difficult unless you have a well-established amphetamine habit, the second best thing is to maintain the appearance of consciousness at all times. In conference, always sit next to the wall, always lean on one elbow, and never put your head down. Avoid sitting next to the attending in conference, as he has probably had seven hours of sleep the night before and will, unlike your colleagues, notice if you snore.

Remain oriented at all times. Your residents will help you with this, orienting you to your location with comments such as "This is the pits," "Compared to this, the Black Hole of Calcutta looks like Club Med," and "No, this isn't Kansas and you aren't Toto—you are a scutpuppy." Your entire team may orient you, as mine once did, with a harmonious and rousing rendition of "Dodedodo dodedodo you are now entering . . . The Toilet Zone!" They will also help orient you to time. Time on medical services is not based on changes in day and night. Everything centers on "Rounds Time," such as in "We have a three blood gases to do and a chest x-ray to find, and it's two hours to rounds."

Keep your thoughts collected. This can be difficult when your mind is blank. However, when the inevitable happens, and you are awakened from a deep sleep by the jolting voice of an attending asking, "Dr. Ricks, what is the usual pathogenesis of this encephalopathy?" keep calm. Stall for time, Say, "AAAaaaaaaah. . . . wellllll." Don't say "What? Who? Is this a joke?" Rely on the kindness of your residents; if a member of your team is whispering *anything*—from "branched chain amino acids" to "guacamole dip"—repeat it loudly and confidently. Of course, you do have to trust your team.

Avoid maligning the field in which you are ro-tating. Statements such as "This is the most disgusting thing I have ever seen," or corollaries such as *"Touch* it? Are you joking?" are bound to antagonize your residents and hurt their feelings. Remember, they have chosen, for whatever unfathomable reason, to do this for their whole lives. So don't say it. Of course, you are free to think anything you want.

Be ready for the $64,000 question: What are you going into? Watch out for this. People will ask you for different reasons and have different responses, but remember that this is a foreign place, analogous to prewar Germany, with many fiercely warring provincial duchies, and you are a simple pawn. People leap to all kinds of conclusions about your competence, intelligence, moral character, personality, and avariciousness based on your reply, and you can't even predict which erroneous assumption to which they will leap. However, if you tell the medicine man that you are going into medicine, he will assume that you are an ally and that you are like him. Tell a medicine man you are going into surgery, and you are a willful ignoramous until proven otherwise.

I would tell people what I was going into, but quickly add statements to counteract the reflex prejudice; e.g., to the medicine people, "I'm going into surgery; but I really want to learn medicine and I think it's very important, and, really, I know how to read and I sometimes even *like* to read! Honest!" On psychiatry: "I'm going into surgery but I really do see patients as whole people and I'm not an insensitive oaf. At least not most of the time." What a relief it was to be on surgery. I was delighted when anyone asked me, and always effusive: "Yes, I'm going into surgery! I love this! I want to be just like you!" One woman who is going into psychiatry felt obligated to repeatedly explain that, although her primary interest was the mind, she was interested in all of medicine and wanted to learn as much as she could during her short exposure to the rotations.

Of course, you can be like one scrofulous S.O.B. with whom I worked, who wormed his slimy way through every rotation with brazen flattery, which worked very frequently to smooth his way: from "Why, I think pediatric oncology is without doubt my primary interest," to "I've wanted to be an obstetrician since high school," to "Cardiovascular surgery, just like you, Sir!" I had to up my dose of Compazine when working with him. Although doing this will probably curry the favor of one's attending, you may well become a social pariah. There might, as well, be a few tough ethical questions somewhere down the line.

Probably the easiest thing to do, if you don't want to get involved, is tell everyone you don't know. You may come off as colorless or indecisive, but at least no one will make unwarranted assumptions.

Stay Cheerful. This last rule is probably the most important and the hardest to follow. You really are in a foreign country; remind yourself that you are there by choice. You can always leave, permanently or for a breather. Seek out your fellow students no matter how incompetent, abused, or lost you may feel. Someone else invariably has a story to top yours. No one knows what is going on, and you've got to take your ego off the line. It's hard after decades of academic excellence to feel dumb and foolish every morning, but you can take it.

Even though you have entered a foreign country, you are there to stay.

A Glossary for the Wards

Communication is a major problem for medical students. It's not the writing of the history and physicals nor the deciphering of those ophthalmology consults, nor even understanding the bizarre endocrinology laboratory jargon that's the problem. The real issue is communication between residents and third-year medical students. For instance, most medical students do not understand that when the chief resident in neurosurgery says, "Take those bloods down to lab as soon as possible," he means, "*Run* them down *now*." Or when the team captain on medicine says to the third-year student, "Do we have an EKG on Mr. Morris?" he means, "Go do an EKG on Mr. Morris, interpret it, and bring it back to me—before attending rounds."

Of course, the average medical student is reasonably bright and will pick up these nuances throughout the third year, with only a few major embarrassing and ego-shattering incidents.

But the following phrases, and their usage maybe helpful:

1. **"You have to learn to do this sometime."** This generally refers to a menial piece of scut that is important only in that completion of medical school is predicated on its accomplishment and not because of any intrinsic value; i.e., disimpacting a 101-year-old nursing home resident who has been frozen in a comatose fetal position since the Truman administration, or starting an I.V. in an ex-heroin addict who quit the habit because *he* couldn't find any more veins. But no resident will ever understand that mastery of starting an I.V. in an ex-heroin addict will not help you one bit in your child psychiatry practice in Scarsdale. So just learn to do it.

2. **"Medicine is an art, not a science."** Doubles as a phrase to be used with patients, especially when something has gone wrong, is about to go wrong, or is wrong without medical solution. It is best used with the patient who has just completed the $64,000 work-up for his chronic fatigue, from spinal tap to ultrasound, without arriving at a diagnosis. Also used by out-of-date attendings who haven't kept up their biochemistry and pharmacology and wish to stifle upstart residents who threaten to expose their knowledge deficit.

3. **"All bleeding stops."** Best used by hardened surgical chief resident in dire straits, i.e., when the multiple trauma patient rolls in from St. Elsewhere with a sucking chest wound and exposed entrails on the E.R. stretcher. Should be said only by the surgeon in charge and stated with absolute confidence. It is considered entirely inappropriate for the medical student to say this, or anything, in this situation.

4. **"Everyone has blood."** Most frequent comment made by interns to third-year medical students after unsuccessful attempts at phlebotomy. Statement is generally made in a patient's room, where the student is surrounded by syringes, 4 × 4s, tourniquet, wrappers, tubes, lab slips, and at least seven used needles and six blown veins on one irate patient.

5. **"What are you going to specialize in, psychiatry?"** This is a flashing red warning sign if said to a medical student by anyone other than a psychiatrist. If a surgeon says it, he thinks you're nuts, or he caught you actually talking to a patient. If a medicine doctor says it, he thinks you're lazy. If an ob/gyn doctor says it, he simply noticed that you fainted at your first screaming-through-the-E.R.-door-with-a-baby-between-the-legs-and 2,000 cc-blood-loss (mostly on your clothing) delivery.

6. **"No, I'm not a nurse."** Most frequent state-

ment uttered by women residents and medical students. Explaining that you are the Nobel Laureate in endocrinology or the TV repair lady will fall on deaf ears. No matter what you tell the patient hollering "Nurse! Nurse!" at you on rounds, he will then say, "Well, anyway, whatever you are, my bedpan needs emptying." Take it with grace and humor. It will happen often. It will amuse your colleagues and add levity to rounds (which is generally in sore need). It isn't the patients' fault: most people don't realize the number of women in medicine, and 90 percent of the time they're right if they call a woman in white a nurse. Besides, if you get upset every time someone calls you nurse, you're going to need lifelong maintenance cimetidine therapy.

7. "Maybe it's not too late to go to law school." Frequently used by students, residents, and attendings alike. Most often heard during disasters and when icky unidentified things are discovered on one's clothing, or in response to any of numbers one through six above. This is never seriously meant and is usually just a wish for a job in which icky unidentified things don't routinely wind up on one's clothes.

8. "I can't do it. I'm too tired. This is disgusting." No. No. No. These phrases do not exist for the medical student nor the resident. They are not in your vocabulary. Besides, even if you are really, honestly, too exhausted to do something, they're going to make you do it anyway, be it hold retractors for a renal transplant from 3 AM to 7 AM or completely work up your seventh E.R. admission with diabetes, renal failure, schizophrenia, and a medical record that comes up Volume 6 of 7 (but 7 is missing). Since you're going to do it anyway, save your energy for the task at hand instead of wasting it on futile protestation.

So on the wards, keep alert for the difference between what is said and what is meant. Sure it's scary to be in the hospital without any real sense of what you are supposed to be doing or how you should be doing it, but it's not that bad an experience. It'll only hurt a little. Really.

Doctors should never talk to patients about anything but medicine. When doctors talk politics, economics or sports, they reveal themselves to be ordinary mortals—you know, idiots like the rest of us.

Andy Rooney

THE STUDENT'S DILEMMA *

Howard J. Bennett, M.D.

The play takes place at 7:30 PM at a Roy Rogers Restaurant. Dennis Miller, a third-year medical student, is hunched over a partially eaten bacon cheeseburger. His face is unshaven, and his eyes look like crushed sardines. Sitting across from Dennis is Dr. Simon, a man in his mid-forties with an open tweed jacket and buttons straining to keep his abdomen out of the coleslaw. Dennis obviously was on call the night before. Dr. Simon, on the other hand, has no excuse for his appearance.

DENNIS: Thanks for inviting me to dinner, Dr. Simon. I really needed to talk to someone.

DR. SIMON: My pleasure Dennis. You certainly sounded distraught on the phone. Tuition problems?

DENNIS: Worse. My fourth-year schedule is due next week, and I still don't know what I want to be when I grow up.

DR. SIMON: Oh, that. All you need to do is set up an appointment with your advisor. He'll straighten things out for you.

DENNIS: You are my advisor, Dr. Simon.

DR. SIMON: Am I really? In that case, tell me what's on your mind.

DENNIS: Well, in the first place, it seems like everyone else knows what they want in life but me.

DR. SIMON (lighting his pipe): Uh-huh.

DENNIS: For example, did you always know what you wanted to be?

DR. SIMON: Not until the sixth grade.

DENNIS: You knew you wanted to be a doctor in the six grade!

DR. SIMON: Fifth actually. In the sixth grade, I decided on neuropsychiatry as a subspecialty.

DENNIS: Oh great—just what I needed to hear.

DR. SIMON: Sorry, Dennis, but I've always been precocious. Why, I even had my midlife crisis before I was 30.

DENNIS: Then I'm not alone?

DR. SIMON: Of course not.

DENNIS: But what about my classmates? A lot of them seem to know what they want to do.

DR. SIMON: Sure they do. And a lot of them eat sushi, but that doesn't mean it tastes good. You've got to stop comparing yourself with everyone else.

DENNIS: You're right. I know you're right. But tell me, what should I do?

DR. SIMON: First, you should realize that you're probably approaching the decision all wrong.

DENNIS: I am?

DR. SIMON: Well, the mistake most students make is trying to base decisions on their third-year clerkships. That never gets you anywhere.

DENNIS: How so?

DR. SIMON: Most students use what Freud called the laundry-list approach.

DENNIS: You mean making a list of what they do and don't like about the various specialties?

DR. SIMON: Exactly.

DENNIS (reaching into his pocket): I have mine right here.

DR. SIMON: List making may work for buying underwear or getting married, but it's rarely helpful with career counseling.

DENNIS: Maybe not, but what else can I do?

DR. SIMON: You've got to tap into your unconscious.

DENNIS: My what?

DR. SIMON: Your unconscious. You know, that little voice that slips out after nights on call or when your blood alcohol level rises above your IQ.

DENNIS: But I thought you were a neuropsychiatrist. Why all this interest in the unconscious?

DR. SIMON: It's just a hobby.

DENNIS: Well, you picked a good night for it. But what does my unconscious have to do with choosing a career?

DR. SIMON: Everything. The best way to determine true compatibility is to look for the deeper associations. For example, going into surgery just because you like tying knots isn't enough.

*Reprinted with permission from Postgraduate Medicine, © 1986; 80(5):266–274.

DENNIS: But how do I go about tapping into my unconscious?

DR. SIMON: It's quite simple, actually. I'll ask you four questions that relate to some everyday situations. All you have to do is answer with the first thing that comes to mind.

DENNIS: That's all there is to it?

DR. SIMON: That's all. Now, why don't you sit back and relax.

DENNIS (leans back and closes his eyes): Okay, I'm ready.

DR. SIMON: Here's the first question. Tell me which bodily fluid is least offensive to you?

DENNIS: Hmmm, let me see . . .

DR. SIMON: Quickly now, the first thing that pops into your head.

DENNIS: Urine.

DR. SIMON: Good! That's one for pediatrics.

DENNIS (sitting up in his chair): Peds—are you sure?

DR. SIMON: It's a start, but we've got more to go.

DENNIS: But peds? I haven't even done my pediatrics rotation yet.

DR. SIMON: You're thinking like a third-year student again.

DENNIS: Okay, okay. But what if I had said blood?

DR. SIMON: Then I would have said surgery.

DENNIS: Sweat?

DR. SIMON: Family practice.

DENNIS: And tears?

DR. SIMON: Psychiatry.

DENNIS: Hmmm. What about Ob/Gyn? What's least offensive to them?

DR. SIMON: No one knows for sure.

DENNIS: And medicine? You didn't give me a choice for medicine.

DR. SIMON: All bodily fluids are offensive to internists.

DENNIS: Well, you're right about that. And I do like children, but . . .

DR. SIMON: No buts, Dennis. Let's move on to question two.

DENNIS: If you say so.

DR. SIMON: What card games do you like to play?

DENNIS (sits up in his chair again): Card games! You can't be serious.

DR. SIMON: Dennis, you're going to block your unconscious if you get excited. Now, why don't you sit back and relax.

DENNIS: Okay, I'll try. . . . Well, I do like playing cards with my niece.

DR. SIMON: And what do you and your niece play together?

DENNIS: Go fish.

DR. SIMON: There we go again.

DENNIS: You mean peds?

DR. SIMON: You said it, Dennis. I didn't.

DENNIS: That's true, I did. But I also play bridge with my roommate. Doesn't that count for anything?

DR. SIMON: What does your roommate do?

DENNIS: He's a fourth-year student.

DR. SIMON: And?

DENNIS: And he's going into medicine.

DR. SIMON: I see. Do you like bridge?

DENNIS: Not really.

DR. SIMON: I thought so.

DENNIS: But what about the other specialties? What associations would you draw for them?

DR. SIMON: Good question. I'll tell you what. I'll mention the other specialties, and you tell me the connections you would make. After all, you may be an advisor yourself someday.

DENNIS (self-consciously): I'll try.

DR. SIMON: Surgery?

DENNIS: War—at least for general surgeons. urologists probably play pinochle.

DR. SIMON: Mine certainly does. But let's stay away from subspecialists tonight. Remember, it's only our first session. How about psychiatry?

DENNIS: Crazy eights.

DR. SIMON: Ob/Gyn?

DENNIS: Poker.

DR. SIMON: Family practice?

DENNIS: Hearts.

DR. SIMON: That's pretty good, Dennis. I think you're getting the hang of it. What's your favorite candy?

DENNIS (leaning forward): Is this part of the session, or do you just want to buy me dessert?

DR. SIMON: You're wavering again.

DENNIS: Candy! What can I possibly learn from candy?

DR. SIMON: Plenty. Now quick, who do you think likes Life Savers the most?

DENNIS: Surgeons?

DR. SIMON: Right! When's the last time you saw a surgeon eat a Butterfinger bar?

DENNIS: Oh no, I can't believe this is happening.

DR. SIMON: Believe it, Dennis.

DENNIS: I know, but . . .

DR. SIMON: But what?

DENNIS: But Dr. Simon, I love Baby Ruth bars. Does that mean . . .?

DR. SIMON: Yes, Dennis.

DENNIS: And all that time I thought I was eating candy because I liked the way it tasted.

DR. SIMON: Now you know.

DENNIS (looking a little bewildered): It's just . . . all those Baby Ruths I've eaten. Big ones. Small ones. Miniatures on Halloween (becoming excited). I love the little ones, Dr. Simon. Do you think I'll end up in neonatology?

DR. SIMON: Perhaps, Dennis. Do you care to make some other predictions?

DENNIS: Okay . . . I'm ready.

DR. SIMON: Psychiatry?

DENNIS: Good & Fruity.

DR. SIMON: Ob/Gyn?

DENNIS: Mounds.

DR. SIMON: Family practice?

DENNIS: 3 Musketeers.

DR. SIMON: Medicine?

DENNIS: Hmmm, medicine's tough. I never see internists eating candy in the hospital. Wait a second. I've got it—Godiva, right?

DR. SIMON: Perfect!

DENNIS (obviously pleased with himself): This is fun, Dr. Simon. Maybe I should skip residency and go right into medical education.

DR. SIMON: Well, at least wait until tomorrow. We have one question left.

DENNIS: Shoot.

DR. SIMON: If you had to live inside a comic strip, which one would you choose?

DENNIS: Let me think for a second.

DR. SIMON: Not too long, now.

DENNIS: Oh, I already know my answer. I'm just thinking about the other specialties.

DR. SIMON: Okay, Dennis.

DENNIS: I've got it. Go ahead, quiz me.

DR. SIMON: Medicine?

DENNIS: Either *Crock* or *The Lockhorns*.

DR. SIMON: Surgery?

DENNIS: *Prince Valiant*.

DR. SIMON: Psychiatry?

DENNIS: *The Wizard of Id*.

DR. SIMON: Ah, my favorite!

DENNIS: I thought so.

DR. SIMON: How about family practice?

DENNIS: *For Better or For Worse*.

DR. SIMON: Ob/Gyn?

DENNIS: *Grin & Bear It*.

DR. SIMON: Very nice, Dennis. Now tell me, which comic strip would you choose to live in?

DENNIS: The one with my namesake, of course.

DR. SIMON: You mean the little menace?

DENNIS: You bet. He was my role model as a child.

DR. SIMON (laughing): I'm not surprised. Any questions left for me?

DENNIS: Not really. I think I'll go home and have a talk with my roommate, though. I'm dying to find out if he really wants to go into medicine.

DR. SIMON: Let me know how things work out.

DENNIS: Oh, I will. I just hope his advisor will be as good as mine.

DR. SIMON: I'm sure he will be, Dennis—at least the one he's got tonight.

DENNIS: Well, I've got the secret now. If you want things to work out right, just follow what Simon says.

DR. SIMON: It's as simple as that.

Additional Readings

1. Bennett HJ: Diary of a third-year med student. J Fam Pract 1993;37:192.

The author reflects on things he learned when he began his clinical rotations. For example, "Ward clerks are an odd bunch. They don't seem to do much, and they do it very slowly," and "Getting an x-ray done before noon is about as likely as making it through attending rounds without being pimped."

2. Bluestone N: Coffee break. New Physician 1980; 29(10):5,8,12.

3. Bluestone N: Percolation test. New Physician 1980;29(11):7,10,14.

In this two-part article, we meet Mary Louise, a premed student who suffers from a severe case of medical admissions anxiety. Mary reacts to this stress by adopting the appearance and behavior of a coffee pot.

4. Bluestone N: An empathy test. New Physician 1981; 30(2):7,16.

According to the author, medical students are bewildered individuals who are never sure what they should be doing. For example, "Am I supposed to toss the breast over her shoulder or listen right through it?" She then presents a miniquiz which demonstrates that the rest of us aren't always sure what we should be doing either.

5. Bluestone N: Labor and delivery. New Physician 1982; 31(3):37–38.

Suzy Kew is a third year student at Healthyself Medical School. Despite efforts to orchestrate her pregnancy and delivery with aplomb, Suzy goes into labor one week early. With her entire support system out of town, Suzy is left in the hands of the chairman—Dr. Spike.

6. Ricks AE: Making the grade: how to evaluate medical students. Resid Staff Physician 1985;31(6):65–66.

Rather than using standard forms, the author suggests a more practical approach to medical student evaluations. For example, when asked if a student is responsible, decide whether you would trust the student with (a) Correctly collecting lab data? (b) Correctly transcribing your orders? (c) Correctly transcribing your orders in the ICU? (d) Correctly transcribing your orders for takeout at the Szechaun Palace?

7. Smithline F: Up the bronchial tree. Perspect Biol Med 1982;25:436–443.

A fantasy about a medical student named Alice who wanders through the hospital. She meets a number of characters more likely to know the Cheshire Cat than the Chief of Medicine.

From 1979 to 1982, Naomi Bluestone published a column in *The New Physician* called "Picking Bones." Although most of her articles dealt with the trials of medical school and residency, she occasionally ventured into other territory.—H.B.

INTERNSHIP & RESIDENCY

The main difference between medical school and residency is that with one you pay to become sleep deprived and with the other, someone pays you. There are other advantages to being a resident, however. Now you can really call yourself "Doctor," no one grades you anymore (at least not officially), and you're the one who gets to make out the scut list. But best of all, you can finally say goodbye to all those organ systems that used to make you nauseous. Now, at last, you can concentrate on what you have always wanted to do—like starting IVs at 3 AM on pudgy toddlers, disimpacting patients in the emergency room, and obtaining histories from patients whose silences rival those of psychiatrists. As the title of one of the following selections states, "Real Interns Don't Have Time to Eat Quiche."

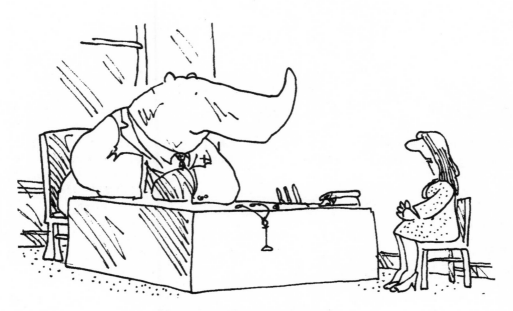

"Are you a resident or an attending?"

KEEPING FIT AFTER RESIDENCY*

Howard J. Bennett, M.D.

Most residents are not aware of the aerobic conditioning that is built into their training. Whether it's stonewalling an admission from the ER or procrastinating over incomplete medical records, residency training takes a lot of energy. Consequently, it's easy to put on weight once you leave the hospital for a cushy job in a clinic or private practice. This is especially true if you start eating real food instead of the *cuisine* that's served in most hospital cafeterias.

To help you stay fit and trim, I spent the last two years researching how many calories it takes to carry out the most common activities on the wards (Table 1). By reviewing this information, you'll be able to choose an appropriate strategy for keeping your waistline in check. Although some of you will have to cut back drastically on your intake of Ben & Jerry's Heath Bar Crunch, others will get by with less sacrifice. For example, many ex-residents stay in shape by taking up a sport like watching the Pro Bowler's Tour on television. Another option, of course, would be to do a second residency.

Table 1. Caloric Expenditures During Residency Training

Activity	Calories Per Occurrence
Answering a page—3 PM	50
Answering a page—3 AM	250
Turfing a patient	325
Disappearing from conferences	150
Staying awake during Grand Rounds	275
Throwing your beeper against the wall	10
Putting your foot in your mouth	25
Removing your foot from your mouth	250
Waiting on hold for lab results	150
Trying to schedule x-ray procedures	175
Arguing over the call schedule	425
Maintaining a high index of suspicion	75
Sitting on a patient overnight	25
Treating your relatives	125*
Quoting the literature	75
Stacking unread articles	150
Talking with patients	200
Doing a discharge summary:	
From a private hospital	100
From a teaching hospital	500
From a VA hospital	1500

*In most cases, this number triples after residency.

*Reprinted with permission from Resident & Staff Physician, © 1994; 40(5):76.
Cartoon reprinted with permission from *Stitches* © June 1993.

THE GENERIC H & P*

Frederick L. Brancati, M.D.

8 AM—the end of another long call night and time for attending rounds. Your team awaits you.

"Gee, you look terrible. How many did you get last night?"

"Seven. Actually, eight if you count that ICU transfer. Not too bad."

Not too bad for an intern like you, but a killer call night for a lesser house officer. You know it and they know it—you're Chief Resident material.

You reach into your pocket for that stack of index cards, your notes from last night. Instead, you discover a Hemoccult card, some Kleenex, and a gum wrapper. No note cards. Your cheeks flush. Beads of sweat collect on your upper lip. You feel your esophagus twist like a rubber band in a model airplane. You spent most of last night learning the intricacies of your patients' lives and illnesses, but right now your mind's a blank. How can you honestly present seven cases without a shred of detail and still preserve your stellar reputation? How indeed. Only one approach can preserve your dignity without making a total mockery of the truth—the generic history and physical.

In presenting the traditional, personalized H & P, the intern strives to focus his or her audience on what is special or different about each particular case. By necessity, the personalized H & P is chock-full of detail. The chief complaint is analyzed exhaustively, minutiae of medical history are scrutinized, dates and times are checked and rechecked. In contrast, the generic history fosters a broader outlook, emphasizing what is common to all cases.

Your voice crackles as you cautiously begin to present your first patient:

Mr. Jones is a middle-aged man with a long history of multiple medical problems who was admitted last night with an exacerbation. We don't have old records, the patient's a poor historian, and no family was available, so most of the history comes from the ER sheet and his nameplate. He was in his usual health until recently, when he noticed that "something wasn't right." He said he used to have spells like this once or twice a year, then he developed longer bouts, and now he's having very frequent episodes. He was seen by an outside physician who told him he had the "flu" and started him on a third-generation cephalosporin. When his symptoms persisted he was admitted to an outlying hospital. Records were not available. Reportedly, they ruled him out, performed an MRI, and sent him home on thyroid extract. He continued to do poorly at home and finally called the paramedics last night.

Current medications include a tiny white pill, a larger pink pill, and a foul-tasting powder.

Most of his family have been ill at one time or another, and several of them have died.

There's a question of alcohol and tobacco use. He used to work and currently lives at home.

His medical history includes several inconsequential surgical procedures when he was younger. About 10 years ago he was admitted to another hospital with an acute illness. After a number of tests they told him he might get this again and to call his doctor immediately if he did.

So far, so good. The generic physical examination is, however, a little harder to finesse. Of course, salient findings are easily recalled and apt to be mentioned even without the aid of note cards. What really gives texture and depth to the presentation, though, are the subtle nuances that are virtually irreproducible on successive examinations. Your confidence waxing, you resume:

Mr. Jones is found lying in bed. The vital signs are stable. There are several small, ill-defined, pig-

*Reprinted from JAMA © 1989; 262:3338, with permission from the American Medical Association.

mented lesions of the skin that he says have always been there. A 5-mm, soft, movable, nontender lymph node is palpated in the submandibular area. Subtle anisocoria is appreciated. The thyroid is top-normal. Basilar rhonchi are heard to clear after coughing. There's a 1/6 systolic murmur at the base and a question of an intermittent S3. An ill-defined firmness is palpated by some examiners in the epigastrum. Genitalia are present, with prominent scrotal rugations. Last night there was trace ankle edema, which was absent this morning. The neurological examination is grossly nonfocal.

The generic physical examination reminds your audience that each patient is a little different without bogging them down in a quagmire of nit-picking details. Moreover, it soothes your attending to the point of somnolence. Fully satisfied that a thorough examination was performed, the attending can settle back and doze off until you reach the assessment. (You can deepen the slumber by carefully enumerating every negative finding and by frequently repeating the phrase "regular rate and rhythm.") Contrast this with the so-called normal examination. Every attending knows that nobody's exam is completely normal. If you imply that your exam is normal, even the most docile conference room couch potato is bound to become a rabid diagnostic pit bull who will drag you and your team all the way to the bedside just to prove you wrong. Fortunately, you know better. You can see in their faces that they're buying the whole presentation. Emboldened, you close with a concise assessment and plan:

In summary, Mr. Jones is a middle-aged man with an exacerbation of a chronic illness. His course is complicated by several underlying conditions, some of which are poorly controlled. Our plan is as follows:
1. To perform some specialized blood work.
2. To obtain high-resolution images of the involved organs.
3. To consult a subspeciality service for an invasive procedure.
4. To follow his clinical course closely after a trial of empirical therapy.
5. To get support services involved and start discharge planning. If there's been no progress after 1 or 2 weeks, we'll reassess and consider further therapy using modalities with a higher risk-benefit ratio. If there's still no improvement at that point, we'll pursue a code status and arrange transfer to the rehabilitation service.

There you have it—the generic history and physical. It's a tried-and-true approach to presenting under fire, recommended by experienced interns in all 50 states. So sit down, straighten your coat, take a deep breath, and relax. With no sleep, no notes, and no wealth of knowledge, you can still present like a star. Yes, indeed. You are Chief material.

But do wipe that sweat from your lip.

After two days in the hospital, I took a turn for the nurse.

W. C. Fields

MORNING DISTORT*

Frederick L. Brancati, M.D.

You're a proud new second-year resident. You've tackled internship and you've prevailed. You're a giant, a marine, a pillar of granite. Okay, so you overcame anxiety, anger, and depression. But you have not yet faced terror—not until this morning. Today you face the terror of morning report for the first time. In the eerie morning light you see the long, ponderous oak table like some sacrificial altar; the pantheon of former chief residents judging you from portraits on every wall; the icy stares of the attending and the chief resident, their hands folded as if in contemplation before an ancient ritual. You notice that your cardiac rhythm has jumped from a traditional march into progressive jazz. Coffee splashes out of your Styrofoam cup as an adrenergic surge rattles your forearm. Yet, as you look around the table, the senior residents are smiling, some with their feet up, others leaning back with hands clasped behind their heads. Why are they so relaxed? It so happens they've been there. They've lived it, they've learned the rules. Yes, they've learned the rules of morning distort.

Rule #1. Make it pat, but not too pat. Morning report is not a forum for sorting out hundreds of unrelated facts. That's a job for naive third-year medical students and compulsive attendings. The resident who wallows in messy details and multiple diagnoses is soon bound to feel the cold edge of Occam's razor against his or her neck. After all, the chief resident wants to hear a story. Make the story short and pat, aiming for what Poe called the "unity of effect." Each word should point unerringly to one diagnosis and create a mood of solemn certitude. You may even wish to drop verbs from your presentation: For example, "Middle-aged man, tobacco, dyspnea, wheezing, sputum, barrel chest, COPD exacerbation." But too many pat stories will arouse suspicion. After presenting several pat cases, present an open-ended, confusing case, just to appear earnest.

Rule #2. Be bold. Nobody likes a wimp. Nowadays medical schools offer so many courses on humanism and ethics that many graduates quiver like gelatin in the face of real disease. Internship should have already taught you to think less like Schweitzer, more like Schwarzkopf. Your chief resident will want to hear that you've driven a needle deep into every lump, space, and swelling. Or better yet, a trochar. To highlight your courage, call in an interventional radiologist from home for an emergency procedure after 2 AM. Whatever you do, don't say "We observed the patient carefully" or "We waited watchfully." Even if you've done nothing beyond taking the H&P, say something like "We monitored him aggressively and sat on him hard."

Rule #3. The best defense is a good offense. Some mornings even the best residents are unprepared. If you feel weak, go on the attack. For example, say the attending taking report is a crackerjack endocrinologist and you have a case of multiple endocrine neoplasia to present, but you're unprepared. Why not present a cardiomyopathy case first, stress the patient's unusual rhythm disturbance, and corner the attending into interpreting a 10-foot-long rhythm strip? Or, if you believe that the chief resident might attack, launch a preemptive strike. Within earshot of the attending, turn to the chief resident and say, "Gee, you look tired. Must be all that moonlighting, huh?" Just don't try to hide at the far end of the table. The chief resident, bred to smell fear, will lunge at you like a Doberman.

Rule #4. Image is everything. Your superiors are going to put you in a pigeonhole, so you might as well choose which hole is yours. One effective image is the hardworking, straightlaced grunt look. Garb is the same for men and women: white polyester coats and slacks accented by pressed scrubs. White tennis shoes and a synthetic pocket protector complete the look. When presenting, play it straight: no jokes, no colloquialisms, just facts read directly from note cards. It's functional, but tedious. Another image is the uptown intellectual, dolce-vita look. Women wear dresses, light makeup, and heels. Manicures are optional, but recommended. Men wear light wool slacks and Italian ties. The presentations are lyrical and witty, often presented from memory (note cards are so bourgeois, n'est-ce pas?). Foreign eponyms are properly accented. It's fun, but it takes work to look the part, and it doesn't play well in the Midwest. A third choice is the look of total desperation. The resident doesn't shave or bathe and rushes into every morning report 10 minutes late wearing oversized scrubs. The aim is to recreate the image of Jimmy Stewart on the verge of collapse at the climax of *Mr. Smith Goes to Washington*. It's okay for sympathy, but doesn't garner much respect.

Rule #5. Stay calm. They are going to rattle your cage and they are very good at it. Don't act like a trapped animal; collect yourself and stand straight. For example, they are going to ask whether you sent some fancy test last night: an $alpha_1$-antitrypsin level maybe, or a urine for porphobilinogen. Of course, they figure that you didn't send it. It's your choice. You can nervously whimper, "Shoot, I didn't think of that. I'm awfully sorry. Please forgive me, I'm a worthless slug. I'll send it right away." Or you can confidently declare, "Sent." You see, "Sent" is really short for "I'll send it so fast, you can consider it sent" or "It's as good as sent," and it makes a much better appearance at report. They are also going to ask you to summarize cases that you don't remember. You can sweat and make excuses or you can calmly explain that "After a thorough assessment, we rounded up the usual suspects and took the traditional measures." Finally, they are going to ask you for laboratory results that you didn't write down. If you take a blank index card from your pocket, scrutinize it, flip it over a few times, and say "Nothing remarkable here," you've learned your lesson.

Whether you call it morning report, morning retort, or morning distort, the rules remain the same around the country. The bottom line is style above substance. It worked in the 80s and it can still work for you in the 90s. Go ahead, then. Lean back, put your feet up, and smile. Be happy. Now you know what the seniors know. You know the rules of morning distort.

———— ❦ ————

A woman accompanied her husband to the doctor and waited for him during his checkup. After the examination the doctor came out and said, "I don't like the way your husband looks."

"Neither do I," said the woman, "but he's good with the kids."

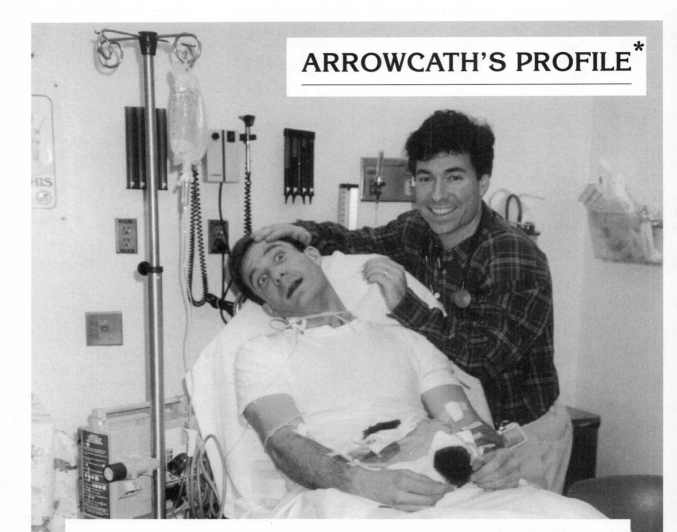

ARROWCATH'S PROFILE[*]

Molybdenum Smith, M.D.

HOME: The hospital.

AGE: 26 (going on 42).

PROFESSION: First-year resident.

HOBBIES: Sleep, dinner, showers.

LAST BOOK READ: *The Place for Euthanasia in Emergency Room Visits*, by Tungsten Holmes, M.D.

LATEST ACCOMPLISHMENT: Successfully put an IV into a patient at 2 AM without leaving Stage 4 sleep.

WHY I DO WHAT I DO: "It beats me."

QUOTE: "You woke me up for what!"

PROFILE: Lethargic and ambivalent with a low sex drive.

HIS IV: Arrowcath's Red Label.

Howard J. Bennett, M.D.

AT LAST! BLESSED RELIEF FOR THE PAIN AND DISCOMFORT OF PERCENTORRHEA*

Michael A. LaCombe, M.D.

House officers bored by endless percentages and professors prone to recite them will benefit alike by committing to memory the indispensable rule presented in this article.

LaCombe's Rule of Percentages (my name is LaCombe) will, when properly applied by house officers, force rounders and attendings to teach rather than perpetuate what Orr calls "shifting dullness." The rule is: *The incidence of anything worthwhile is either 15–25 per cent or 80–90 per cent.*

With this rule in mind, you need only know whether something is common or uncommon in order to affect profound medical knowledge when replying to percentage questions. Thus, you'll force those who want to teach you to deal in pathophysiology rather than percentages, and you may learn something.

Let me illustrate with a clinical example.

ROUNDER: What percentage of patients with Hodgkin's Disease experience pain at the site of active foci following the ingestion of alcohol?

HOUSE OFFICER (thinking of himself): I remember hearing about this once as I was falling asleep in a hematology lecture. . . . He's smiling at me as if I should know, so it can't be too rare. (Aloud, loudly): About 15 per cent to 25 per cent, depending on the study.

ROUNDER: Excellent! Actually, it's 17 per cent. Would you like to become an Associate Professor of Medicine like me?

HOUSE OFFICER: I'm afraid I don't know enough percentages yet, sir.

Now, don't get the idea that the house officer was being dishonest, specious, or glib. He was using LaCombe's Rule as a weapon, fully aware of the tremendous power of the phrase "depending on the study," which can mean anything upward from "I know as many references as you do."

There exist, naturally, exceptions to my rule, and two corollaries must be remembered. The first, called the Scrinch Amendment, refers to that instance when the rounder screws up his face (scrinches) and searches from student to intern to resident before asking for a really bizarre percentage. The corollary: *A scrinch is less than 1 per cent.*

The second, called Dudenhoefer's Corollary after an intern who used it twice, is: *An answer of 50 per cent will suffice for the 40–60 range.* It is to be applied rarely, and only by a master at reading nonchalance in facial expression, verbal nuance, and voice inflection. Why? It takes rare cool for a rounder to ask a percentage question when the answer desired is in the 40–60 realm. Lucky and blessed is the man who once in his lifetime successfully executes Dudenhoefer's Corollary.

With practice, LaCombe's Rule will prove indispensable. Like "The Barnes Manual of Medical Therapeutics," it is an acquaintance that once made will never be shunned.

*Reprinted from Hospital Physician, © 1971; 7(2):102. With permission from Physicians World Communications Group. Edited from the original.

THE INTERN: A FANTASY*

Harold K. Gever, M.D.

It was another bright, cheerful morning of Internship as I rolled out of bed in my suburban apartment. I had to hurry to make the 9 AM commuter train to University Hospital. "Make sure you get home on time today, honey. I hate when you drag yourself in at four in the afternoon," my wife mildly scolded as she warmed the Mercedes to take me to the station.

"Of all the hassles of Internship, this must be the worst," I thought as I fought my way through the end-of-rush-hour crowds to the hospital.

"Good morning, Dr. Gever," spoke the security guard at the entrance. "Shall I tell the telephone operators you're in?"

"Please do, Jenkins. I'm already a little late for attending rounds. It's my first day on the new service, so I better get up there right away. Thanks a lot."

The elevator attendant spotted me from a distance and held the door for me while I was talking to Jenkins. As I walked in, I could tell that some of the other riders didn't appreciate my tardiness, despite my status as Intern. There were several visitor types among the nurses, aides, and respiratory technicians. In the far corner, dressed in wrinkled, blood-stained surgical blues, stood a couple of weary looking attendings.

"Bad night on call, doctors?" I asked, trying to be friendly. I always hated to address attendings that way because it seemed so impersonal. Furthermore, I found that attendings always appreciated it when I knew their names; it must give them a feeling of self-esteem to be noticed by an Intern. But these guys were clearly a couple of the many attendings that seem to come and go so randomly at University.

In response to my question, they simply smiled at me servilely and muttered, "Not too bad, sir, just a couple of codes and a handful of admissions."

"Well," I chuckled, "could have been worse," as I strolled out of the elevator onto my floor. It always made me feel good to say a few encouraging words to attendings, especially after their nights on call.

I made my way briskly to the back room of the fifth floor to meet with my own new attendings, who no doubt were assembled around the conference table, x-rays already hanging on the viewbox. As I entered, I realized I had forgotten to bring the box of doughnuts I usually offered my attendings. I might have started off on the wrong foot with these sullen fellows, I thought. At University, sometimes the difference between being judged a good Intern and a bad one is in the quality of doughnuts one brings to rounds.

I looked around at my new team. It was a ragged crew, ranging in age anywhere from 28 to 76. Some of them, perhaps, could even remember the Great Medical Economic Revolution when third party payers realized it was cheaper to fund Interns and Residents for services rendered than to pay exorbitant attending rates. Most attendings were forced to either take down the shingle for good or come to subsist in the hospitals. Fortunately, they weren't allowed to unionize. The law was very clear in this regard; regular hospital employees could enter into collective bargaining, not those who merely subsist in the hospital.

My attendings proved to be fairly conversant with the literature. I've always enjoyed being involved with their teaching since it proves to be a mutual learning experience that even the best of Interns can profit from. Right in the middle of my lecture on how to insert IVs, however, the head nurse, Mrs. Phillips, exploded into the room.

"Dr. Gever, I'm so sorry for interrupting, but Mrs. Jones in 21A is short of breath. Can you send one of your attendings to see her?"

"But Mrs. Phillips, this lecture is important. Where are the medical students?"

"Union meetings," she said impatiently.

"Oh, I see. Well then, why don't you, doctor, take a look at her," I said said, pointing to one of the attendings who had just awakened from his nap during my talk.

When the lecture finished, I was still feeling bad about not having brought doughnuts, so I invited my attendings to join me for lunch. The r.s.v.p. was unanimous. It's not often attendings get a chance to eat in the Intern's Dining Room.

I quickly called University Food Services to make a reservation for six at noon. The maitre d' asked me to choose between filet mignon or lobster tail, because with such short notice, only these two items could be properly cooked to order.

Lunch in the Intern's Dining Room was delightful as always. My attendings appeared to be suitably awed. "I'm not impressed by the wine list, though," one of them said boldly. "It's a lot better at City General where my Intern took me when I was doing my surgery rotation there."

Lunch would have passed otherwise uneventfully, if it hadn't been for the obvious gloom of my other colleagues who were flagrantly trying to get drunk on Chateau Lafite Rothschild at the next table. "What's the matter?" I asked, turning my chair in their direction.

"It's time to start looking all over again," one said sorrowfully.

"What do you mean?" I asked. "Leaving University?!"

"We have no choice," he said. "We all just got our letters today from the program director. We're being promoted to Residents."

The whole idea was frightening. Being promoted to Resident meant not only less salary, but longer hours and probationary union privileges. It really left few alternatives. One was to apply for Internship at some other hospital. The best bets were some of the smaller community hospitals that didn't recognize University's Internship as creditable service. But those plums were few and far between and extremely difficult to match into. The only other alternative, of course, was to apply for Internship in some other specialty . . .

Mercilessly, the beeper startled me out of my slumber—a cruel return to the real world. In piercing monotone, it directed me to call my floor to find out about my new admission. As I stumbled to the elevator in the main lobby, the doors shut in my face. It would be another 15 minutes before it would come down again. Too tired to do anything else, I stared at the closed doors, my eyes burning from fatigue. When the doors opened again, I found myself face to face with a well-dressed woman. It was Nurse Phillips.

"Up all night, doctor?" she asked. I nodded in the affirmative. "Here," she said, shoving an opened cardboard box in front of my nose. "Have a doughnut. I don't know why the third party payers keep giving these to us. They know we're all on diets."

From the corner of my eye, I could see Jenkins helping Mrs. Phillips into her Mercedes in front of the hospital. Confidently, she tipped the valet parking attendant and drove off.

"What I wouldn't do to be a Nurse," I heard an older man's voice say wistfully from within the elevator. He looked like an attending.

"I know what you mean," I heard myself say. "Ever since the third parties put Nurses in charge, it's been a thankless job being a physician. Oh well, I'm really just in it to supplement the allowance my wife gives me."

"And I couldn't stand to watch another soap opera," the older man said. "This fills up my day. By the way, when do you get off?"

"I'm doing a double today, the night shift and now the day shift. I finish at three," I responded.

"Me too!" he said. "Hey, how about joining me for a beer afterwards. We'll drink to old times."

THE PEDIATRIC INTERNSHIP SCREENING TEST*

Howard J. Bennett, M.D.

Each year, some 16,000 students graduate from medical schools in the United States. Having finished four years of grueling education, these young doctors now begin an experience euphemistically known as "postgraduate training." Unfortunately, residency training is to medical school as a blown pupil is to anisocoria.

In the past, residency was seen as a rite of passage, and a "sink or drown" philosophy was adopted at most teaching hospitals. Recently, however, the plight of overworked housestaff has been significantly eased. Today's interns and residents are better paid, have fewer nights on call, and, in most hospitals, are given time off for major illness and death.

The Pediatric Internship Screening Test (PIST) was developed to provide a simple method of testing an intern's adjustment to his or her residency. The PIST focuses on interns for two reasons. First, the internship year requires the skills most like Freud's anal stage and is therefore the easiest to measure and follow. Second, we all know what happens if something goes amiss in that arena.

During the pilot phase of the study, I spent approximately four years wandering the halls of teaching hospitals, talked with hundreds of interns, and underwent analysis in order to relive my own internship experience. The test was then standardized on 1,036 pediatric interns. All subjects volunteered, more or less, for the study, which takes only 15 minutes to complete and thus could not be used as an excuse to refuse an admission or to get out of attending rounds.

In order to avoid type I and type II errors, no effort was made to examine the subjects statistically. It is interesting to note, however, that some subjects had been tested two decades ago in the classic developmental work by Frankenburg and Dodds (The Denver Developmental Screening Test. J Pediatr 1967;71:181). Despite this observation, any similarity between the PIST and the DDST is purely coincidental.

The PIST has been designed so that interns can be tested on a monthly basis from July until the following June. The examiner draws a line through the corresponding month and then administers those items intersected by the line. Footnotes that accompany the form provide additional directions for testing.

How to Score the Test

Each item is scored P for pass, F for fail, or S for asleep. The PIST is then interpreted as normal or abnormal depending on whether the majority of items are passed or failed. An intern is considered questionable if he spent more time sleeping than responding to the examiner.

The PIST is not an intelligence test. It is intended solely to help program directors monitor the progress of the youngest members of their housestaff. The indications for testing include arguing over schedules, failing to change out of scrubs after a night on call, not wanting to come back to work after vacation, and calling home more than once a week. In addition, all interns should be tested between February and March.

When the test is used as directed, interns can be counseled more effectively than in the past. In particular, they can be reassured that they are developing well and should not be overly concerned with their physiologic celibacy. Those with abnormal results on the test might consider switching to a radiology residency or opening a gourmet ice cream parlor. Interns with a questionable PIST can either spend an extra month in the nursery or agree to be retested in four to six weeks, whichever they prefer.

The author is now completing work on a revision to be called the PIST-R, which is designed for use with PL-2 and PL-3 residents. It remains to be seen whether they will take this sitting down.

*Reprinted with permission from Contemporary Pediatrics, © 1987; 4(5):96–99. Edited from the original.

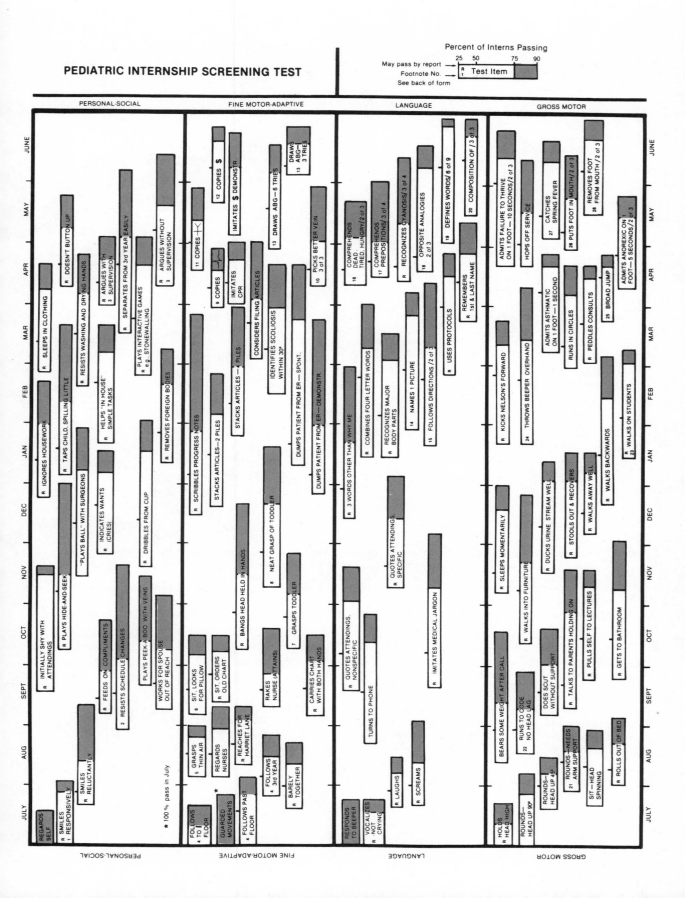

PEDIATRIC INTERNSHIP SCREENING TEST

1. Try to get intern to smile by smiling, waving or offering to take the next admission. Do not touch him.
2. When intern is getting ready to go home, tell him there's been a schedule change and he's on call. Pass if he threatens to quit.
3. Intern does not have to be able to win arguments to pass.
4. Give intern his schedule. Pass if he makes it to the assigned ward.
(Forgets the next day; follows 3rd year)
5. Pass if intern tries to bluff when asked questions in attending rounds.
6. Pass if intern looks for a pillow when he sits down to take test.
7. Pass if intern keeps toddler still by holding any part of his body.
8. Pass if intern keeps toddler still by saying it won't hurt, offering a bribe or by sitting on him.

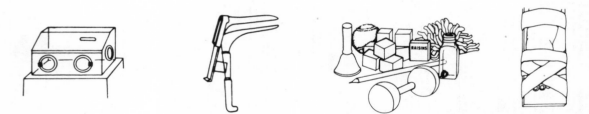

9. Pass normal rhythm. Fail any escape beats or aberrant rhythms.
10. Which vein is better? (not bigger.) Turn paper upside down and repeat. 3/3 or 5/6)
11. May be oriented in either direction.
12. Have intern copy first. If failed, do not recommend private practice.

13. When scoring, needs ½cc of blood to pass. Each jab counts as one try.
14. Point to picture and have intern name it. (No credit is given for sounds only.)

15. Tell intern to: Write up student evaluations; prepare a case for grand rounds; finish incomplete medical records. Pass 2 of 3. (Do not help by prodding, growling or withholding paycheck.)
16. Ask intern: What do you do when you are dead?...tired?...hungry? Pass 2 of 3.
17. Tell intern: Write your number on the slip; leave the requisition in the box; lab results will be ready by noon; close the door behind you. Pass 3 of 4.
18. Ask intern: If a horse is big, your salary is? Fire is hot, your sex life is? You are sensitive, chief residents are? Pass 2 of 3.
19. Ask intern: What is a weekend?...a black cloud?...QNS?...a novel?...an LMD?...turfing?...an off service note?...an infiltration?...a slough? Pass 6 of 9.
20. Ask intern: What is an HMO made of?...a PPO made of?...an IPA made of? Pass 3 of 3.
21. During work rounds intern leans on chart rack for support.
22. Intern runs to code. Pass if his head follows.
23. Intern may use third or fourth year students, preferably third year.
24. Intern must throw beeper overhand into the hall or at the chief resident.
25. Intern must perform standing broad jump over nursery flow sheet. (36½ inches)
26. When questioned on rounds, intern argues about workup then realizes he knows less than he thought he did.
27. Take intern outside on a sunny day. Pass if he forgets he's on call.
28. Intern stops arguing.

DATE AND BEHAVIORAL OBSERVATIONS (How intern feels at time of test, last meal eaten, recent Fri/Sun call, state of consciousness, etc.):

The following point-counterpoint* was written by two residents and an attending. Although the residents went first, considering all the ribbing that goes on in hospitals, it could just as easily have gone the other way around.—H.B.

Real Interns Don't Have Time to Eat Quiche

Real Interns . . .

- don't wake up their residents at night
- don't request cardiology consults
- don't admit patients from the emergency room
- do their own scut work
- change diapers
- treat meningitis as an outpatient disease
- can stay awake during X-ray rounds
- answer equally well whether awake or asleep
- answer questions they don't know the answer to with "Yawn, I don't know, I was up all night on call"
- can find something to complain about in the morning even if nothing went wrong on call
- circumvent their attendings and do things the right way.

Steven Blatt, M.D. and Rita Ryan, M.D. (Former Real Interns, now Real Residents)

The Attendings Strike Back

If "Real interns don't have time to eat quiche" then real attendings don't know what quiche is. The whimsical list submitted by two interns cries out for a rebuttal. Thus, real attendings:

- always sound awake when the intern calls at night
- play tennis with the cardiologist
- admit their patients right to the floor
- find more scutwork for the intern to do
- recommend against the use of diapers
- can cite every article that supports *their* way of treatment
- come late to radiology rounds and insist the films be reviewed from the beginning
- always have one more pearl
- call on the one medical student who can answer questions the intern missed
- tell about the good cases they saw on call during their residency
- call the nurse to circumvent the intern.

Michael Martin, M.D.

Be careful about reading health books. You may die of a misprint.

Mark Twain

*Reprinted with permission from Contemporary Pediatrics, © 1985; 2(4):76 and 1985; 2(8):12.

THE YOUNG BOYS NETWORK*

Naomi Bluestone, M.D.

"John, dear, you're going to have to do something about little Johnny." The senior resident braced himself. "O.K., what is it now?"

"He's been playing doctor again."

"Oh, no. How many times do I have to tell that kid to keep his hands to himself. If I've said it once, I've said it a hundred times: 'Never Lower Tillie's Pants, Mother Might Come Home.'"

"No, dear, that's not what I meant. I mean he's *really* playing doctor."

The usually cheerful face turned grim. "All right, honey, give me a drink and let's have it." He threw his bag on the table and opened his necktie.

"Well, it was a rainy day and he was feeling ornery, so at first I thought it might work when I heard him say to his little sister that the felt like being a doctor, and that she had to be his nurse since he really didn't trust any of the other little girls in the neighborhood. He promised her a huge salary and lots of time off and even said he'd start a tax-deferred annuity for her. So she called up to the white cape on the corner and asked the little Wilkins girl if she'd come over and play because they needed a patient. Well, the Wilkins's baby sitter was only too glad to dump her, so the next thing I knew the three of them had taken over the game room and were starting to divvy up the roles.

"I must say it started amiably enough. Johnny said he needed some experience cutting, and since he wants to be an orthopedic surgeon, he thought the Wilkins girl should have an open fracture of the femur so that he could reduce it and get some nice mattress sutures into place. But then Martha decided to assert herself and let Johnny know that that didn't suit *her* needs at all. She told him that she'd had all the med-surg nursing she wanted under her belt and she was damned if she was going to give another anesthetic or even start an I.V. again. She said Wilkins needed intensive care and she was just a floor nurse, and besides, they only had an hour or two until Wilkins had to go home for her nap, and

she didn't want to get in over her head. She said she wanted to practice her OB, and that if Wilkins wasn't going to be in the third stage of labor, she wasn't going to play. Then Johnny started yelling that with his luck, Wilkins would probably turn out to be a breech, and how could they possibly get a breech out before naptime?

"Well, just when it looked like they were coming to blows, the little Wilkins girl decided to put her two cents in. She has three older brothers, you know, so she's used to fighting her way through a screaming mob. She told Johnny and Martha that she was damned if she was going to break her leg for them, and that she wasn't going to let them stick her after what they'd done to her veins the last time. She said she was still sick from the *last* time they'd given her anesthesia. You remember how they dropped that wine vinegar on an old sponge and tried to tie it to her nose with her mouth stuffed full of old nylons? Well, they asked her why she was being such an uncooperative patient and advised her that if she didn't stop interfering, they'd send her over to the Johnson boy down on Fifth Street, and between you and me, dear, he really is a butcher.

"So then she got a little meek, and asked them (rather nicely, I thought) if they wouldn't consider letting her be a dotty little old lady who couldn't remember her own name. That way they could just do a brief mental status and then leave her be. She tried to point out that they both would get a chance to study for their exams while she was napping.

"Well, right about then the phone rang, and it was Mrs. Smith across the street. She'd just lost a filling and had to run to the dentist and could I please take the twins for an hour? I had to say yes, because you never know when the favor will be returned. So in they waltz, and both decide that there's a place for them in all of this. Phil decided that he wanted to be the consultant, which was fine with Johnny because he knew he could count on him for support, through the young boys' network. Rose, on the other hand, decided that what the group needed was a high-powered social worker, someone who could see the reality of placement problems and who knew how dispensable physicians really are. And that's when it all started, dear."

"Oh, God, Alice, are you really sure you want to tell me this? I really had a lousy day. Don't you think you're exaggerating? Give me another drink." He elevated his feet onto the coffee table and rearranged the cushions behind his rhomboid of Michaelis. "I'm ready."

"The twins are generally quite tractable, John. But whenever Phil gets to play consultant, he starts carrying on like Hannibal Homer. He wears his grandfather's pocket watch, and he keeps clearing his throat, and no matter what diagnosis Johnny makes, he always has a better one. He's fond of prefacing everything with, 'As the students at the Mass General feel . . .' and then he gives some esoteric syndrome that no one ever heard of before.

"Rose, on the other hand, has made a career for herself showing everyone that no one cares about the patient but Rose. She acts as if diagnostic procedures were performed for the sole purpose of delaying or destroying her placement procedures, and no matter what a doctor writes on a chart, she faults the wording, the sentiment, or the timing. I've told her mother she is going to be in a bad way when she reaches middle school, but she feels that Rose was destined to marry young and so none of this has any meaning anyway.

"Well, to make a long story very short, Phil decided that the patient could not have anything but a bad sprain, as much as he knew that his colleague had his heart set on an open, clean break. And Rose decided that placing a crowning multigravida was easier than placing a female organic brain syndrome. The patient decided that she didn't want to be interviewed by either the social worker or the consultant, and that she thought the nurse was being pretty damned callous and clumsy. Martha said that no social worker was going to interfere with her nursing responsibilities, and that since no official consult request form had been filled out by Johnny, Phil had no right opening his mouth and upsetting the apple cart.

"I was just about on my way in to break it up, because I saw Phil pick up a small rock, and he had a pretty ugly look in his astigmatic eye. But then Johnny let loose. Dear I wish I could have taped it. I mean, he just went berserk. He started screaming

that he was the captain of the team. He said that God had given the captaincy of the healing team, and that while he respected the right of every person in the room to have his opinion and his competency, he was damned if he was going to let them take over as if they owned the joint. He told the patient to shut up and that she was going to have whatever disease he thought was in her best interest. He told Martha that he would put her on report with the nursing supervisor if she made one more reference to childbirth. He told Phil that his services were no longer required, nor would they ever be again, since when was the last time he'd referred a patient to *him*? And he told Rose that she was a pain in his gluteus maximus, and why hadn't *she* gone to medical school? Then they all said they were sick of playing doctor, and they were going home."

"How awful for you, honey, how did you handle it?"

"Well, I told Phil and Rose that perhaps it really *was* time that they went home, and that they should try to be forgiving because they had gotten into fights with *their* little playmates, too."

"And the Wilkins kid?"

"She's traumatized, dear. She's supposed to go for her pre-school vaccinations soon, and now there's no way her mother will be able to drag her in. I've heard that the Smith girl is a pretty good shrink, though, and they have a good relationship, so maybe she'll work it out. I'm not too worried about Martha. I gave her some milk and cookies, and she just treated it all philosophically and said she really wanted to be an astronaut."

"But what about Johnny?"

"Please talk to him, dear. I sent him up to his room to cool down, but for hours he was just ranting on and on about how he always wanted to be a captain, and medicine just wasn't the tight ship it used to be, and how is he supposed to pass his Boards if he doesn't get the kind of clinical material and professional support he thinks is necessary? He has no insight, I'm afraid. He still can't see why no one wanted to play it his way. He's starting to obsess about what a bad doctor he is, and how his father won't be proud of him. A boy needs his father at a time like this."

"Of course, I'll talk to him honey. It's not so terrible. He just got carried away a little bit. I think it's because he's presenting at Grand Rounds tomorrow. Do you know if he worked up his case?"

Additional Readings

1. Bluestone N: Hired hands. New Physician 1979;28 (10):10–14.

This is an amusing story that suggests a novel way to survive your internship—hire a maid to do all of your scutwork.

2. Cilley RE: There are many ways to kill a resident: try house officer's headache or intern's neck. JAMA 1985;254:1905–1906.

As house officers advance in rank, the paraphernalia in their white coats decreases in weight from an average of 2.0 to 1.0 kg. Residency, it would seem, is a pain in the neck both figuratively and literally.

3. Joynt RJ: A note for interns and residents: a new law and advice on its circumvention. Perspect Biol Med 1981;25:144–147.

No matter how well you follow your patients, your attending will always want to see the one you didn't have time to check. The author provides some techniques to help residents keep their noses above water.

4. Lurvey AR: How to live with house officers without strangling them. Med Economics 1983;60(Apr 4): 141–148.

This article is for attendings only. Keep it handy the next time you admit a patient to an academic medical center.

5. Morrell RM: Sequelae to roundsmanship. New Physician 1964;13(1):A77–79.

The author suggests a number of ways for residents to outmaneuver attendings ("frontrowmen") during Grand Rounds. For example, how to block pearls before, during, or after delivery.

6. Ricks AE: All the right moves. Resid Staff Physician 1985;31(8):59–60.

The author muses about the hordes of Muppies (medical urban professionals) that move every July in search of the best education and training.

7. Sapira JD: Rules and guidelines for house staff involved in general medical rounds with attending physicians whose own training predated the present era of educational consumerism. South Med J 1981;74:866–867.

A satire which presents 16 tips on how to avoid learning anything during bedside rounds. For example, "Be late for rounds. If this is not possible, be punctual but be in the wrong place."

ACADEMIA

When patients read articles on "How to Choose a Doctor," one of the most common suggestions is to find out whether the physician is affiliated with a medical school. Ostensibly this means the individual will be up on the latest advances and therefore will give better medical care. In reality, of course, being a faculty member means something entirely different. It means having no control over the hiring and firing of employees, having to go to endless meetings and serve on countless committees, remembering to show up for lectures (giving them, not hearing them), worrying about promotion and tenure, having to evaluate students continuously, avoiding the chairman when quarterly reports are due concerning research in progress, and last but not least, having to accept a lower salary for the privilege of putting the word "professor" after your name. Although the following articles do not address all of these issues, they do shed light on some of the oddities in academic medicine. A few should be suitable for your next staff meeting.

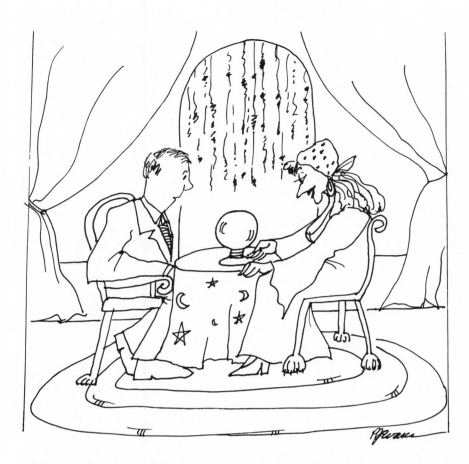

"Tenure looks pretty good, but what did you say your wife does on Thursday evenings?"

DEAR _____
(A) SIR (B) MADAM (C) DR.*

Melvin Hershkowitz, M.D.

Last year our 45 house officers asked for 310 letters of recommendation. What can be done about the need to produce this mass of correspondence, admittedly important for the credentials of medical trainees, but so substantial a drain on the time and energy of department directors and secretaries? While I contemplated another letter for one of our house officers, a fantasy brought forth the following:

*Reprinted with permission from The New Physician, © 1981; 30(8):24–25. Copyright by American Medical Student Association. Edited from the original.

_____
_____
_____
_____
_____

_____

This letter supports the application of Dr. X for _____ *(a) internship (b) residency (c) fellowship (d) moonlighter* in your _____ *(a) department (b) emergency room (c) ambulatory plastic surgery center (d) stress testing facility (e) executive health clinic.*

I have observed Dr. X during his/her _____ *(a) period of training (b) tour of duty (c) clinical rotation (d) liver rounds* here and have had _____ *(a) abundant (b) sufficient (c) very little (d) hardly any* opportunity to evaluate his/her performance. I can therefore report that Dr. X is _____ *(a) a Nobel Prize contender (b) highly competent (c) average (d) hopelessly incompetent* and that his/her fund of knowledge and familiarity with the literature is _____ *(a) encyclopedic (b) average (c) below average (d) typical for one who cannot read.*

His/her clinical judgment is _____ *(a) exceptionally mature (b) satisfactory (c) erratic (d) consistently unreliable.* Dr. X is also _____ *(a) unusually industrious (b) diligent (c) lazy (d) rarely seen in the hospital* and shows what may be considered _____ *(a) a deep and genuine interest (b) only casual interest (c) a general lack of interest (d) sincere avoidance* in his/her work. In addition, Dr. X's charts and medical records are _____ *(a) well organized, thorough, and legible (b) a bit careless (c) disorganized and illegible (d) brief and uninformative* because Dr. X's command of the language is _____ *(a) excellent (b) fair (c) poor (d) utterly unintelligible.* Dr. X's personality is _____ *(a) outgoing and pleasant (b) passive and silent (c) grouchy (d) nonexistent* and his/her moral character is _____ *(a) beyond reproach (b) apparently good (c) flawed and untrustworthy (d) typically political.* We have confirmed this by observing his/her relations with _____ *(a) attending physicians (b) fellow house officers (c) medical students (d) nurses (e) morgue attendants.*

We may add that Dr. X's participation in teaching activities has been _____ *(a) catalytic and stimulating (b) active (c) minor (d) to attend and sleep (e) to not attend* and his/her response to emergencies is _____ *(a) rapid and efficient (b) slow and uncertain (c) anxious and unpredictable (d) to faint.* When asked to work under stress, Dr. X's response is _____ *(a) to try hard and adjust well (b) to decompensate (c) to request an immediate vacation.*

In view of the above, we recommend Dr. X _____ *(a) with unreserved enthusiasm (b) with a heavy heart (c) with fear and foreboding,* and we are certain that he/she will be _____ *(a) an invaluable addition to (b) a valued member of (c) a grave handicap to* the already outstanding program you are supervising.

Yours sincerely,

_____

A Weary Faculty Member

Now that Dr. Hershkowitz has made writing letters of recommendation as easy as popping dinner into the microwave, Barry Kirkpatrick shows us how to interpret those unwieldy missives known as dean's letters. For those of us who actually have to write (or read) these letters, this piece will have an unmistakable ring of truth beneath the laughter. Dr. Kirkpatrick wrote his letter in response to an editorial that criticized the way students are currently evaluated in U.S. medical schools (Friedman RB: Fantasy land. N Engl J Med 1983; 308:651–653).—H.B.

What the Dean Really Means*

To the Editor: I submit the following guide for interpretation of what the dean really means:

The Dean's Letter	What the Dean Really Means
Sensitive	Cries easily
Very sensitive	Cries on rounds
Very cooperative	Easy; will work extra nights
Relatively good	Would not want him for my doctor
Sensitive to patients' needs	Steals food from their trays
Extremely capable	A little better than average
Well-liked	His mother always spoke well of him
Extremely conscientious	Probably paranoid
Assertive	Real S.O.B.
Self-motivated	Obnoxious
Outstanding integrity	On parole; is watching every step
Enthusiastic	Hebephrenic
Grasps new concepts quickly	Basically stupid, but flexible
Highly satisfactory	About average
Compulsive, goal-oriented drive	Obnoxious, but no more so than the self-motivated individual
Recommended to you with confidence	Glad to get him out of our school
Recommended to you without reservation	Glad to get him out of our school
Look forward to watching this individual as he matures in his career	Hope the turkey improves
Will be an asset to your program	Don't call us, we'll call you

Barry. V. Kirkpatrick, M.D.
Medical College of Virginia
Richmond, VA

The next selection was taken from an essay published in *JAMA*'s weekly column, "A Piece of My Mind." Like the editorial just referred to, Dr. Schneiderman was concerned with the problem of communicating a student's performance in written reports. Though his essay was serious, he ended on a light note by providing the following whimsical adjectives to describe medical students' performance in just the right word.—*H.B.*

Le Mot Juste*

Performance Percentile	Descriptor
99	Magnificent
98	Superlative
93	Extraordinarily strong
88	Notable
83	Wonderful
80	Terrific, radiant, and humble
78	Accomplished
75	Nonsteroidal anti-inflammatory
70	Well read
65	Capable
60	Intermittent
55	Well above the mean
50	Strong
45	Hearty
40	Friendly
35	Well groomed
30	Attentive and respectful
25	Pleasant
20	Punctual
15	Imminently about to blossom
12	Present and fully continent of all excreta
10	Normocephalic and nonfelonious
8	Claudicative
6	English speaking
5	Ambulatory
3	Respirating and well perfused
1	Charmingly fresh in outlook
0	Eukaryotic and possibly diploid

Henry Schneiderman, M.D.
Farmington, CT

*Reprinted from JAMA, © 1988; 259:87, with permission from the American Medical Association.

THE ART OF PIMPING*

Frederick L. Brancati, M.D.

It's hard work becoming a revered attending physician in a university hospital. The task daunts the newly appointed junior attending as he strides down the corridor of his first ward with his first team. Oh, he's made some changes in anticipation of his new position. He's wearing a long coat now, an all-cotton coat with razor-sharp creases and knit buttons. The stained, shrunken polyester white pants and tennis shoes have given way to gray, light wool slacks with a cuff and polished loafers. Framed certificates bear testimony to his intelligence and determination. He should be ready to take the helm of his ward team, but he's not. Something's missing, something important, something closer to art than to science. When physicians talk about the "art of medicine" they usually mean healing, or coping with uncertainty, or calculating their federal income taxes. But there's one art this new attending needs to learn before all others: the art of pimping.

Pimping occurs whenever an attending poses a series of very difficult questions to an intern or student. The earliest reference to pimping is attributed to Harvey in 1628. He laments his students' lack of enthusiasm for learning the circulation of the blood: "They know nothing of Natural Philosophy, these pinheads. Drunkards, sloths, their bellies filled with Mead and Ale. O that I might see them pimped!"

In 1889, Koch recorded a series of "Pümpfrage" or "pimp questions" he would later use on his rounds in Heidelberg. Unpublished notes made by Abraham Flexner on his visit to Johns Hopkins in 1916 yield the first American reference: "Rounded with Osler today. Riddles house officers with questions. Like a Gatling gun. Welch says students call it 'pimping.' Delightful."

On the surface, the aim of pimping appears to be Socratic instruction. The deeper motivation, however, is political. Proper pimping inculcates the intern with profound and abiding respect for his attending physician while ridding the intern of needless self-esteem. Furthermore, after being pimped, he is drained of the desire to ask new questions—questions that his attending may be unable to answer. In the heat of the pimp, the young intern is hammered and wrought into the framework of the ward team. Pimping welds the hierarchy of academics in place, so the edifice of medicine may be erected securely, generation upon generation. Of course, being hammered, wrought, and welded may, at times, be somewhat unpleasant for the intern. Still, he enjoys the attention and comes to equate his initial anguish with the aches and pains an athlete suffers during a period of intense conditioning.

Despite its long history and crucial importance in training, pimping as a medical art has received little attention from the educational establishment. A recent survey reveals that fewer than 1 in 20 attending physicians have had any formal training in pimping. In most American medical schools, pimping is covered haphazardly during the third-year medical clerkship or is relegated to a fourth-year elective. In a 1985 poll, over 95% of program directors admitted that the pimping skills of their trainees were "seriously inadequate." It comes as no surprise, then, that the newly appointed attending must teach himself how to pimp. It is to this group that I offer the following guide to the art of pimping.

Pimp questions should come in rapid succession and should be essentially unanswerable. They may be grouped into five categories:

1. Arcane points of history. These facts are not taught in medical school and are irrelevant to patient care—perfect for pimping. For example, who performed the first lumbar puncture? Or, how was syphilis named?

2. Teleology and metaphysics. These questions lie outside the realm of conventional scientific inquiry and have traditionally been addressed only by medieval philosophers and the editors of the *National Enquirer*. For instance, why are some organs paired?

*Reprinted from JAMA, © 1989; 262:89–90, with permission from the American Medical Association.

3. Exceedingly broad questions. For example, what role do prostaglandins play in homeostasis? Or, what is the differential diagnosis of a fever of unknown origin? Even if the intern begins making good points, after 4 or 5 minutes he can be cut off and criticized for missing points he was about to mention. These questions are ideally posed in the final minutes of rounds while the team is charging down a noisy stairwell.

4. Eponyms. These questions are favored by many old-timers who have avoided learning any new developments in medicine since the germ theory. For instance, where does one find the semilunar space of Traube? Or, whose name is given to the dancing uvula of aortic regurgitation?

5. Technical points of laboratory research. Even when general medical practice has become a dim and distant memory, the attending physician-investigator still knows the details of his research inside and out. For instance, how active are leukocyte-activated killer cells with or without interleukin 2 against sarcoma in the mouse model? Or, what base sequence does the restriction endonuclease *Eco*RI recognize?

Such pimping should do for the third-year student what the Senate hearings did for Robert Bork. The intern, in contrast, is a seasoned veteran and not so easily rattled. Years of relentless pimping have taught him two defenses: the dodge and the bluff.

Dodging avoids the question, wasting time as well as a valuable pimp question. The two most common forms of dodging are (1) to answer the question with a question and (2) to answer a different question. For example, the intern is asked to explain the pathophysiology of thrombosis secondary to the lupus anticoagulant. He first recites the clotting cascade, then recalls the details of a lupus case he admitted last month, and closes by asking whether pulse-dose steroids are indicated for lupus nephritis. The experienced attending immediately diagnoses this outpouring as a dodge, grabs the intern by the scruff of the neck, and rubs his nose back in the original pimp.

A bluff, unfortunately, is much more damaging than a dodge. Allowed to stand, a bluff promulgates a lie while undermining the academic hierarchy by suggesting that the intern has nothing more to learn from his attending. Bluffs weaken the very fabric of American medicine, threatening our livelihood and our way of life. Like outlaws in a Clint Eastwood movie, bluffs must be shot on sight—no due process, no Miranda Act, no starry-eyed liberal notions of openness or diaglogue—just righteous retribution.

Bluffs fall into three readily discernible categories:

1. Hand waving. These bluffs are stock phrases that refer to hot topics in biomedicine without supplying detail or explanation. For example, "It's a membrane transport phenomenon" or "The effect is mediated by prostaglandins." In many institutions, they may evolve directly from the replies of Grand Rounds speakers to questions from the audience.

2. Feigned erudition. The intern's answer, though without substance, suggests an intimate understanding of the literature and a cautiousness born of experience. "Hmmm . . . to my knowledge, that question has not been examined in a prospective controlled fashion" is a common form. Frequently, the bluff is accompanied by three automatisms: clearing of the throat, rapid fluttering of the eyelids and tongue, and chewing on the temples of the eyeglasses. This triad, when full-blown, will make the intern bear a sudden resemblance to William Buckley and is virtually pathognomonic.

3. Higher authority. The intern attributes his answer to the teaching of a particular superior. When the answer is refuted, the blame of ignorance comes to rest on the higher authority, not on the obedient, accepting intern. The strength of the bluff depends on just whom is quoted. An intern quoting a junior resident about pathophysiology is every bit as cogent as Colonel Qaddafi quoting Ayatollah Khomeini about international law. An intern from an Ivy League medical school quoting the "training" he received on his medical clerkship goes over like Dan Quayle explaining the Bill of Rights at an ACLU convention. The shrewd intern, however, will quote his Chairman of Medicine or at least a division chief, pushing the nontenured attending to the brink of political calamity. Did the chairman actually say *that*? The attending is powerless to refute the statement until he is certain.

Indeed, a good bluff is hard to handle. Sometimes the intern's bluff sounds better to the ward team than the attending's correct answer. Sometimes it sounds better to the attending himself. Ultimately, the cunning intern is best discouraged from bluffing by aversive training. Specifically, each time he bluffs successfully, the attending should counter by inducing Sudden Intern Disgrace (SID). SID is induced in two ways:

1. Question the intern's ability to take a history. This technique depends on the phenomenon of historical drift. That is, a patient's story will reliably undergo a significant change in the 8- or 16-hour interval between admission and attending rounds. The attending need only go to the bedside and ask the same questions the intern did the night before. Now the entire case is seen in a light different than that cast by the intern's assessment. Yesterday's right upper quadrant cramping becomes right-sided pleuritic chest pain. Yesterday's ill-defined midepigastric "burning" becomes crushing substernal heaviness radiating to the arm and jaw. Suddenly, the intern is disgraced. He will never bluff again.

2. Question the intern's compulsiveness. In less rigorous programs, this is easy. Did the intern examine the peripheral blood smear and the urine sediment himself? If the intern does routinely examine body fluids, a more methodical approach is required. In this case, results of the following tests, procedures, and examinations may be requested in rapid succession: Hemoccult slide test, urine electrolytes, bedside cold agglutinins and serum viscosity, slit-lamp examination, Schiøtz's tonometry, Gram's stain of the buffy coat, transtracheal aspiration, anoscopy, rigid sigmoidoscopy, and indirect laryngoscopy. Once the attending discovers a test or examination left unperformed, he asks the intern why this obviously crucial point was neglected. (The tension may be heightened at this point by frequent use of the word "cavalier.") The intern's response will generally revolve around time constraints and priorities in diagnostic evaluation. The attending's rejoinder: did the intern eat, sleep, or void last night? The scrupulous intern at once infers that he has placed his own needs before the needs of his patient. Suddenly, he is disgraced. He will never bluff again.

Clearly, pimping—good pimping—is an art. There are styles, approaches, and a few loose rules to guide the novice, but pimping is learned in practice, not theory. Despite its long and glorious history, pimping is in danger of becoming a lost art. Increased specialization, the rise of the HMO, and DRG-based financing are probably to blame, as they are for most problems. The burgeoning budget deficit, the changing demographic profile of the United States, the Carter Administration, inefficiency at the Pentagon, and intense competition from Japan have each played a role, though less directly. Against this mighty array of historical forces stands the beleaguered junior attending armed only with training, wit, and the determination to pimp. It won't be easy to turn back the clock and restore the art of pimping to its former grandeur. I only hope my guide will help.

———⋙•⋘———

If there's one thing I've learned over the years, it's that not all doctors appreciate the value of medical humor. While it's obvious that Dr. Brancati's article is a satire, some people took him seriously and were offended by what he had to say. This is not the only time that Dr. Brancati has ruffled a few feathers, and anyone interested in the debate should see "Pimper Pimped" (JAMA 1989;262:2541–2542) and "Morning Distort: We Are Not Amused" (JAMA 1992;267:807–808). For more on the origin of the word "pimping," see JAMA 1990;263:1632–1633.—H.B.

Medical one-upmanship has been around for a long time. Nowadays, it takes place primarily in hospitals where attendings and residents compete to see who can quote the most references on rounds. In the past, physicians tried to outdo each other by presenting unusual cases and miraculous cures that often bordered on fiction. William Osler was particularly miffed by this behavior and satirized the practice through his fictitious alter ego, Egerton Yorrick Davis (see p. 127). In one instance, the elusive Dr. Davis was supposed to present a case about the bizarre obstetrical practices of an obscure Indian tribe from northern Canada.[1–3] Davis never showed up, of course, so Osler (who was secretary of the medical society) read the paper to the assembled body. It was all a fabrication, but once Osler finished, doctor after doctor stood up to tell his own inflated tale. The following article is undoubtedly a parody of the same practice that befuddled Osler. Although it's over 90 years old, the theme has aged quite well.—H.B.

1. Holmes B: The relation of medical literature to professional esteem. Lancet-Clinic 1915;114:113–115.
2. Robb-Smith A: Egerton Y. Davis and placentophagy. Bull NY Acad Med 1980;56:258–259.
3. Bean WB: Osler, the legend, the man and the influence. Can Med Assoc J 1966;95:1031–1037.

REPORT OF A MEETING OF A MODERN MEDICAL SOCIETY*

F. E. Bunts, M.D.

FIRST SURGEON (DR. JONES): I am pleased to bring before the members of this society the following case report. A 42-year-old man was accidentally kicked over a fence by a mule and landed with his right side on a pig's head. No symptoms developed for twenty-four hours. When the family became alarmed at the absence of symptoms, I was called in to see the case and at once diagnosed a rupture of the liver. The signs were somewhat obscure, but an operation made thirty-six hours hence proved the accuracy of my observations. The liver and portal vein were carefully sutured and the abdominal wound was closed with four rows of sutures—catgut, silk, silkworm gut, and silver wire, respectively. The patient made an uneventful recovery and returned to his occupation as a mule driver nine days after surgery. In conclusion, I would say that the chief points of interest in this case are the accuracy of the diagnosis and the excellent results following a most hazardous and desperate operation.

CHAIRMAN: This interesting paper by Dr. Jones is now open for discussion.

OPHTHALMOLOGIST: I'm sure we are all indebted to Dr. Jones for his valuable contribution to surgical knowledge. In fact, it reminds me of a case I was called in to see about a well known man who ruptured his eyeball while attempting to watch a troupe of ballet girls all at once. The treatment consisted of prompt removal of the eye. The cure was immediate and uneventful, and the patient has never again attended a ballet performance. In conclusion, I again congratulate the author for his paper.

GYNECOLOGIST: The subject under discussion is somewhat out of my line of work; however, its brilliant result reminds me of a case of endometritis fungoides complicating a Bartholin's cyst in a 96-year-old patient. In this case I removed the uterus and appendages per vagina after excision of the cyst. The patient made an uneventful recovery, has since remarried, and now feels as young as she did seventy years ago. I would like to thank Dr. Jones

*Reprinted from the Fort Wayne Medical Journal, 1902; 22:288–290. Edited from the original.

for the opportunity his paper has given me to present this case.

OTOLARYNGOLOGIST: I cannot allow this opportunity to pass without referring to a case which Dr. Jones' paper has brought to mind. Some years ago, a patient of mine snuffed a bean up her nose. A careful inquiry at the time failed to reveal the bean, but yesterday (two years from the date of the first examination), there appeared an unmistakable beansprout extending from the anterior nares. I at once diagnosed a sprouting bean and removed it under cocaine anesthesia. No untoward effect was produced and the patient made an uneventful recovery. I congratulate Dr. Jones for his most excellent paper.

NEUROLOGIST: Rupture of the liver should remind all of us that sudden jars may also cause rupture of the cerebral sinuses or hemorrhage into the spinal canal. In a case similar to the one by Dr. Jones, motor paralysis was present from the moment a patient sustained the shock of receiving a doctor's bill. I made the diagnosis without any difficulty. Fortunately, the patient recovered in time to make the races the very next day. I wish to congratulate Dr. Jones on his very elaborate and painstaking paper.

SECOND SURGEON: I can endorse everything that Dr. Jones has said and appreciate fully the value of his paper. I wish to take exception, however, with his means of diagnosis and to say that from the symptoms related in the history, there could not possibly have been a rupture of the liver. Nor could he, in my estimation, have sewn up the portal vein without seriously interfering with the functions of the liver and bringing on an attack of the piles. In all cases of this kind, I have made it a point to also dissect out the pile-bearing area. In conclusion, Mr. Chairman, I hope that no one will think from my remarks that I differ in any essentials from the practice of my distinguished confrere.

CHAIRMAN: As there is no further discussion about this paper, Dr. Jones will now close the meeting.

DR. JONES: The field of surgery has been so fully covered this evening that it's impossible for me to add anything to that which has already been said.

———— >◦◦◦< ————

A surgeon, an internist, and a family physician go duck hunting.

The surgeon sees a duck, shouts "Duck!" and shoots it down.

The internist sees a duck, shouts "Duck! Rule out quail! Rule out pheasant!" and shoots it down.

The family physician sees a duck and blasts it out of the sky with a burst of machine-gun fire. As the tattered carcass falls to the ground, he remarks, "I don't know what the hell it was, but I sure got it!"

THE FINE ART
OF DISAPPEARING FROM MEETINGS*

Harold J. Ellner, M.D.

As my hospital-staff presidency neared its end, my awareness of the expertise of some of the medical staff in prematurely departing from meetings had finally crystallized. During ascendancy to this position, I could not fully appreciate the extent of this ingenuity. As secretary, I was too busy trying to record the minutes. As vice-president, I had an understudy's engrossment in the president's predicaments and could observe little else. But after the torch was passed and, upright, I faced my seated colleagues at staff meetings, I had a talent scout's view of this venerable art form.

The Telephone Gambit: This classic maneuver deserves mention as the forerunner of all the innovative techniques that follow. The phone calls begin shortly into the meeting, each one summoning a specific physician to a brief but earnest conversation. The callee strides out purposefully, not to return. Practitioners of this method have usually scheduled the call themselves or, serendipitously receiving any call whatever, hit upon it as a cause to leave. The same doctors seem to get called at roughly the same time during each meeting. In fact, one of our former members was called away regularly by his wife for 17 years in this manner.

The Page: A variation of the Telephone Gambit, this method requires an intrahospital page to extricate the doctor from a staff meeting. It is more difficult to orchestrate than the Telephone Gambit, but fortunately often occurs by chance. A good relationship with the page operator doesn't hurt, however. The adaptable staff member, once out, does not return.

The Indignation Ploy: This method requires a certain amount of boldness to succeed. The staff member professes his displeasure soon after the meeting begins. He advises the president that he expected to use his valuable time to transact certain hospital business (whatever is not on the agenda). He then strides off—to the cocktail lounge.

The Fidgetary Finesse: In this maneuver, escape velocity is gradually achieved by the more timid members in attendance. It starts when one of them begins to get restless. Next, the doctor makes the first of many trips to the coffee urn (the one near the door). A final effort propels him through the portal when escape velocity is reached. As the year progresses the staff member usually gains confidence and requires fewer trips for coffee. He may eventually omit the formality of stopping at the urn altogether.

The Direct Approach: With this method, the doctor stands, glances at his watch (optional), purposefully adjusts his head slightly downward, and exits.

The Intermission Exit: For those too reticent to use the Direct Approach, it helps to remain until halftime and to exercise a modicum of timing. A clear advantage of this technique is that it is compensated by refreshments, conversation, and fellowship. After these have all been enjoyed, but before the first sign of the recall to order, one oozes out a nearby door.

Early Surgery: This is a special situation that requires a breakfast meeting to work. The surgical schedule is traditionally set back to allow the staff to meet. The practitioner of this maneuver claims to have gotten a complicated patient on his service at an inconveniently late night hour. The doctor schedules emergency morning surgery from his bed. He then comes to the meeting, has a leisurely breakfast, preempts the scheduled cases, and does his "emergency."

The foregoing summarizes only the basics in a field where there is great opportunity for those with talent and imagination. Doubtless, much has been omitted. Each practitioner has his own style, and methods must be studied in order to determine which ones will best serve an individual's needs.

*Reprinted from JAMA, © 1982; 247:508, with permission from the American Medical Association. Edited from the original.

And now, for the final word on academia . . .

MALEVOLENT CHOCOLATE FROSTING*

To the Editor: In November 1971, 35 members of the medical house staff at a university medical center experienced an explosive outbreak of acute diarrheal illness lasting for approximately 12 hours. Undaunted epidemiologic investigation has now shown a surprising association between those in whom the malady developed and attendance at a birthday party for the chief medical resident. Further inquiry has implicated a chocolate cake served at this occasion, and it is strongly suspected that the cake in question was frosted with a phenolphthalein compound (chocolate-flavored Ex-Lax, Ex-Lax Corporation, Brooklyn, New York). Medical house officers and physicians in general should be aware of this potential cause of gastrointestinal illness within institutions of higher learning.

CHARLES SCOGGIN, M.D.
University of Colorado
Denver, CO 80220   Medical Center

———————

A man who was having trouble with his sink called a plumber to his house. After the plumber examined the pipes, he leaned back and said, "I can fix the problem, but I want you to know that my fee is $150 per half hour."

"$150 a *half* hour!" said the startled man. "Why I'm a neurosurgeon, and I only get $150 for a full hour."

"Hey, don't feel bad," the plumber said sympathetically. "When I was a neurosurgeon, I only made $150 an hour myself."

*Reprinted with permission from The New England Journal of Medicine © 1977; 296:233.

Additional Readings

1. Abrahamson S: Diseases of the curriculum. J Med Educ 1978;53:951–957.

Although this article is not humorous per se, the author uses wit and satire to make his case. For example, some of the "diseases" he describes are curriculosclerosis (hardening of the categories), curriculoarthritis, and iatrogenic curriculitis. (For a commentary on this article, see Davis WK: Abrahamson's Disease. Academic Med 1991;66:532.)

2. Bluestone N: Signing out. Resid Staff Physician 1986;32(10):85–88.

After 18 years of service to Farethewell Hospital and the Healthyself Medical School, the Chief of Surgery gets a letter telling him he is subject to mandatory retirement soon after his 62nd birthday. The letter details the protocol he must follow, including such items as being sure all of his library fines are paid in full.

3. Copple PJ: Conferencemanship. New Physician 1961;10(5):A80–81.

The author presents 15 tips for organizing and running a case conference. For example, "Schedule the conference for those hours when people are at their best, such as 8 AM Monday, 1 PM any other day, 4:30 PM Friday, or 11 AM Saturday."

4. Coulter DL: The academic oedipal crisis. J Polymorphous Perversity 1987;4(2):17–19.

This article examines a developmental milestone not mentioned in most standard psych textbooks: the need of assistant professors to kill their department chairmen.

5. Eisman B, Thompson JC: The visiting professor. N Engl J Med 1977;296:845–850.

A satirical essay on the visiting professorship. It includes a universal form letter that is complete with blank spaces for the visiting professor's name, the choice of lecture topics, and dates, etc.

6. Markivee CR: Rating of speaker performance. AJR 1985;144:864–865.

The author presents a system for rating medical speakers. Points are added or subtracted depending on ones proficiency or ineptness in several areas: the use of a microphone and light pointer, the quality and quantity of medical slides, etc.

7. Marshall GS, Rabalais GP: The pediatric infectious disease screening test. Pediatr Infect Dis J 1995:14:317–318.

This article pokes fun at advancement in academic medicine. Although it's written for those in pediatric infectious disease, it should appeal to anyone who works in a university setting.

8. Pauker SP: Grand rounds whiplash. N Engl J Med 1970;283:600.

The author suggests the use of Thomas collars to prevent complications that might occur when tired house officers attend grand rounds.

9. Rose I: Lectureshipmanship. Can Med Assoc J 1969;101:114–116.

The author provides some tips on how to present a medical lecture. For example, "Slides must be confusing and in the smallest possible print," and "Never use a simple sentence when a complex one will do."

10. Smith RP: Conference coma. Obstet Gynecol 1983;61:647–648.

A formula for figuring out how much sleep you can expect during a conference. It takes into account the number of slides to be shown, the distance the speaker had to travel, and other variables.

11. Stanton GK: Medical education upgraded. J Irreproducible Results 1981;27(3):17.

The author presents a rating scale for picking the best teaching cases at grand rounds. For example, a patient who voids on an attending gets 10 points, whereas hitting a medical student only earns 2 points.

MEDICAL LANGUAGE

When medical students begin their education, they have no idea that half of medicine is learning the language. Within days, however, they discover that an armpit is no longer an armpit but really an axilla and that the belly button, that long contemplated dimple in our midriff, is now called an umbilicus. Then, after a two year crash course that teaches them the nouns, verbs, and adjectives in medicine, they hit the wards to learn the grammar. Patients, they find, are not merely taken care of, but "followed," "digitalized," and "covered with antibiotics." In addition, they learn that a major goal in medicine is to cram as much as possible about a patient's life onto a 3 × 5 card. The jargon, the initials, and the other conventions are only a means to that end. The selections that follow take a humorous look at this area by showing some of the ways that medicine dislocates how we speak and write.

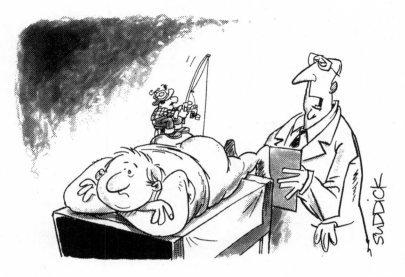

"It would seem you have a small anal fisher, Mr. Duffy."

A DICTIONARY OF MEDICAL PUNS*

Howard J. Bennett, M.D.

A few weeks ago, I had a wonderful time visiting with a 6-year-old named Molly. At the end of her physical, Molly asked me if I wanted to hear a joke. I said yes, of course, at which point she sat up to deliver her comic morsel.

"When is a door not a door?" she asked, barely able to contain herself.

"I don't know," I answered. "When is a door not a door?"

"When it's ajar!"

After Molly's visit, I began thinking about the ubiquitous nature of puns. Although they come in many sizes and shapes, one of my favorites is something called a "daffynition," an amusing definition of a word from the pundit's point of view. Examples of some well-known daffynitions include *pasteurize* (too far to see), *crocodile* (a jar of soap), and *illegal* (a sick bird).

Since most punsters have directed their attention to everyday speech, I decided to explore the hidden humor in our medical vocabulary. To do this, I spent a weekend flipping through the 1990 edition of *Stedman's Medical Dictionary*. Like regular puns, some of these will make you smile, and some will make you groan.

- **aerobe:** a garment worn around the house
- **alimentary:** what Sherlock Holmes said to Dr. Watson
- **apparent:** one who changes diapers
- **atonic:** a drink that goes with gin
- **attenuate:** what Bo Derek says to less attractive women
- **barium:** what you do to a patient if surgery fails
- **bowel:** a letter like a-e-i-o- or u
- **buccal:** something that holds up your pants
- **bullae:** a tough guy
- **carpal:** someone you drive to work with
- **castrate:** the going price for setting a fracture
- **chiropractor:** an Egyptian doctor
- **chorea:** where Hawkeye and Trapper John operated
- **cystogram:** a wire sent to your sister

*Reprinted with permission from Postgraduate Medicine
© 1994; 95(4):25–27. Edited from the original.
Cartoon reprinted with permission from Bill Suddick © 1995.
Originally appeared in *Stitches*, April 1995.

- **decapitate:** to cancel a contract with an HMO
- **denial:** where Cleopatria used to swim
- **dilate:** to live long
- **elixir:** what a dog does to his owner when she gives him a bone
- **emetic:** someone who drives an ambulance
- **fibula:** a little white lie
- **fundi:** what Princess Diana was before Charles
- **genotype:** the kind of girl Gino likes
- **hippocampus:** where a hippopotamus gets a degree
- **inbred:** the best way to eat bologna
- **innuendo:** where an Italian gastroenterologist puts his proctoscope.
- **intern:** one after the other
- **intubate:** what a fisherman is
- **isodense:** what a med student says after taking the national boards
- **kerion:** what you take with you during a flight
- **migraine:** what a Russian farmer now says about his harvest
- **nitrate:** what AT&T charges after 5

- **paradox:** two physicians
- **platelet:** a saucer
- **pleural:** more than one
- **pons:** a popular facial cream
- **porphyrins:** acquaintances who ask to borrow money
- **psoas:** in order that
- **rabid:** fast
- **rectum:** what being up all night did to the intern
- **sacral:** holy
- **sella:** a good place to keep wine
- **serum:** what you do when you barbecue steaks
- **testes:** what you order when you don't know what a patient has
- **tolerance:** what you get if you give growth hormone to ants
- **tumor:** an extra pair
- **urinate:** what a nurse might say if a patient asks what room he's in
- **vertigo:** how foreigners ask for directions
- **vitamin:** what you do when friends stop by for a visit

From 1952 to 1959, John Hayes published a monthly column called "Pro Re Nata" (PRN) in the *Journal of the American Hospital Association.* In addition to jokes, anecdotes and poetry, Mr. Hayes liked medical puns. Here are some of his best.—H.B.

PRO RE NATA*

John H. Hayes

- **annular:** occurring once a year
- **antibody:** no one in particular
- **aseptic:** one who doubts
- **caustic:** expensive
- **currette:** a partial recovery
- **dislocation:** here
- **duct:** avoided being hit
- **ester:** a girl's name
- **ether:** one or the other
- **ethyl:** another girl's name
- **fahrenheit:** very tall

- **fester:** quicker
- **friable:** can be cooked
- **influenzal:** having a lot of power
- **lobar:** a tavern for midgets
- **miscible:** not easy to hit
- **node:** was aware of
- **orifice:** a place of business
- **protein:** in favor of teens
- **serous:** not funny
- **thorax:** weapon of a Norse God
- **vein:** conceited

*Reprinted with permission from the American Hospital Association, © 1954–1958.

CALLING DR DOCTOR*

Howard J. Bennett, M.D.

A few months ago, I read a funny article about people who take poetic license with their use of the title "Doctor." (DePaolis M: Paging the rug doctor. *Postgrad Med* 1992;91(4):47.) In his travels through the phone book, the author found not only a "Pet Doktor" and a "Bike Doctor," but he also discovered someone who billed himself as "The Rug Doctor."

After reading this article, I began thinking about the humorous implications of people's names. For example, although Joseph Heller created a fictional character named Major Major in his novel *Catch-22*, there actually are physicians in this country named Doctor (18 to be exact). Realizing that this was probably just the tip of the iceberg, I decided to find out how far this Dr Doctor thing might go. So, with pen in hand, I spent a weekend flipping through the 1990 edition of the *American Medical Directory of Physicians in the United States.*

The first thing I learned during my research is that there are a lot of doctors in this country. Although I did not get page turner's tendinitis, I did need a stiff drink by the time I reached the Zs. I also learned that doctors' names often bear an interesting relationship to what they do for a living.

There are 22 doctors in the United States named Needle, Probe, Lance, and Ligate. Not to be outdone by such simple procedures, there are another 20 named Drill, Scope, Bolt, and Pin. I couldn't find anyone name Cut or Clamp, but there are three doctors named Drain.

Many doctors have names that are more generic and, I might add, quite appealing from the patient's point of view. I found 19 physicians named Fix, Cure, or Heal. If any of them formed a group with those named Brilliant (6), Able (6), or Best (62), there's no telling how popular their practice might be. It goes without saying that they would have a clear advantage over the 9 doctors named Klutz, Croak, Blunt, and Blewitt.

Doctors' names often say a lot about the type of medicine they practice. I found a dermatologist named Rash, a rheumatologist named Knee, and an orthopedic surgeon named Bone. My favorites, however, were a psychiatrist named Couch and an anesthesiologist named Gass. Nevertheless, a doctor's name does not always correspond with his or her specialty. There are 10 doctors named Blood, but none of them are hematologists. Similarly, of 11 doctors named Dust, Mold, and Pollen, none are allergists. I also discovered a handful of doctors named Eye (3), Nose (2), Tongue (2), Kidney (1), Stool (4), and Surgeon (1), none of whom work in the area suggested by their name. The best in this category belong to Drs Briss (1) and Stream (4), who, I'm sorry to say, are not urologists.

Sometimes a doctor's initials can be more revealing than his name. I found an obstetrician with the initials R.O.A., a cardiologist with the initials E.C.G., and a neurologist with the initials C.N.S. There is also a surgeon out there who can sign his orders N.P.O. On the other hand, there are no internists with the initials F.U.O., and I couldn't find anyone, not even a pathologist, with the initials Q.N.S.

Given my affiliation with a medical center, I was interested in those names that had an academic ring to them. Although I didn't find anyone named Publish, there is a physician in this country named Perish. This is fitting, I suppose, because I couldn't find anyone named Tenure either. I did find lots of Grants, however, something my colleagues say are in short supply these days. I also found 3 Deans, 1 Teacher, and 48 doctors named Pearl. Given that medical students often complain about their preceptors, the abundance of Pearls seems to balance out the 20 doctors named Bicker, Gripe, Fuss, and Grill.

Some doctors have names that might create a little confusion in the places where they work. Imagine what people think when an operator pages Dr

*Reprinted from JAMA © 1992; 268:3060, with permission from the American Medical Association. Edited from the original.

Page (140) or when the ER puts in a stat call for Dr Stat (1). And how would patients react if they shout "Nurse!" and Dr Nurse (3) is the one who shows up as they're fumbling with their bedpan? Other names that probably raise a few eyebrows from time to time include the 65 doctors named Flesh, Gore, Ache, and Looney. Finally, should you develop chest pain in the middle of the night, whom would you rather meet in the emergency room, Dr Code (5) or Dr Crump (29)?

Finally, the next time you send in a check to cover your escalating malpractice insurance, consider the irony in this: There are 43 doctors in the United States named Judge or Jury. I couldn't find any Attorneys, but that shouldn't be a problem since they never have any trouble finding us.

If all this is giving you indigestion, perhaps you should give your own doctor a call. However, if his name is Placebo, just take some Maalox and call it a night.

For an amusing response to this article, see "Dr Doctor calls back" (JAMA 1993;269:1637)—H.B.

———

Tina Kenyon and Stephen Davis recently published an article on medical malapropisms (Kenyon TM, Davis SW: Medical malapropisms: the sequin (sequel). J Fam Pract 1995;41:193–194). Here are some of the best:

- "The pain was so bad, I got a bottle of Jack Daniels and drank myself into *Bolivia*." (oblivion)
- "We decided not to have an autopsy because he was already dead."
- While speaking to the triage nurse about a genital rash, a patient said, "I just want you to know that I'm married and we're *monotonous*." (monogamous)
- "Look at that sunset—it has all the colors of the *rectum*." (spectrum)
- A pregnant patient called to say that she was having *erotic* contractions. (erratic)
- "Will I need a *resurrectomy?*" (hysterectomy)
- In a discharge summary, "no papilledema" came out, "no papal edema." In another, "perennial asthma" came out as "perineal asthma."
- A medical student's note stated, "The patient claims she got pregnant in Boston, which is impossible."
- A Welch-Allyn sigmoidoscope was transcribed as a "well-challenged sigmoidoscope."

For more on medical malapropisms, see pp. 259–260.—H.B.

A LESSON IN MEDICAL LINGOISTICS*

Justin Dorgeloh, M.D.

Scene: A classroom filled with eager medical students. As the curtain rises, Dr. Jaargon, Professor of Medical Lingoistics, enters.

DR. JAARGON: Good morning, students. Today we'll review some of the terms you will be required to use as doctors. First, what must patients do before they die?

CLASS *(in unison):* Go downhill.

STUDENT: Or pursue a downhill course.

DR. J: Very good. Now, to demonstrate diagnostic acumen, what must one have?

CLASS: A high index of suspicion.

DR. J: Right again. Normal lungs are always—

STUDENT: Clear.

DR. J: And a flat abdomen is—

STUDENT: Scaphoid.

DR. J: And a pharynx is—

STUDENT: Clear or injected.

DR. J: To look up published medical articles we—

STUDENT: Review the literature!

DR. J: *What* literature?

CLASS: *The* literature!

DR. J: Excellent. Now tell me what is wrong with the following statement: "There is no history of rheumatic fever, malaria, or syphilis."

STUDENT: A patient must always *deny* syphilis.

DR. J: Correct. Now, I overheard one of you saying yesterday that the treatment given one of our hospital patients was "ineffective." The required phrasing is, "The patient responded poorly to treatment." Please note the subtle shift in responsibility. That brings us to a related subject. What may a drug manifest?

CLASS: (No answer)

DR. J: Side effects. Not drawbacks or poisonous properties (heaven forbid!), but *side effects*. Now to go on. Feeding a patient is—

CLASS: Alimentation.

DR. J: And how about intravenous feeding?

STUDENT: Parenteral alimentation.

DR. J: And a patient excreting less or more nitrogen than he absorbs is in—

STUDENT: Nitrogen imbalance.

DR. J: No! The patient is always in *balance*. Positive balance or negative balance, but never imbalance. Remember that. Here's another question: Available remedies form a doctor's—

STUDENT: Therapeutic armamentarium.

DR. J: Right. Now, diseases of which we don't know the cause—

CLASS: Diseases of obscure etiology.

DR. J: And such a disease may be called—

STUDENT: Idiopathic.

DR. J: Or?

STUDENT: Cryptogenic.

DR. J: Ah! *There's* a word to inspire respect in the listener. And casual reference to such items as polyploidy, hamartomas, the Kell factor, and the chi square formula can be similarly effective . . . A disease capable of causing varied signs and/or symptoms is invariably known as—

STUDENT: A disease of protean manifestations.

DR. J: And a congenital or familial disease of metabolism is—

STUDENT: An inborn error of metabolism.

DR. J: Right. Now to proceed: An antibiotic affecting a variety of bacteria is a—

STUDENT: Versatile antibiotic.

DR. J: No.

STUDENT: Broad-action antibiotic.

DR. J: No, but you're closer. The proper term is broad-*spectrum* antibiotic. One might think that iridescent, multicolored, or rainbow would do, but they won't. It must always be *broad spectrum* . . . Now, class, a serum which will affect a variety of bacteria is a—

STUDENT *(confidently):* Broad-spectrum serum.

DR. J: No. You have fallen into my trap. It is a *polyvalent* serum. At this point a few more warnings may be in order. You can proctoscope, cystoscope, or bronchoscope a patient, but you cannot *stethoscope* him. For that matter, you cannot sphygmomanometer him, either. The internist is clearly at a disadvantage in this regard but has retaliated by adopting *digitalize* before that term could be claimed by the proctologist.

STUDENT *(breaking in):* Pardon me, sir, but how did we do in our written examination?

DR. J: Let's see. You were asked to rephrase, in a form suitable for medical publication, the statement: "The patient's nose was large and red." Mr. Jones' composition was the best. His translation is as follows, and I quote: "The case presented an erythematous blush of the nasal region, superimposed upon a process which had induced changes associated with a size at or just beyond the upper limit of the range generally considered the physiologic norm." Congratulations, Mr. Jones. You can really roll those syllables around.

(Here the curtain falls momentarily to indicate a short recess. As it rises again, Dr. Sinktest, a pathologist, enters.)

DR. J: Students, I have asked Dr. Sinktest to address you on Pathological Lingoistics. Dr. Sinktest, will you say something?

DR. SINKTEST *(startled):* The body is that of a well-developed, well-nourished—

DR. J: No, no. Dr. Sinktest. That's a microphone, not a dictaphone. Suppose, instead, you answer questions. What do you call a lump in the body?

DR. S *(promptly):* A tumor mass, of course.

DR. J *(to the class):* Dr. Sinktest is an expert in tautology.*

DR. S *(defensively):* There might be some doubt about a tumor, or a mass, but with a tumor mass you've got something.

DR. J: And a tumor mass always shows something on—

DR. S: Cut section. Sometimes the clinicians claim I forget to section the tumor masses. *Cut* section emphasizes the matter. "Cut section slicing" might convince those bums even better—

DR. J: Thank you, thank you very much, Dr. Sinktest! . . . Class dismissed.

CURTAIN

For the past 18 years, *Diversion Magazine*† has published a monthly feature called "Wit's End." The feature is actually a contest that tests an individual's flair with puns, malapropisms, and other forms of word play. For example, a recent contest asked readers to come up with some novel reworkings of medical terms. As a result, "Charcot's joint" became "Charcot's disreputable gathering place" and "cribriform plate" became "cribriform saucer." These contest provide a great outlet for those of us who enjoy juggling medical terminology.—H.B.

*The needless repetition of an idea, statement, or word.
†1790 Broadway, New York, N.Y. 10019

ACRONYMICAL CORRECTNESS*

Kim Shaftner, M.D.
David V. Meehan, D.O.

Doctors love abbreviations. So much, in fact, that much of what we write is couched in compact precision: "46 y/o WM admitted w/CP, DOE, PND. PMH: s/p ASMI, CABG, ACEI, and ASA."

These days we have a new love—acronyms. This penchant is especially acute in the research arena from which new studies (complete with their acronymic identifiers) emanate daily. We have MRFIT, STOP, MIDAS, a plethora of TIMIs and TAMIs, and others.

What we see here is a whole new specialty area of science and medicine, wherein a really good study has to have a really good name in order to make a splash on the scientific horizon. Picture the huddled masses in medical school basements: they sit around tables illuminated only by a single overhead bulb, thumbing through their dictionaries and racking their collective brains for that elusive good study name (one might wonder whether they sometimes pick a name and *then* dream up a suitable study, but that is another question altogether). Entire careers could be enhanced or trashed upon the power of one good word.

Such an arduous task is not without peril. Consider the hapless researcher who might have proposed that the Multicenter Diltiazem Postinfarction Trial be called MUDPIT. That fellow would likely spend the remainder of his career tending rats at a community college. Just imagine walking down the hallowed halls of your alma mater and overhearing a distinguished professor expounding upon the "unequivocal results of the MUDPIT study." Highly unlikely indeed.

Worse yet, otherwise excellent trials might have received a tepid response if they had been misnamed. What if the TIMI trials had been called Therapeutic Windows in Thrombolysis? "Hello, Dr. Jones. This is Dr. Smith from the Ivory Tower Medical Center. I'm recruiting co-investigators for the TWIT study." *Click.* "Hello?" Enrolling patients would be another obstacle: "Aw, heck, doc, why would you wanna give me a drug for twits? I ain't as dumb as I look, ya know."

Furthermore, the TEAM study (Thrombolysis with Eminase in Acute Myocardial Infarction) might have been billed as the CHEAT study (Cohort Study of Eminase in Antithrombosis) and the LATE trial (Late Assessment of Thrombolytic Efficacy) might have turned up DEAD (Dynamic Effect of Antithrombotic Delay). Horrors!

Here are a few of the Acronyms that Didn't Make It from our own research in this area (Shaftner K, Meehan DV: The ADMIT study. *Annals of Initials* 1995;14:208–294):

- MUTTS: Multidisciplinary Thrombolysis Treatment Study
- NERD: Nifedipine Effect in Reducing Death
- BUBBA: Broad-based University Study of Beta Blockers in Angina
- RATS: Risk of Antithrombotic Therapy Study
- HAHA: Hypertensive Adaptations in Heart Attack
- PORNO: Prospective Outcomes Research of Nifedipine in the Old

Having thus established the critical importance of acronymical correctness, we may soon be obliged to designate specialty training and perhaps certification in this area. An appropriate title for these new specialists would be derived from their degrees. Those awarded a Masters of Acronymics and those who become Doctors of Acronymics would be MIAs and DOAs respectively.

For another article that takes a pot shot at medical acronyms, see McMillan R, Longmire RL: Crisis in oncology—acute vowel obstruction (with apologies to oncologists everywhere). N Engl J Med 1976;294:1288–1289.—H.B.

*Reprinted from The Journal of Family Practice ©1996; 43:12, with permission from Appleton & Lange, Inc.

TRANSLATING MEDICAL IDIOM*

To the Editor: We hope the following guide will help medical students struggling with the foreign verbiage of medical language while attempting to assimilate new skills and knowledge.

IDIOMS OFTEN USED AT MEDICAL GRAND ROUNDS

Idiom	Meaning
"In my experience. . . ."	I have seen ONE such patient.
"In my series. . . ."	I have seen TWO such patients.
"In case, after Case, after CASE. . . ."	I have seen THREE such patients.
"I haven't had a lot of experience with this. . . ."	Well, ah, actually, never seen one before.

James Dolezal, M.D.
James Plamondon, M.D.

Iowa City, IA

NOTES FROM A MEDICAL LEXICOGRAPHER'S WASTE BASKET†

A-bor'-tion: 1. The quantity usually served to one person; as, "Give me abortion of potatoes." 2. A serving of beetflavored soup; as, "All I had for lunch was abortion a couple of bagels."

A-or'ta: Proper or required behavior; as, "If there's nothing more to drink maybe aorta go home."

Ap'-ne-a: Form of greeting to one whose arrival has been unduly delayed; as, "We was wondering what apnea."

Cau'-ter-ize: To become the object of observation by a third party; as, "He kept looking at her until he finally cauterize."

Co-ry'-za: Manifestation of emotional disturbance; as, "Everytime I hafta go out on a night call, she sits down and coryza eyes out."

Dig'-i-tal'-is: Introductory phrase of inquiry; as, "If we weren't supposed to know about it, why digitalis?"

Hem'-or-rhoid: Transportation afforded a third person; as, "He didn't have his car so I offered hemorrhoid."

Myx'-e-de'-ma: Transitive verb, past tense, for having combined fluids for the ingestion of the third person; as, "I knowed he was thirsty, so I myxedema martini."

Su'-pi-nate: Departure from the usual dietary practice at the beginning of a meal; as, "I passed up the supinate the salad."

U'-ri-nal'-y-sis: Relating to the environment of a second person with respect to the lodgings of a third person; as "I'm in Mary's room and urinalysis."

Ur'-ti-car'-i-a: Indicative of a desire to be manually transported by a third person; as, "The only reason that kid is screaming at her mother is that she wants urticaria."

Xiph'-o-cos'tal: An estimate of value; as, "It ain't pretty but it looks as xiphocostal lot a money."

H. S. Grannatt

*Reprinted with permission from The New England Journal of Medicine, © 1976; 295:176. Edited from the original.
†Reprinted from JAMA, © 1961; 176(8):A236 and 178(3):A246, with permission from the American Medical Association. Edited from the original.

During my research, I ran into a number of authors who poked fun at medicine's obsession with initials. The following letters, published 20 years apart, say it best.—*H.B.*

SORRY
(SO OUR RIDDLES RILE YOU)*

To the Editor: After glancing through the June 12 issue of the *Journal* I wonder about my ability to keep up with the language—let alone the pace—of modern medicine. I think I can follow the role of EBV in PTM—not to mention CMV. But when one does a CF for CMV does one require C$\overline{1}$, C' or merely C2? Perhaps my comments are NA—but even though I can tell DNA from RNA I am floored by MTX, dU, HTdR and CGD. I thought (see above) that I knew what "CF" meant, but I'm wrong—it's "citrovorum factor"! If this keeps up I'll be DOA before they can get me to the EW.

Chestnut Hill, MA

Geoffrey Edsall, M.D.

ABBREVIATIONS
IN THE MEDICAL LITERATURE†

To the Editor: There is a recent trend (RT) in the medical literature (ML) to abbreviate previously unabbreviated phrases for the sake of efficiency (PUPSAE). Although it makes good sense (GS), the frequency with which it is used can tax the inexperienced reader (IR). Sometimes repetition can actually be beneficial (RCABB) by allowing the reader to retain words he does not constantly have to refer back to (WOHCREBT).

I would like to suggest to the Editor (ED), that for the IR who doesn't wish to have PUPSAE, he have the GS to change the ML so that RCABB and he can eliminate WOHCREBT.

Steven G. Mann, M.D.
Santa Cruz Radiation Oncology
Medical Group
Santa Cruz, CA

ED's reply: We agree with Dr. Mann, but protest our innocence (POI). We do not ordinarily abbreviate PUPSAE because we also believe RCABB and we know that the IR needs WOHCREBT. But it makes GS to allow some previously abbreviated phrases (PAPS) when they are in widespread use (WU), and we occasionally even allow abbreviation of PUPSAE when repeatedly spelling them out would be unusually cumbersome (STOWBUC). We admit, however, that WU of PAPS and PUPS in the ML, even when STOWBUC, often raises the IR's and the ED's BP and HR.

*Reprinted with permission from The New England Journal of Medicine, © 1969; 281:223.
†Reprinted with permission from The New England Journal of Medicine, © 1989; 320:1152.

Additional Readings

1. Bennett HJ, Ratner JB: How common is common? South Med J 1991;84:903.

Since doctors never agree on anything, the authors set out to standardize the terms we use to describe disease frequency. They provide a table with 20 adjectives ranging from extremely common to extremely rare. For example, a "common" ailment is one that is seen weekly, whereas a "rare" disease will turn up once in a career. If a disease is "uncommonly rare" it would only be seen in another life, assuming of course that you were unlucky enough to be reincarnated as a physician.

2. Brickner WM: Acute anatomy. Amer J Surg 1921; 35:67.

This article satirizes some recent abuses of medical language—recent that is for 1921! It seems we are not the first generation of physicians that has had to contend with muddled terminology.

3. Christy NP: English is our second language. N Engl J Med 1979;300:979–981.

In this amusing satire, the author takes a scalpel to Medspeak—that inbred and sometimes pretentious language of the hospital. Among other things, he scoffs at the use of big words (symptomatology, armamentarium) when small ones would do and the use of verbal screens to dodge questions on rounds: "Was the man anemic PTA?" Answer: "Not really."

4. Cranefield PF: Diagnosis and treatment of book collecting. JAMA 1964;188:274-275.

The article pokes fun at book collecting by discussing it as though it is a disease. For example, although the history and physical exam are usually nonspecific, an elevated CBC (complete book count) and RBC (rare book count) make the diagnosis highly probable.

5. DePaolis M: Closing in on jargon. Postgrad Med 1994;95(1):17–18.

Doctors are always getting blamed for using too much jargon with patients. But what about other people? In this article, the author squares off with a closing attorney during the refinancing of his mortgage. For example, when the lawyer says, "Of course, personal mortgage insurance is required for any transaction involving a federally approved lender," Dr. DePaolis fires back with, "Well, ascending cholangitis can be ameliorated through parenteral antibiotic therapy." This exchange goes on for a couple of paragraphs.

6. Dorgeloh J: Milkman's syndrome? You mean Dr. Milkman. Med Economics 1966;43(Oct 31):190–197.

The author has some fun with medical eponyms and the confusion they cause in day-to-day medical practice.

7. Fitzgerald FT: A doctor's glossary (Part II). The Pharos 1982;45(winter):18.

The author presents a series of amusing definitions that relate to the physical examination. For example, **de•ferred** (di-fûrd) *adJ* Not done, and not likely to be done.

8. Freedman, Bernard J: Just a Word, Doctor. New York: Oxford Medical Publications, 1987.

A collection of witty essays on the origins of medical words and usages. The essays were originally published in the British Medical Journal between 1977 and 1986.

9. Gaño SN: Deficiencies in the English medical vocabulary. JAMA 1964;188:278.

The author describes some amusing inadequacies of language as it applies to clinical practice. For example, when getting a history on a patient with dyspnea, wouldn't it be more concise to ask, "Does she dysp?" Or, if a patient is having ventricular extrasystoles, can it be said that he is "extrasystolizing"?

10. Johnson RJ: A guide to emergency room jargon. Plast Reconst Surg 1993;92:173.

When emergency physicians call for a plastic surgeon, their comments often need to be interpreted. The author provides some examples of how to do this: "I have a real nice gentleman here." (He has no insurance.) "The family is real anxious." (They're looking up attorney listings right now.)

11. Newman TB, Browner WS: The epidemiology of life and death: a critical commentary. Am J Public Health 1988;78:161–162.

Using a style that satirizes epidemiologic writing, the authors present their analysis on the state of the art in life and death research. For example, death is defined as ". . . the ultimate state of the final common pathway that emerges subsequent to a terminal morbid event culminating in the eventual biocessation of animate bioprocesses."

12. Robb J: Medspeak made simplifax. Br Med J 1981; 283:1683–1684.

This is another article that takes some pot shots at Medspeak. The essay has fewer barbs than Dr. Christy's, but is just as amusing. For example, "One often sees on a haematology report 'essentially normal film'—a type of Haemspeak. Does this mean that the film is 'perfectly normal,' or 'more or less normal?'" The author concludes that it doesn't matter what we say to each other as long as we "layspeak" to the patient.

13. Scott RS, Myles WM: Ophthalmic diction-err-y. Survey Ophthalmol 1994;38:570.

This article is similar to the ones on pp 57 & 58, only here the daffynitions are ocular in nature. For example, *blind spot* (a dog that can't see), *fundus* (grant application plea), and *hyaloid* (a greeting for Lloyd).

WRITING & PUBLISHING

Physicians write a lot, some because they like to and others because they have to. While the former are certainly in a better position than the latter, I suspect they exist in smaller numbers. In fact, as one of my old professors used to say, "The only thing doctors do more than write is procrastinate about writing." Despite all the fuss, the articles still manage to get written, and the medical literature is healthy, if not somewhat corpulent, as a result.

During my research, I found a number of articles that took a swipe at the process of writing and publishing. I also ran into a few with amusing titles. The award for the funniest title goes to an article published in 1881 by Dr. Rufus Griswold (Clin News 1881; 2(15):199–200). Although the article itself is not that funny, the title is perfect: "Medico-Literary Tenesmus."

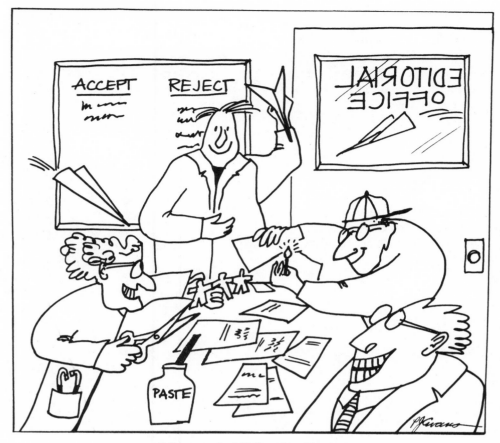

Manuscript Selection Process

HOW TO WRITE NIFTY TITLES FOR YOUR PAPERS*

Berril Yushomerski Yankelowitz, M.D.

General Principles

1. When you're up for promotion, the committee will most likely not read anything you have written. This is especially true if your titles are so esoteric that the promotions committee would not dare to peek at the text.

2. All of your titles should "sound" like original contributions.
3. If your study is not particularly good, make the title catchy or timely to help get it accepted.
4. If your study is decidedly dull, use the longest possible title you can invent.

*Reprinted with permission from the British Medical Journal, © 1980; 1:96. Edited from the original.

When to Write Titles

1. If you have not thought of a project and a title comes to mind, use it and work a paper around it.
2. Titles are best written with a brandy after dinner. Titles written on an empty stomach are likely to be dull and witless.
3. Some great titles have been done while sitting on the john. This is an excellent time to engage in title creation.

Examples of Titles for Your First Papers

1. "A patient with pimples and coronary occlusion—case report of a new association."
2. "The association of pimples and coronary occlusion—a case report."
3. "Concurrence of coronary occlusion and pimples in a patient—a new observation."

Examples of Titles for Follow-up Papers

1. "Two patients with pimples and coronary occlusion."
2. "A second case of pimples in coronary occlusion and review of the literature."
3. "Pimples and coronary occlusion—a historical perspective."

Catch Words and Phrases to Make Your Study Sound "Sound"

1. Starting phrases—try to use statistical terms: "A randomised trial of . . ."; "Multiple linear regression analysis of . . ."; "The frequency of the occurrence of . . ."; "The association of . . ."; "The rarity of the occurrence of . . ."
2. Phrases to make you sound honest and reliable

(insert whatever you like in the blank spaces): "The failure of _____ to influence _____"; "_____, an important negative study"; "The unreliability of _____ in assessing _____"; "The implausibility of _____ in understanding _____"; "The total and utter ineptness of _____ to comprehend _____."

3. Phrases to make you sound innovative: "Creating life, starting with one and two carbon compounds and rare earths—a progress report"; "The pathophysiologic relationship between pimples and coronary occlusion—a hypothesis." "The omega factor, a critical new parameter in examining the (*choose a body organ*)". The omega factor can be anything you like.
4. Phrases to make you sound timely: "The relationship of the omega factor to *urban health care*"; "*Medically underserved* patients with pimples and coronary occlusion"; "*Peer review* in assessing the quality of care of patients with pimples, with *special emphasis on the subpopulation* with coronary occlusion." (The length of this alone is catchy; do not mind the content.)
5. Ending phrases you can use (insert your study in the blank spaces): "_____, an essential tool in evaluating _____"; "_____, a preliminary report"; "_____, a statistical analysis and consideration for the future"; "_____, a negative study"; "_____ in New York City between 1921 and 1922."
6. Middle phrases you can use: "_____ in a population with _____"; "_____ in a family with _____"; "_____ in the senile great aunt of a patient with_____."

These title suggestions should get you off to a proper start. Happy writing, and enjoy the promotion.

Except for an occasional heart attack, I feel as young as I ever did.

Robert Benchley

PARSE ANALYSIS:
A NEW METHOD FOR THE EVALUATION
OF INVESTIGATORS' BIBLIOGRAPHIES*

Paul J. Davis, M.D. 0.92
Robert I. Gregerman, M.D. 0.08

During the past five years our laboratory has been concerned with the development of a quantitative system for describing the relative contributions of authors to multiple-author manuscripts. The concept that has evolved is termed "parse analysis" and has been logically broadened to include the measurement of manuscript quality. This report reviews the basic principles of parse analysis and describes their recent application to the evaluation of scientific careers. We emphasize the point that the principles outlined here are the product of cooperative efforts of a host of scientists—many of them from abroad and elsewhere—working in our laboratory. Without the imagination and insight of these investigators, the concept of parse could not have been formalized.

The system of parse analysis was created to meet the following specific needs: evaluation of relative contributions of authors to papers with more than one author; determination of the order of authors listed on title pages of manuscripts; weighting of the degree of difficulty of the scientific problem under investigation in a given manuscript; quantitative evaluation of the quality of execution of the study described; and indication to prospective employers of the net worth of a set of publications to which a prospective investigator has contributed.

The first principle of parse is the assignment of decimal fractions to each author of a given paper to indicate contribution to overall effort. These fractions in all cases follow each author's name, as in the example, "'Beta-adrenergic Blockade,' by R. L. Fernley 0.24, P. L. Pritchard-Grant 0.08, T. Bates 0.36 and R. G. Ferguson 0.27."

This is not a particularly good example because the sum of the decimal fractions is only 0.95, a parse analysis finding indicating that the work is incomplete or is significant only at the 5 per cent level, or includes work (about 0.05 worth) performed by a visiting investigator no longer affiliated with the laboratory. However, the basic idea is clear. In this particular example, the blame for the work must be fairly evenly apportioned among Fernley, Bates and Ferguson. Pritchard-Grant was probably the senior author[1] of the paper, in the light of his negligible contribution. This distribution of decimal fractions devolves as a unique responsibility upon the authors, themselves, and can, conceivably, result in serious delays in the submission of manuscripts. Occasionally, manuscripts might not even be submitted for publication because of the authors' inability to agree upon a parsing; when this happens the literature has most probably been done a service. An alternative solution is the submission of decimal assignments agreed to by a majority of the authors but not unanimously approved. In these cases the decimal fraction that is contested is followed by the notation, U.P. ("Under Protest"), as in the example, "R. G. Ferguson 0.27 U.P." In no case should the sum of the fractions be greater than 1.00. The independent studies of F.R.C. Johnstone,[2] of Vancouver, have recently been pointed out to us, and readers may note certain similarities that are gratifying in the development of his work and the first principle of parse analysis.

The second principle of parse is the determination of the order of authors on a manuscript according to the method of Pecks.[3] Experience has shown that the following factors may be considered in determining author order: number of pa-

*Reprinted with permission from The New England Journal of Medicine, © 1969; 281:989–990. Edited from the original.

pers previously published by each of the collaborators (the so-called reciprocal factor of Pecks); responsibility for the basic concept of the work; responsibility for the actual work done; duration of stay of each of the collaborators in the senior author's laboratory (the so-called tenacity factor of Pecks); and alphabetization of collaborators' last or first names. Tables of natural Pecks factors are available from our laboratory, if not from Pecks himself. In general, we point out that high Pecks scores are the reward of the devoted, underpublished collaborator but seldom influence author sequence on manuscripts. The splendid work of Harriet A. Zuckerman[4] can hardly be overlooked in this context and should be of interest to scientists and others.

The third and fourth principles of parse are designed to provide casual readers with easy methods of evaluating at a glance both the difficulty of the subject matter attacked by investigators and the quality of the attack made on the problem. For example, in the study of "Beta-adrenergic Blockade" by Fernley et al., it is obvious that everyone nowadays is working on beta-adrenergic blockade, and the degree of difficulty of the subject is only about 1.6 out of a possible 3.0. Careful reading of the paper by Fernley, however, indicates that whereas the subject matter was rather easy, the design of the experiment was complex, ingenious, novel and yet somehow carried out within the guidelines set by the Declaration of Helsinki. The execution of the study therefore rates a 2.3 out of a possible 3.0. We will not go into the interesting derivation of such scoring at this time. The product of the degree of difficulty and the execution is called by convention the "parse product." In this case it is (1.6) (2.3), or 3.68. The parse product divided by the parse potential—a perfect score of 9.0—represents the "parse index" (usually expressed $\times 100$), in this case 40.8. Since the overwhelming majority of papers in the literature parse index at slightly better than 10.5, the paper by Fernley et al. can be seen at a glance by the casual reader to be a very good paper indeed. The parse index is assigned by journal referees and is usually printed immediately after the title of the paper, as in the example, " 'Beta-adrenergic Blockade 40.8,' by R. L. Fernley 0.24, etc."

The final virtue of parse analysis is its uncanny and inherent capacity to sum up an investigator's career in one or two easily manipulated numbers that obviate job interviews and the reviewing of a great many dull bibliographies. These numbers may be the basis for the tendering of academic offers. This penultimate parse is called "career parse." Like many of the other principles elaborated by the computer, the career parse is composed of two factors and their product. The factors are the *sum* of decimal fractions of relative contributions to all papers on which the author's name appears and the *mean* parse index of all the papers to which he contributed. The product (career parse) has been determined by R. L. Fernley, who has kindly lent his bibliography to our laboratory. Fernley, who is now engaged in the private practice of medicine in upstate New York, is one of the authors of the well known paper on beta-adrenergic blockade, and his career decimal-fraction sum—obtained from a series of twelve papers published between 1955 and 1964—was 1.76, which is not much of a sum. However, because during that period Fernley worked on a number of extremely complex, ingenious and novel projects, his mean paper parse index was a whopping 43.7. It takes only a parsing knowledge of mathematics to see that Fernley acquired a career parse of 76.91. This was not enough, we are sorry to report, to acquire tenure at any of the seven institutions at which he worked. He also barely passed his State Board Examination.

Conclusions

Responsibly applied, parse principles have immense potential for defining academic success in easy-to-understand, mathematical terms. At present in our laboratory we are investigating parse at both the theoretical and practical levels. These investigations include the building of a multicompartment, journal-specific mathematical model to describe the kinetics of parse indexing,* and a parse-or-fail system for computer matching of academic positions and prospects on a countrywide basis (National Data Bank for Career Parses or NDBCP).

References and Notes

1. Two definitions in absolute terms of "senior author" are current: where no collaborator has an office, the

author with fewest desks in his laboratory is senior; where several collaborators have offices the collaborator whose office is farthest from the laboratory is senior.

2. Johnstone FRC: The true publication index. A measure of scientific endeavor. JAMA 202: adv p 371, Nov 20, 1967.

3. P.I. Pecks, a former collaborator in our laboratory who is remembered primarily for his cream cheese sandwiches and shrill countertenor.

4. Zukerman HA: Patterns of name ordering among authors of scientific papers: a study of social symbolism and its ambiguity. Amer J Sociol 74:276, 1968.

5. So far, and this is tentative, it looks like 11 compartments will do it (unpublished observations).

As with all ground breaking articles, the one by Davis and Gregerman generated a flurry of responses (see NEJM 1970;282:170–171.) For additional satires on author inflation, see the following:

1. Hecht F: Et al gets the Nobel prize. N Engl J Med 1977;296:234.

2. Scheible W, Resnick D, et al: Author inflation and cv creep. AJR 1985; 144:863.

3. Sobal J. Ferentz KS: Abstract creep and author inflation. N Engl J Med 1990;323:488–489.

In their desire to keep current, Drs. Davis and Gregerman have written a new treatise, *Parse Analysis II* (NEJM 1995;332:965–966), that retracts their original assumptions and goes in a different offbeat direction. If you enjoyed *Parse Analysis I,* you will definitely like the sequel.—H.B.

GET INTO PRINT!*

John Larkin, M.D.

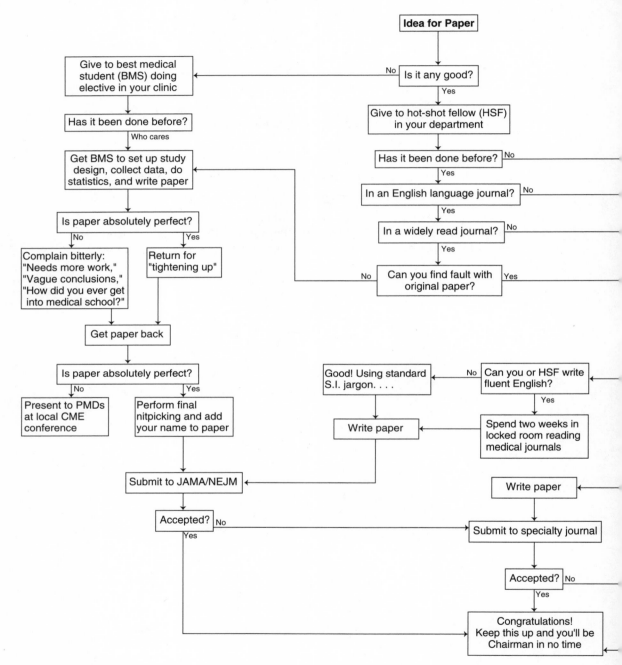

*Reprinted from World Medicine © 1984; 19(12):24-25. with permission from the author. Edited from the original.

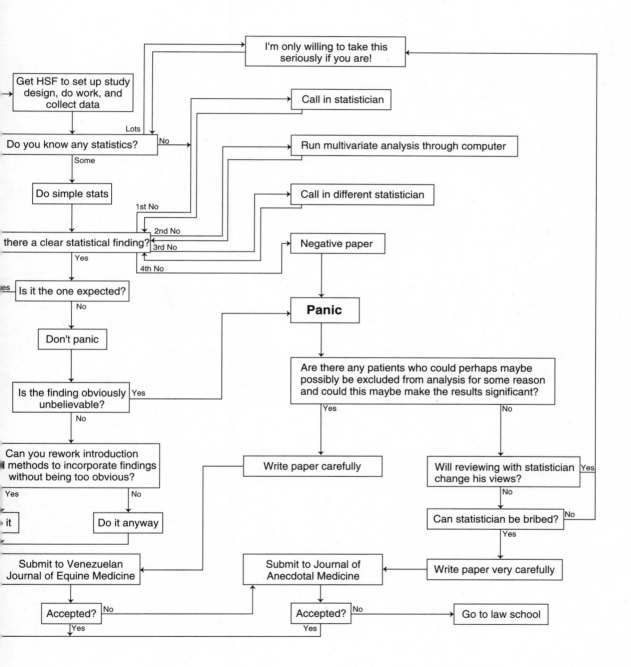

HOW TO CREATE A LONG CV FROM A SINGLE DATA BASE*

Berril Yushomerski Yankelowitz, M.D.

In this day when fame and academic promotion depend on the dry weight of a curriculum vitae rather than its content, it is important to get as much out of a piece of work as one can. This article shows the principle of amplification to achieve success.

1. It is usually wise to have a data base to start with.
2. Never write one paper when you can write two—that is, split your data base. Each split will hereafter be referred to as a "study."
3. In addition to local journals, publish each study in at least three foreign publications.
4. Change the title and submit each study to another journal.
5. Change the way the authors are listed and resubmit the study to another journal.
6. Change a few words in each paragraph and resubmit the paper to yet another journal.
7. Add a data point and submit to the original journal as a follow-up.
8. Repeat steps 3–5 with a new data point.
9. Add a second new data point and resubmit the study again.
10. Write a paper entitled: "Final Results of (list your study here)." This paper should look a lot like your last follow-up study.
11. Repeat steps 3–5.
12. Write a review article about the study.
13. Repeat steps 3–5.
14. Write a book chapter entitled (name your study here). Repeat as often as you are asked.
15. Write an article called, "An historical perspective of (list your study here)."
16. Repeat steps 3–5.

You should now have at least 24 papers, four book chapters, four review articles, and four historical perspectives for a total of 36 listings on your CV. If you also buy stock in a paper company, you'll not only be promoted, you'll be rich—so good luck and happy writing.

After breaking away from a patient who sought his advice for a medical problem, a doctor finally got to his restaurant table.

"Do you think I should send her a bill?" the doctor asked the lawyer who was sitting next to him.

"Why not?" the lawyer said. "You rendered professional services by giving advice."

"Thanks," the doctor said. "I think I'll do just that."

When the doctor went to his office the next day to send out the bill, he found a note from the lawyer. It read, "For legal services, $50."

*Reprinted with permission from the British Medical Journal © 1979; 2:1139.

LETTERS TO THE EDITOR THAT I'D LIKE TO SEE*

Howard J. Bennett, M.D.

To say that doctors sometimes disagree about clinical or research matters is most certainly an understatement. Nevertheless, despite all the lampooning that goes on in hallways, bedrooms, and the hospital cafeteria, you would never know how brash physicians can get by reading the correspondence sections of our medical journals. Just once, I'd like to see what my humble colleagues would write about if propriety did not stand in their way.

Who's Quoting Whom?

To the Editor: At first with skepticism and then with growing dyspepsia, we read the recent article by Todd and Williams. These physicians should have spent a little more time reviewing the literature and a little less time at parties trying to get their research funded. Perhaps then they would have noticed that we published a similar paper (over five years ago) in the *Journal of Irrefutable Research.* Although their discussion lacked the complexity that ours had, a citation was clearly in order.

> *Daniel Jennings, M.D.*
> *Angela Wood, M.D.*

In Reply: Get a life, you guys! Just because our paper made *Time Magazine* and all the major networks is no reason for you to be mad at us. We would have cited your article, but it's getting a little old by now, and we already had enough references showing the wrong way to approach this problem.

> *Stacy Todd, M.D.*
> *Greg Williams, M.D.*

Envy Has Me in Its Grip

To the Editor: We read the recent report by Anderson and Lee with interest. Actually, it wasn't so much with interest as curiosity. Well, not actually curiosity, but with a degree of awe because of the volume of research they publish. Come to think of it, we're not sure awe is the right word either because that implies respect or adulation. And the truth is, these guys really steam our socks! All they do is sit in their lab day after day churning out articles while we have to see patients. You know, it's really hard to be a full-time clinician and a researcher too. But does the university understand that? Noooooo! All they care about are publications, publications, publications. So people like Anderson and Lee get the credit while we do all the work.

By the way, can we add this letter to our CVs?

> *Mark Peters, M.D.*
> *Sarah Trust, M.D.*

Editor's Reply: No.

Where There's a Pill There's a Way

To the Editor: How can we believe the recent report by Crane and colleagues when it was funded by the same company that makes the drug they studied? Isn't that a conflict of interest or something? Obviously, these guys knuckled under when the pharmaceutical industry waved a few million bucks under their noses. The only way the medical community will accept this research is to have it validated at another center.

It just so happens that my lab is pretty quiet right now, and I might be able to do this for them. In fact, I know I'll be able to do it. So give me a call, okay? Please. My mice are losing weight, my grants have all run out, and I'm up for tenure in less than a year.

> *William Moore, M.D.*

In Reply: Don't call us, we'll call you.

> *Jonathan Crane, M.D.*
> *Barbara Crane, M.D.*
> *Henry Crane, Ph.D.*

*Reprinted with permission from Resident & Staff Physician, © 1992; 38(7)72–74

Sticks & Stones

To the Editor: I was quite surprised when I saw that Miller and Jones made the lead article in a recent issue of the journal. Not only were there some obvious flaws in their research design (my 12-year-old son picked these up), but their use of creative statistics was intriguing to say the least. Believe me, I went to med school with these guys, and to them, positive predictive value meant how likely you were to pick someone up at a local bar. And if that isn't enough, I know they never really understood the Krebs cycle.

Frank Watson, M.D.

In Reply: Considering that Dr. Watson got through medical school by the skin of his teeth (ask him to show you his National Board scores), one wonders where he gets the gumption to pan our article. What Frank forgot to mention, of course, is that he applied for the same grant we did and lost. And not only that, ask him whose notes he borrowed to make it through biochemistry.

Benjamin Miller, M.D.
Lauren Jones, M.D.

That's a Boy

To the Editor: I read the recent article by Thomas with great enthusiasm. The author not only did a thorough review of the literature, but his research design and statistical analysis were brilliant! I just wish all the papers that appeared in your journal were of the same caliber.

Sharon Thomas, M.D.

In Reply: Thanks, Mom.

James Thomas, M.D.

Doctors aren't the only ones responsible for the humor that appears in our journals—the literature is also filled with amusing advertisements. My favorite appeared in *JAMA* in 1948 (July 24, p. A13). In the same issue that featured articles on Streptomycin and The Pressor Effects of Epinephrine, there was a full page ad for ice cream. The manufacturer wanted doctors to know that ice cream is a flexible dessert, that it's made up of highly digestible proteins, and that it can be used with patients who are on either a low calorie or a high calorie diet. Now that's flexible!—H.B.

THE EDITORIAL ORDEAL
OF DR. JOB PLODD*

Alvan G. Foraker, M.D.
A. E. Anderson, JR., M.D.

Podunk General Hospital
Podunk, Missabama

January 2, 1975

Fritz Dingleburr, M.D., Editor
Northeast Journal of Medicine
Northeast City

Dear Dr. Dingleburr:

Please consider the enclosed manuscript for publication.

Sincerely,

Job Plodd, M.D.

Northeast Journal of Medicine
Northeast City

March 17, 1975

Job Plodd, M.D.
Podunk General Hospital
Podunk, Missabama

Dear Dr. Plodd:

The Editorial Board has voted not to accept the paper by Dr. Button and yourself, entitled, "Omphalo-sarcoma: A Clinical and Histochemical Review." This nonacceptance does not imply major criticism, since the Journal receives thousands of manuscripts each year and can publish less than one percent of these. For your interest, we have enclosed one reviewer's comment. We do not, however, suggest that you return this manuscript to us after revision, since the decision of our Editorial Board is final.

Sincerely,

Fritz Dingleburr, M.D.
Editor

*Reprinted from Pathology Annual, © 1976; 11:189–199, with permission from Appleton & Lange, Inc. Edited from the original.

February 16, 1975

    I do not recommend acceptance of the paper by Plodd and Button. They reviewed 37 cases of omphalosarcoma from their hospital and applied certain basic histochemical tests. The work is adequate, on a low-level scientific and intellectual plane, but not inspiring. It is not likely to appeal to the majority of readers of the *Northeast Journal*. In addition, the horrible misuse of the subjunctive mode renders this opus unattractive, although doubtless this conforms to the linguistic practices among the denizens of Missabama.

Memorandum

March 19, 1975

To: B. Button, M.D., Attending Omphalologist
From: J. Plodd, M.D., Pathologist

    This rejection was anticipated. I'll redraft the manuscript, trying to be more correct with the subjunctive mode, whatever that is. Then we'll try the next journal on our list.

J. Plodd, M.D.

Podunk General Hospital
Podunk, Missabama

April 16, 1975

Esau Terrick, M.D., Editor
Journal of Investigative Biomolecular Omphalology
Metrocolossal University Medical Center
Metrocolossal City

Dear Professor Terrick:

    Please consider the enclosed manuscript for publication.

Sincerely,

Job Plodd, M.D.

Metrocolossal University Medical Center
Metrocolossal City

June 28, 1975

Job Plodd, M.D.
Podunk General Hospital
Podunk, Missabama

Dear Dr. Plodd:

I regret to inform you that our editorial advisors are uniformly opposed to acceptance of your manuscript, which is returned with one reviewer's comment. Be assured that we are always willing to consider investigative papers which conform to our scientific and intellectual standards.

Sincerely,

Esau Terrick, M.D.
Editor and Research Professor

(Anonymous Reviewer's Comment)

May 6, 1975

The paper by Plodd and Button is indeed plodding and should be pigeon-holed if not button-holed. The histochemical techniques are simplistic and obsolete. They applied the ancient chi square test to their data, rather than the more modern zeta-beta techniques. There may be a place for studies on human omphalosarcoma, but not in the *Journal of Investigative Biomolecular Omphalology*. Studies of this type should be considered only if currently accepted scientific technics are applied, such as four-dimensional interference-ferrito-electron microscopy.

Memorandum

July 1, 1975

To: Be. Button, M.D.
From: J. Plodd, M.D.

There isn't much we can do about these scathing criticisms, but I'll redo the manuscript to emphasize general pathology and try it on one of my own trade journals.

J. Plodd, M.D.

Podunk General Hospital
Podunk, Missabama

August 4, 1975

Strikk Lee Beynall, M.D., Ph.D.
Editor, Annals of Omphalic Pathology
Burgeon University
Burgeon City

Dear Dr. Beynall:

Please consider the enclosed manuscript for publication.

Sincerely,

Job Plodd, M.D.

Burgeon University
Burgeon City

October 15, 1975

Job Plodd, M.D.
Podunk General Hospital
Podunk, Missabama

Dear Dr. Plodd:

Our Editorial Board has recommended rejection of your manuscript, which is returned herewith. A reviewer's comment is enclosed.

Sincerely,

Strikk Lee Beynall, M.D., Ph.D.
Editor

(Anonymous Reviewer's Comment)

September 30, 1975

This puerile piece is far below the standards of the *Annals*. It is rather illegitimate, to speak kindly, being too surgical for a pathology journal, and not good enough for us, although it might be accepted in a journal of *clinical* surgery. There are entirely too many old fashioned H & E photomicrographs, and absolutely *no*, repeat *no* electron microscopic illustrations. Fancy that in 1975! Virchow might have written this piece himself, although he would have done it better. In my view, physicians from Podunk should treat their patients, check their cotton fields, and not try to be scientists.

Memorandum

January 7, 1976

To: J. Plodd, M.D.
From: B. Button, M.D.

I've had it up to here with these "Longhairs." There's just one shot left in my locker. This guy will take anything—believe me—anything.

B. Button, M.D.

Podunk General Hospital
Podunk, Missabama

January 11, 1976

Boyy Biggvoyce, M.D., Editor
Missabama State Medical Society Journal
Chief, Service of General Practice
Gladesdale Community Hospital
Gladesdale, Missabama

Boyy, you old son-of-a-gun:

How are ya, Boyy? Here's a real scientific piece for your monthly rag. This is good surgical stuff, with a dose of science added by my path man, Job Plodd. Don't say I never did anything for you.

When we get together at the spring meeting, I'll show you some great pictures I took sailfishing off the coast of Latinonia. I'm telling the IRS I went to a meeting. The fish were great.

Your old drinking buddy,

Bill B.

Gladesdale Community Hospital
Gladesdale, Missabama

March 13, 1976

B. Button, M.D.
Podunk General Hospital
Podunk, Missabama

Dear Bill:

Your piece is way too scientific for us Missabamian medicos. I don't understand most of that guff, and those pictures by Plodd are real yawners. Everybody knows you're the best belly button cutter in the state anyway, so you don't need to blow your horn with us. Why don't you try this mass of mush on some egghead publication like the *Northeast Journal?* It should be just their cup of tea.

Why don't you write a piece for us about your recent sailfishing trip?

Your good friend,

Boyy Biggvoyce, M.D.

Memorandum

March 29, 1976

To: J. Plodd, M.D.
From: B. Button, M.D.

I give up. Cut this piece into paper dolls, stuff it in File X—do what you wish. I'm giving up research to concentrate on my new hobby—writing fishing stories for doctors.

B. Button, M.D.

Podunk General Hospital
Podunk, Missabama

April 18, 1976

M. Y. Opick, Ph.D., Editor
Western Missabama Quarterly Journal of Science
Assistant Professor of Biology
Podunk Junior College
Podunk, Missabama

Dear Milt:

Please consider the enclosed manuscript for publication.

Your friend,

J. Plodd, M.D.

Podunk Junior College
Podunk, Missabama

April 26, 1976

Job Plodd, M.D.
Podunk General Hospital
Podunk, Missabama

Dear Dr. Plodd:

I'm delighted to accept your excellent article, "Omphalosarcoma: A Clinical and Histochemical Review," for publication in the *Western Missabama Quarterly Journal of Science.* As you know most of our publications are by junior college and high school biology teachers, such as classifying the snakes in Chattahoochie Creek.

You will be expected to pay publication costs of $75 per page, and to purchase 500 reprints for about $275. We appreciate your maintaining membership in our Science Teachers Association at $100 per year, and your continuing support of science education in Western Missabama.

Thank you for allowing your outstanding research paper to appear in our journal.

Respectfully,

M. Y. Opick, Ph.D.
Editor

———⋙●⋘———

One of the most difficult things to contend with in a hospital is the assumption on the part of the staff that because you have lost your gall bladder, you have also lost your mind.

Jean Kerr

The following selection was compiled from seven articles published in the *Southern Medical Journal* between 1983 and 1993. The full citations are listed on p. 89.—H.B.

DIZZY MEDICAL WRITING*

Herbert L. Fred, M.D., Patricia Robie, Mark Scheid, Ph.D.

After completing his glorious pitching career, Dizzy Dean became a popular baseball announcer. In response to a listener who accused him of not knowing the King's English, Dizzy said, "Old Diz knows the King's English. And not only that. I also know the Queen is English."

Old Diz may have known the King's English, but you couldn't prove it by how he spoke. Similarly, many physicians and scientists may know the King's English, but you couldn't prove it by how they write. We decided, therefore, to present the "Dizzy Awards" for outstandingly dizzy medical writing. Only recent articles in prominent American medical journals were eligible (references available upon request).

The Batty Title Award (three-way tie)

"Early Gastric Cancer in a United States Hospital"
—Presumably the hospital's chief complaint was pain in the middle of the corridor on the ninth floor.

"The Ectopic Kidney in the Emergency Department"
—Unless accompanied by their owners, kidneys should never enter the Emergency Department.

"When Should Patients with Lethal Ventricular Arrhythmia Resume Driving?"
—When they are reincarnated.

The Extra Innings Award

"The epicardium, cardiac valves, and endocardium appeared normal. The epicardium, cardiac valves, and endocardium appeared normal."
—But what about the epicardium, cardiac valves, and endocardium?

The Knot-Hole Award

". . . subsequent reports suggest that colonoscopy can recognize angiodysplasia."
—But only after they've known each other for a long time.

The Touch Every Base Award

"The proposal that cobalt-induced lung disease might thus at least partly result from 'transitional metal overload' leading to oxygen free radical tissue injury, does not appear to have been hitherto envisaged, and such a mechanism is admittedly still speculative, but this hypothesis merits further experimental investigation."
—Would you care to qualify that statement?

The Cases at the Bat Award

"Only 13 cases have been reported to date in the literature, of which four were pregnant."
—Nine months from now, there should be at least four more cases to report.

The Signs From the Coach Award

"Thus, the initial diagnostic FOB in patients with suspected PCP complicating CTD should include BAL and TBLB."
—SOS.

The Flagpole Award

"The common practice of misdiagnosing deep vein thrombosis clinically should be abandoned."
—Agreed.

*Printed with permission from the Southern Medical Journal, © 1983–1993.

The Sudden Change in the Line-Up Award

"We report a 65-yr-old man with hepatitis B related liver cirrhosis and biopsy-proven hepatocellular carcinoma who has undergone spontaneous regression."

—How far back did he go?

The Extra Innings Award

"Since a prospective study of 50 or more HAPE patients would be very hard if not impossible to plan, we had to accept all disadvantages of retrospective data analysis, such as a limited amount of documented information, varying roentgenographic technique and exposure intervals, and last but not least, the selection of patients needing hospital care, ie, probably a more serious subset of subjects with established rather than nascent HAPE studied at low altitude after evacuation."

—It keeps on going and going and going.

The Switch Hitter Award

". . . the pulmonary function studies of our patients revealed a restrictive pattern, and they had only a few complaints despite widespread radiographic changes."

—Our pulmonary function studies never complain.

The Batted Out of Order Award

"After 10 years as chairman of medicine, the family moved to California, . . ."

—The Papa Chair, Mama Chair, and all the little Chairs?

The Ejected From the Game Award

"The Organism was transported to the Centers for Disease Control. . . ."

—Under heavy guard, no doubt.

The Balk Award

"However, in the absence of a thyroid primary, in view of the ability of carcinoids to form various polypeptide hormones (although not usually as much as was formed by Sweeney, McDonnell and O'Brien's tumour), and the finding of small amounts of amyloid in both our cases, Sweeney, McDonnell and O'Brien's case may be another carcinoid of the larynx forming an unusually large amount of polypeptide hormone and, secondarily to that, large amounts of amyloid."

—We disagree, we think.

The "It Ain't Over Til It's Over" Award (A tie)

"Very obviously, mouse connective tissue is not necessarily human connective tissue. . ."

—Very obviously.

"Shock never developed if the disease was not serious . . ."

—Seriously?

The Removed From the Lineup Award

"Catheter function was preserved in all patients who were completely lysed."

—Isn't it against the law to lyse patients?

The Out in Left Field Award

"However, none of the subjects indicated any localized muscle pain or soreness of the delayed type at these times that they experienced later."

—We, however, wish to indicate diffuse pain and soreness of the immediate type brought about at this time by the statement above that we experienced earlier.

Epilogue

We draw two conclusions, one happy and one sad: The memory of Old Diz will be around for a long, long time. And so will dizzy medical writing.

References

1. Fred HL, Robie P: Dizzy medical writing. South Med J 1983;76:1165–1166.

2. Fred HL, Robie P: Dizzy medical writing: part II. South Med J 1984;77:755–756.

3. Fred HL, Robie P: Dizzy medical writing: concluded. South Med J 1985;78:1498–1501.

4. Fred HL, Robie P: Dizzy medical writing: report on recent relapses. South Med J 1989;82:897–899.

5. Fred HL, Robie P: Dizzy medical writing: will it never end? South Med J 1991;84:755–759.

6. Fred HL: Dizzy medical writing and editing: no relief in sight. South Med J 1992;85:743–745.

7. Fred HL, Scheid M: Dizzy medical writing and editing: a decade of nonprogress. South Med J 1993; 86:705–709.

Additional Readings

1. Abigail: Advice for forlorn medical authors. JAMA 1964;188:A228–229.

This is a medical version of an Ann Landers column.

2. Bennett HJ: Post-rejection paronychia. J Fam Pract 1995;40:122–123.

The author slams his finger in a desk drawer after receiving a rejected manuscript in the mail. He suggests that writers should consider other ways of venting their frustration. For example, yelling at managed care administrators, arguing with drug reps, or refusing to go to any hospital committee meetings.

3. Bigg S: Newspaper fare. JAMA 1968;204:115.

The author conducted a nutritional study in which sheep were fed different sections of JAMA. While all of the sheep gained weight, some unexpected behavioral effects were noted: Those animals who dined on letters-to-the-editor became pugnacious, while a diet rich in editorials led to excessive somnolence. Finally, the ingestion of advertising pages caused a considerable amount of gastrointestinal disturbance.

4. Bing RJ: Withering and the Quarterly Journal of Negative Results. Arch Intern Med 1963;111:143–144.

This is a brief satire on clinical observation and the scientific method. The author postulates that Withering's classic report on foxglove would never have been published if it were submitted in today's medical climate.

5. Hansen M: Lessons of a Figley fellow or how I learned to stop worrying and love the publication game. AJR 1994;162:783–790.

This is a marvelous article that was unfortunately too long for the book. The author makes fun of editors, reviewers, proofreaders and just about everything that happens to a manuscript from the time it leaves your hand until it finally makes it into print.

6. Harlow HF: Fundamental principles for preparing psychology journal articles. Anesth Analg 1976;55:455–458.

Although this paper originally appeared in a psychology journal, it's generic enough for anyone who writes scientific articles. For example, "It's fun to write introductions—one is not constrained by the facts."

7. Hearse D: Of humour, music, anger, speed, and excuses: reflections of an editorial team after one year in office. Cardiovasc Res 1992;26:1161–1163.

The editors present a behind-the-scenes look at what it takes to put a journal together. Among other things, the article includes a letter from an exasperated author: "Some of the reviewers' comments we couldn't do anything about. For example, if (as reviewer C suggested) several of my recent ancestors were indeed drawn from other species, it is too late to change that."

8. Pittenger JB, Whitney P: Reviewerese: a glossary of remarks commonly appearing in articles submitted for publication in psychology journals. J Polymorphous Perversity 1986;3(3):21–24.

Although this article was written for psychologists, the humor transcends disciplines. For example, when a reviewer says "The author is unaware of much of the literature relevant to this topic and neglected to mention Jones' well-known 1978 study," what he really means is, "I'm Jones and I'm miffed."

9. Quay E: Verbal hyperplasia: new thoughts on an old disease. JAMA 1965;192:126–128.

Verbal hyperplasia is one of many disorders that result from an excess or deficiency of those enzymes needed for clear speech and writing. Most of these diseases exist in a heterozygous and homozygous state.

10. Rafal RB: A standardized method for determination of who should be listed as authors on scholarly papers. Chest 1991;99:786.

The author proposes a new scoring system that takes the guesswork out of picking a co-author (the higher the score the better). For example, "The resident who conceived the idea, did the research, and wrote the paper gets a +2, whereas a blood relative gets a +21 and an in-law gets a −25."

11. Reece RL: Space-occupying gambits for medical writers. JAMA 1967;200:162–164.

The author presents 10 techniques for turning clear writing into masterworks of ambiguity. In summary, "Say nothing well and don't stop saying it."

12. Yankelowitz BY: Making visual aids work for you. Br Med J 1980;281:1718.

The author provides a number of suggestions on how to create effective graphs for scientific papers.

For example, "In biology it is good to have at least three data points not lying on the best fitting curve. This gives the reader the impression that you did not fudge the results or 'dry lab' the experiment altogether."

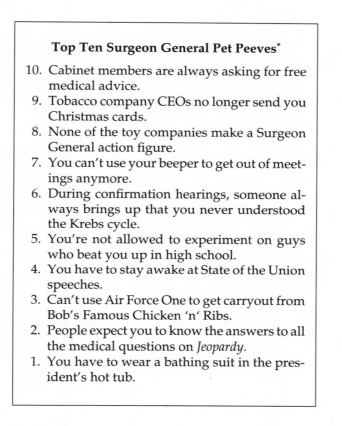

Top Ten Surgeon General Pet Peeves[*]

10. Cabinet members are always asking for free medical advice.
9. Tobacco company CEOs no longer send you Christmas cards.
8. None of the toy companies make a Surgeon General action figure.
7. You can't use your beeper to get out of meetings anymore.
6. During confirmation hearings, someone always brings up that you never understood the Krebs cycle.
5. You're not allowed to experiment on guys who beat you up in high school.
4. You have to stay awake at State of the Union speeches.
3. Can't use Air Force One to get carryout from Bob's Famous Chicken 'n' Ribs.
2. People expect you to know the answers to all the medical questions on *Jeopardy*.
1. You have to wear a bathing suit in the president's hot tub.

POETRY

Physicians like poetry. At least that's what my research shows. Although it is not well indexed, I found a considerable amount of poetry in columns, as white space filler, and in the correspondence section of many journals. Most physicians are not poets, of course, and their technique is usually simple and straightforward. Such simplicity does not interfere with their message, however, particularly in the case of humorous poetry, which makes up about 10% of the verse that is published in medical journals.

I would like to begin with the following limerick which I ran into when I read "The Wit of Medicine," by Lore and Maurice Cowan (see Appendix). The author is unknown.

> A maiden at college named Breeze
> Weighed down by B.A.s and M.D.s
> Collapsed from the strain,
> Said her doctor, "It's plain,
> You are killing yourself by degrees."

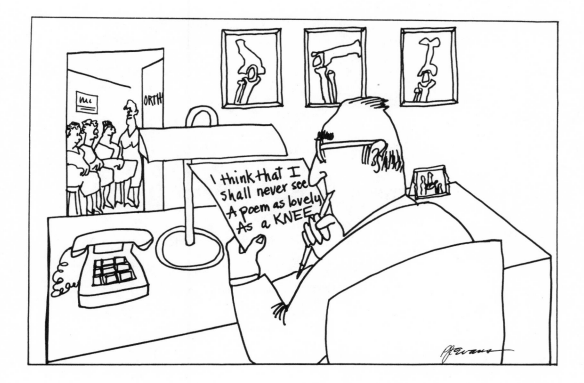

The Diagnosis*

The casualty† was crowded when the patient was
    brought in,
The students gathered round him, their faces all a
    grin.
The patient was unconscious and they rushed all
    round the place
To examine and percuss him—to diagnose his case.
Each gave his own opinion of the patient's present
    state.
I'll quote you just a few and leave the patient to
    his fate.
One shouted to his partner—"Oh, come and listen
    Charles.
He's got whisp'ring pectoriloquy and lots of
    crackling rales.
His stomach is dilated, his clavicles are straight.
His PMI is beating at a rate of twenty eight.
He's got a hemic murmur at the apex and the base.

I think I see a palsy on the right side of his face.
His pupils are unequal which suggests a case of
    tabes,
But he's foaming at the mouth which makes me
    think of rabies."
Another spoke of syphilis, on principle no doubt,
And said a dash of iodide would drive the
    symptoms out.
Some spoke of laparotomy and tumor of the brain,
While others bet on typhoid fever, hemorrhage
    and strain.
The seniors condescended to express their views
    thuswise,
"The man's got meningitis, you can see it in his
    eyes."
But one thing puzzled all of them, 'twas pitiful to see,
His arms and legs and body were as rigid as could
    be.

*Reprinted with permission from The Leech 1931;3(2):35. Edited
from the original.
†This is the British word for emergency department.

They eliminated poisoning and tetanus by degrees,
And spastic paraplegia by the straightness of his
  knees.
At last in desperation, with sad and downcast
  face,
They asked the Senior Houseman to diagnose the
  case.

At first he too was puzzled by the rigid form in bed,
But soon his face lit up with smiles and loftily he
  said,
"This case is very difficult in very many ways,
The man's got rigor mortis, he's been dead about
  three days!"

B.K.

'Twas the Night Before Match Day*

'Twas the night before Match Day, and all through the school
Not a student was certain, not even a fool,
Of the choices he'd put on his match list with care,
In hopes that St. Medicus soon would be there.

Significant other and I in my scrubs
Had just settled down for some starry-eyed love,
When suddenly I rose to the sound of the drone
Of the clamoring ring of my red telephone!

The call gave bad news from a bleary-eyed dean.
I begged him and wailed, "Sir, what do you mean?"
I *had* to have matched at least one or more!
After all, on my list were 104!!"

"There, there now," he soothed, in a tone professorial,
"We've a slot just for you out at Peau-Dunque Memorial!"
"Please, not *there*, sir" I cried, "where each bed has a saddle
And the interns get bruised starting IVs on cattle!"

"Well, we still have a flexible out in Corfu
That comes with a nice on-call room with a view. . . ."
"But *they're* much too cheap to buy beepers or phones—
To wake interns they tug on strings tied to their toes!"

"For ecology fans there's Mount Bogus," he said,
"Where to save paper and trees they keep charts in their heads. . . ."
"Not for me, sir," I wavered, "but thanks just the same—
After one night on call I'd forget my own name!"

"You're awfully picky when put to the test.
But there is something that must be confessed:
As dean of our jovial medical school,
The reason I called was to play April Fool!!"

"The fact is: you matched at Mass General, I heard!
Good luck, there, my boy, you will need it, you nerd!"
"Thanks a lot, sir," I said, "I am proud and relieved.
That's a jolly good joke to be so deceived. . . ."

"You're welcome, my boy. Now rest your swelled head.
For this year is the last you will see of your bed!"
And I heard him exclaim 'fore he hung up the phone:
"HAPPY CAREER TO ALL! AND REMEMBER YOUR LOAN!"

Kevin E. Vitting, M.D.

The following poem was published in *JAMA* between 1966 and 1971. I was unable to track down the original citation, but Dr. Stewart reprinted the poem in a small volume called *Verses 1966 to 1971*.—H.B.

Long Day's Journal Into Night

The race to the top of the medical ladder
Goes to the doctors whose CVs are fatter,
Since building a national reputation
Requires a bibliographic foundation.

So whatever disease is a bee in your bonnet,
Work up a series of articles on it.
Significance rests (in the final analysis)
On research, and footnotes, and typewriter calluses.

Michael M. Stewart, M.D.

See No Evil[†]

A "double-blind" study has merits galore
(Especially one well controlled);
The critics and skeptics are satisfied more
When the story's objectively told.

All unconscious biases will be screened out
(I'm sure conscious ones don't exist).
It's clear there is no valid reason to doubt
The results of a randomized list.

So bear this in mind and you won't be deceived:
If data are worth the pursuing,
Those doctors can be without question believed
Who really don't know what they're doing.

Bronx, NY

Richard A. Rosen, M.D.
Albert Einstein College of Medicine

[†]Reprinted with permission from The New England Journal of Medicine, © 1971;285:975.

I've Read the Journal For Many Years*

To the Editor: I read Michael Crichton's article in the December 11, 1975, issue of the *Journal* regarding the quality of English usage. I took the article for what it was worth until I saw the taunting review of his article in this week's *Time* magazine. Since the criticism received such wide publicity I felt compelled to write this little verse:

I've read the *Journal* for many years
Completely unaware
Of the dreadful English usage,
Nor did I really care.

But now that Michael Crichton
Has pointed out the flaws
As I peruse each article
I find I often pause.

And ask myself these questions:
Is this paper worth my while?
How can I rely upon
An author with poor style?

Is the message crystal clear,
Or is it obfuscated?

Is the man illiterate,
Or is he addle-pated?

How *did* such dismal copy
Pass editorial eyes,
Of Dr. Ingelfinger
And all those other guys?

To improve the *Journal* style
And make it more grammatical,
Perhaps the editorial staff
Should take a long sabbatical.

Of course I write this all in jest.
I'll make a safe prediction,
The *Journal* style will stay unchanged.
And Mike will stick to fiction.

Milton J. Chatton, M.D.
Department of Rehabilitation
San Jose, CA

Keeping Informed†

One thing that is really not difficult, friends,
Is keeping abreast of new medical trends,
New treatments, new gadgets, new antibiotics,
New cures for the ailing, including neurotics.

And if you don't learn from attending a meeting
Or glancing at journals, though glances be fleeting.
Or talking with colleagues, you'll not be without it,
For surely your patient has read all about it.

Richard Armour, Ph.D.

*Reprinted with permission from The New England Journal of Medicine, © 1976;294:564.
†Reprinted from Postgraduate Medicine, 1958;23(2):A154. Copyright 1958 by Richard Armour. Reprinted with permission of John Hawkins & Associates, Inc.

Number 1 et al*

To the Editor: The commentary of Dr. G. M. Bernier et al (New Eng J Med 1969;281:567) entitled "On the phenomenon of having the names of as many as eight authors appearing on a single paper" inspired this gentle rejoinder, humbly submitted.

It's 2 times 4
And 4 times 2
And what is more
Just who is who?

Assuming 1 is the driving force
And number 8 the chief, of course.

The who is 5,
What did he do
That makes him 5
Instead of 2?

Pity poor 7 and 6 and 3
Their place suggests obscurity.

In time's recall
Said paper shall
Be know to all
As such and such by 1 et al.

Donald T. Quick, M.D.
University of Florida
Gainesville, Fl   J. Hillis Miller Health Center

Multiple Authorship
On the *NEJM* COVER†

The outer front cover
May soon not provide
Enough space to list
All the authors inside.

Original articles
Should not as a rule,
Be authored by half
Of a medical school.

It is nice to give credit,
Where credit is due,
But on the front cover
Restrict it to two.

Milton J. Chatton, M.D.
San Jose, CA   Santa Clara Valley Medical Center

*Reprinted with permission from The New England Journal of Medicine, © 1969;281:911.
†Reprinted with permission from The New England Journal of Medicine, © 1980;302:1425.

William Bennett Bean was an important medical figure from the 1950s to the 1970s. His contemporaries described him as a true renaissance man: a humanist, an educator, a scholar, and a superb clinician.[1] Dr. Bean was the editor of the *Archives of Internal Medicine* from 1962–1966. Like Osler (p. 127), Bean appreciated the value of humor in medicine. He also had the unique talent of incorporating light verse into his serious publications.[2-6] The following poems are good examples of Bean's wit. The first appeared in a book he wrote called *Rare Diseases and Lesions*.[5] The second was published at the end of a 13 page article on spider hemangiomas.[6]—H.B.

Borborygmus*

When I sat by the duchess at tea,
It was just as I knew it would be,
Her rumblings abdominal
Were really phenomenal;
And everyone thought it was me.

Mother Goose†

An older Miss Muffet
Decided to rough it
And lived upon whiskey and gin.
Red hands and a spider
Developed outside her—
Such are the wages of sin.

1. Moser RH, Bogdonoff MD (eds): The William Bennett Bean Festschrift. Arch Intern Med 1974;134:823–877.
2. Bean WB, Katz LN, Levin B, et al: Weekly clinicopathological exercise. N Engl J Med 1966;275:44–53.
3. Bean WB, Funk D: The vasculocardiac syndrome of metastatic carcinoid. Arch Intern Med 1959;103:189–199.
4. Bean WB, Felson B, Dolan KD: A nonletter from the editor and a case for all seasons. Seminar Roentgenol 1982;17:153–161.
5. Bean WB: Rare Diseases and Lesions: Their Contribution to Clinical Medicine. Springfield: Charles C Thomas, 1967 p. 30.
6. Bean WB: The arterial spider and similar lesions of the skin and mucous membranes. Circulation 1953;8:117–129.

Tumbling After‡

Jack told Jill to take her pill
    With a glass of water.
Jill forgot, and Jack begot
    A bouncing baby daughter.

Milton J. Chatton, M.D.
San Jose, Calif

*Reprinted courtesy of Charles C Thomas, Publisher, Springfield, IL.
†Reprinted with permission of the American Heart Association.
‡Reprinted from JAMA © 1966;195(Jan):A224, with permission of the American Medical Association.

POETRY
100

Although it's not referenced, the following poem was written in response to a letter by Dr. Melvin Hershkowitz, "Penile Frostbite, An Unforeseen Hazard of Jogging" (see p. 130).—H.B.

Lyophallization*

There exists an MD who jogs
Wearing his everyday togs;
Without care or worry,
'Round the park does he scurry,
A full 30 minutes he logs.

All went well 'til December
(A night I'm sure he'll remember);
He challenged Jack Frost
And undoubtedly lost
As Frostie nipped the doc's member.

Now being a scholarly chap,
He profited from his mishap.
He penned a description
Of this new affliction,
Which had dropped right into his lap.

This syndrome's not rare, I would guess,
And more cases will soon come to press;
I'd say, then, in short,
That this first report
Shows the tip of the iceberg, no less.

Now, our jogger's immortalized,
And always will be recognized
By the medical clan,
As the very first man
Ever to be lyophallized.

Michael Silverman, M.D.
University of Colorado
Medical Center

Frisbee Finger†

To the Editor: The following letter to the editor is in response to the letter to the editor entitled "Frisbee Finger," which appeared in the August 7 issue of the *Journal:*

A frisbee's fun is not as fabled,
In fact, you might become disabled
With bursting blisters on your finger
You'll fail in feigning as a flinger.

Yes, frisbee finger now is put
With tennis elbow, athlete's foot.
Abuses of athletic action—
Will someone's tossing thumb need traction?

I do not argue the contention
Abstention is the best prevention;
So have it printed on each disk:
"You toss this plate at your own risk."

No doubt frisbeers will still flip
Though "flicted flippers" disks may slip;
Still some will say the cautious course is:
"Don't play around with flying saucers."

Minnetonka, MN

Barry S. Levy, M.D.

*Reprinted with permission from The New England Journal of Medicine, © 1977;296:825.
†Reprinted with permission from The New England Journal of Medicine, © 1975;293:725–726.

POETRY
101

Nighttime Rhymes*

One of the things they don't teach you in medical school is that most patients get sick at night. Fortunately, not everyone who gets sick actually calls in (it just seems that way when you're on call). Therefore, to help dull the pain of taking call, I offer the following limericks for your relief. There are eight in all—one for each hour in a good night's sleep.

Said the mother whose babe had been teething,
"He was crying in bed, really seething.
But now he's asleep,
Not making a peep,
Should we wake him to make sure he's breathing?"

There once was a floor nurse named Doodle
Who rarely relied on her noodle.
When temperatures rose,
She'd powder her nose,
And sit on her kit and caboodle.

A dull operator named Sue
Rang my beeper at quarter past two.
It seems Mrs. Fabor
Had gone into labor,
And she hadn't a clue what to do.

Said the doc to the man constipated,
"Don't you think this complaint could have waited?
It's five after three,
So take it from me,
What you need is your head lubricated."

There was a young doctor named Dean
Who had sex with his ex-wife Colleen.
The coroner said
He dropped dead in bed
'Cause he took calls betwixt and between.

There once was a doctor named Fink
Who dreamed he turned into a shrink.
Now taking call
Was no bother at all
'Cause shrinks only lose half a wink.

There once was a patient named Silya
Who asked, "Can insomnia kill ya?"
"That depends," said her doc
As he glanced at his clock,
"On whether you pay when I bill ya."

When I chose to become a physician
I was following family tradition.
But had I a peep
Of how little I'd sleep,
I might have become a musician.

Howard J. Bennett, M.D.

When doctors satirize topics in health care, they sometimes adapt famous poetry for comic effect. As the following references show, Hamlet's "To Be or Not to Be" soliloquy has inspired many doctors over the years.—H.B.

1. Altenburger KM: The tragedy of Ham Let, (a spoof on HMOs). N Engl J Med 1986;315:326.
2. Dimmick EL: Hamlet's soliloquy on allergy. Obstet Gynecol 1962;20:148.
3. Dubik M, Wood B: To "circ" or not to "circ". Contemp Pediatr 1996;13(1):129.
4. Murry RF: Soliloquy on screening. N Engl J Med 1974;291:803.

Help?*

When doctors doctor, and nurses nurse,
Most patients get better, though some get worse.
The system's not perfect, but one of the facts is
That no one is suing the nurse for malpractice:
She knows what her job is, and does it with grace,
While doctors make sure that she stays in her place.

Now nurses start doctoring: Junior Physicians?
Noctors? or Durses? Nurdocs? Nursicians?
What will their work be? And how shall we choose them?
How to be certain the public will use them?
And how to get doctors (traditional, staid)
To accept as their colleague this new Medi-Maid?

Problems aplenty, but what's even worse is:
If one of them's sued, they'll wish they were Nurses.

Michael M. Stewart, M.D.
Rockefeller Foundation

Bangkok, Thailand

A Pulmonologist's Valentine†

To the Editor: Last year my husband, a pulmonary fellow, sent me a valentine; he thought that the cardiac system was receiving far too much attention on that day. I thought that your readers would enjoy the valentine:

Roses are red
Violets are blue
Without your lungs
Your blood would be too.

David D. Ralph, M.D.
(Submitted by Susan Ott, M.D.)

Seattle, WA

*Reprinted with permission from The New England Journal of Medicine, © 1971;285:1384.
†Reprinted with permission from The New England Journal of Medicine, © 1981;304:739.

During my research, I found that humorous poetry generally fell into two categories: either spontaneous reflections on medical topics or responses to previously published articles. The following poems show that the clever author can not only use verse to review a book, but also to review the reviewer. For an "American" review that rhymes, see Dagi TF: N Engl J Med 1972;286:1010.—H.B.

Introduction to Surgery*

An Introduction to Surgery. Edited by David H. Patey, London: Lloyd-Luke (Medical Books) Ltd. 1958.

This useful little book is meant
For those on surgery intent,
To tell them what they ought to know
Before into the wards they go;
Within small compass, too, it packs
Much that the student often lacks,
And stresses well the "human touch"
Which to the patient means so much.
To every dresser‡ then we say—
Read through this book without delay;
The hours in reading it you spend
Will pay a handsome dividend.

Zachary Cope, M.D.

Rhymed Review†

How pleasant to the eye and mind
A lucid book review to find,
So apt and pithy with its rhyme,
Saving a column's reading time.
Such verse appropriately used
Would brighten those who have accused
The *B.M.J.* as dull and glum,
Too vague, prolix, and wearisome.
Then with your grace may we all hope
That others follow Zachary Cope.

Basingstoke   I. Atkin, M.D.

*Reprinted with permission from the British Medical Journal, © 1958;2:958.
†Reprinted with permission from the British Medical Journal, © 1958;2:1106.
‡This is the British term for a surgical assistant.

Laments of a Clinical Clerk*

Dermatology
or
Give Me a Man Who Calls a Spade a Geotome

I wish the dermatologist
Were less a firm apologist
For all the terminology
That's used in dermatology.

Something you or I would deem a
Redness he calls *erythema;*
If it's blistered, raw and warm he
Has to call it *multiforme.*

Things to him are never simple;
Papule is his word for pimple.
What's a *macule,* clearly stated?
Just a spot that's over-rated!

Over the skin that looks unwell
He chants Latin like a spell;
What he's labeled and obscured
Looks to *him* as good as cured.

Julia Bess Frank, M.D.

Laments of a Clinical Clerk—V†

Infectious Disease

Of all my consultants, most easy to please
Is the fellow who comes from infectious
   disease.
His wants are so simple! His needs are so few!
Just gather some sputum, blood cultures
   times two,
X-ray the patient from guggle to zatch,[1]
Examine the urine, both cath and clean catch;
It takes but a moment to do an L.P.,
Swab wound, throat and cervix, yank out the I.V.

When all of the data at last are collected,
The last culture plated, the last slide inspected,
The attending arrives to review and recap
(While intern and student enjoy a brief nap);
He broods with the air of a scribe with papyrus
And gives his opinion: "Most likely a virus.
Don't bother to fix it; can't treat it, can't cure it,
Though superinfection may later obscure it.
Should there be recurrence of fever or pain
Go back to square one and start over again!"

Julia Bess Frank, M.D.

1. For the location of these anatomical landmarks, see James Thurber's
   The Thirteen Clocks, New York, Simon and Schuster, 1950.

*Reprinted with permission from The New England Journal of
Medicine, © 1977;297:660.
†Reprinted with permission from The New England Journal of
Medicine, © 1978;298:1009.

In 1983, the journal *Survey of Ophthalmology* began publishing a poetry column called "Time Oph." Although most of the poems are geared toward ophthalmologists, some have broader appeal.—H.B.

—>●<—

Prostatic Resection, Or Lines for My Urologist*

Now that, at last, I lie so meekly here
   My nether half benumbed, a prey to fear,
Good Doctor, I beseech you, have a care
   As you explore those tubes and ducts down there!
I hope that in your cystoscopic quest
   (As three diplomas on your wall attest)
With sponge, resectoscope, hawk-billed coudé
   You know just what you are about today!
Oh, do be careful as you probe and shove
   With catheter and sound and rectal glove,
While in my dank and murky depths you grope
   With tiny, incandescent telescope,
With practiced eye and craft superior
   To reconnoiter my interior.

I know you have, as yonder parchments state,
   The arcane skills that they certificate.
You dilate, snip, excise and cauterize;
   Such arts unfeignedly I eulogize
I do not doubt your virtuosity,
   But ponder, sir, what this can mean to me!
If you should falter—no offense!—I plead
   To what calamaties can all this lead?
What piercing pangs may we precipitate,
   What surging ecstasies abbreviate?
What dire impairments may your blade inflict,
   What cherished sins in future interdict?
As to the mark your nimble scalpel swoops,
   The word I do not wish to hear is "OOPS!"

Richard Bardolph
University of North Carolina

Greensboro, NC

*Reprinted with permission from the New England Journal of Medicine, © 1980,303:647.

The next two poems are medical takeoffs of the nonsense poem *Jabberwocky*, written by Lewis Carroll. The poem, which appears in his book *Through the Looking Glass*, is felt to be the most famous nonsense poem ever written. After Alice reads the poem she says, "... it seems to fill my head with ideas—only I don't know exactly what they are." Although one needs footnotes to understand all the words in Lewis Carroll's poem, Geniewacky and Gynawocky are a little easier to figure out.—*H.B.*

Geniewacky*

'Twas genic and the acrocents
Did twine and twist and gyrotate
To lub and lubber's recompense
A truly metaphasic plate.

Yes, seek them out, mosaics rare
And non disjunctions panoplied
But of the beast you must beware
Lest you be vittles for his greed.

A thunder through the spital thrums
With bowing nurds on either side
Behold the great Granteater comes
With multiforms upon his hide.

He comes with outstretched geltigrab
Antennae tuned to visiteams
Engorged by a research lab
Fulfilled of fluff and borrowed dreams.

Quick on him cast the potent drug
Oh, cleanish boy with eyes of green
His gulps now steam upon the rug
No man has such a colchicine.

'Twas genic and the acrocents
Did twine and twist and gyrotate
No trace of dollars or of cents
Did there remain to translocate.

Samuel P. Bessman, M.D.
University of Maryland

Baltimore, MD

*Reprinted with permission from The New England Journal of Medicine, © 1968;279:220.

Gynawocky*

From the 1943 University College Hospital, London

'Twas gynig and the slithy vulvs
Did grease and glather in the glare;
The midderstuds, like hungry wolves,
Waved dettol-fingers in the air.
One by one they came to grips
With problems of the Gynaequest;
Caressed the os with sensitips,
As from above they fundiprest.
The Gynaeprof, all fidgetas,
Could feel, he thought, a viscerop.
'Twas but a bulkypelvimass
Projecting 'bove the symphitop.
"Tell me, good Muth, your menstridates:
I fear you have a graviwomb.
You must come up to antenates
That we may test for albimune.
We'll closely watch your pressiblood,
And you will tell us, if you would,
Your foetipulse and fundiheight,
The times you uripass at night.
Your swellifeet, your mornipulse,
Are all of interest to me;
Though trivisympts to you they look,
Preclamptitoxisigns they be."
The months passed by and pendybell
Grew bigger every day.
No toxisympts, and all was well
Until the estiday.

From noctislumb a listiclerk
By telebell was woke:
"Arise, good sir, quick off the mark!
The membribags have broke."
All slumberfull he stumbled down
And flustertripped upon the stair;
He hurriscrubbed and caught the crown
In time to stop a peritear.
"Now rapipant," cried midderstud,
"An foetipush no more."
But with a mighty spurtiblood
A prematinf she bore.
"Now, fundigrip with all thy strength
Before the flacciwomb distend."
The umbicord increased in length—
Placenta came, and 'twas the end.
"Well now, my dear," said Gynaeprof,
"In case your womb descends
I'll fit you with a cervipop;
'Twill not defeat your ends."
"In three months time return to me."
In three months time she came.
"Now let me see what I can see;
Turn on your back again."
The Gynaeprof, all fidgetas,
Could feel, he thought, a viscerop.
'Twas but a bulky pelvimass
Projecting 'bove the symphitop. . .

Anonymous

*Reprinted from JAMA, © 1948;137(7):A38, with permission from the American Medical Association.

Methanosis*

To the Editor: Dr. W. C. Duane freely admits in the paper he co-authored with Dr. M. D. Leavitt, "Floating Stools—Flatus versus Fat" (N Engl J Med 1972;286:973) that his consistently floating stools were fortuitously noted to be associated with "a CH_4 excretion rate of near record proportion." This forthright admission of a high methane rating from one of our professional colleagues inspired the following trio of limericks:

Our thanks to frank Doctor Duane
Who takes the time to explain
Just how he had noted
That his stools often floated
Before they were flushed down
   the drain.

He must have thought first, "Mama mia!
Do I suffer from steatorrhea?

But it cannot be that—
There is no trace of fat."
Which led to another idea.

Well aware of the gas he unloosed
The doctor quite shrewdly deduced,
(Almost clairvoyant)
His feces were buoyant
Because of the methane produced.

San Jose, CA

Milton J. Chatton, M.D.

A month before "Methanosis" was published, Joseph Teller offered his own poetic response to Dr. Duane's article. For an exhaustive review of this subject, see Danzl DF: Flatology. J Emerg Med 1992;10:79–88.—*H.B.*

Floaters and Sinkers†

To the Editor: The recent article "Floating Stools—Flatus versus Fat" inspired me to embrace the Muse as follows:

While safe's the stool that comes a sinker,
The floater's apt to be a stinker.

So it's not fat but, rather, flatus
Imparts the elevated status.

Freehold, NJ

Joseph D. Teller

Urinalysis*

Some bring their sample in a jar,
Some bring it in a pot,
Some bring a sample hardly ample,
While others bring a lot.

Some hide it in a paper bag,
Some wrap it like a treasure,
Some, quite undaunted, proudly flaunt it
As if it gives them pleasure.

Some cork it up so tightly that
It's quite a job to spring it,
Some let it slosh, almost awash,
And some forget to bring it.

Richard Armour, Ph.D.

Ode to Room 459†

They test your blood by pints and quarts
They fill you up with barium,
And watch your blushing innards flip
Like fish in an aquarium.

They puncture you like needlepoint
They steal your clothes and drag you
From whatsiscope and whosiscope
They pummel, thump and gag you.

For there's a test for every ill
To help the doctor cure it.
But few except the well and strong
Are able to endure it!

Gainesville, FL   Leonard Reaves III, M.D.

Plea to an M.D. (any M.D.)‡

The doctor is a worthy gent;
His patients claim he's heaven-sent.
The man is knowing, erudite;
But, holy cats! He just can't write!

The surgeon's hands are deft and skilled;
The surgeon's head is *know-how* filled.
Yet why—since he's so doggone bright—
Cannot the surgeon learn to write?

Dear sons of old Hippocrates
Pray hear a troubled nurse's pleas:
Remember that the gals in white
Have got to *read* the stuff you write!

Your physicals and histories,
Like Dead Sea Scrolls, are mysteries;
Your order sheets make nurses squint;
So please, dear sirs, write *right*—or print!

Cecilia Hargrove, R.N.

*Reprinted from Postgraduate Medicine 1959;26(10):A252. Copyright 1959 by Richard Armour. Reprinted with permission of John Hawkins & Associates, Inc.
†Reprinted from JAMA, © 1963;184(7):A242, with permission from the American Medical Association.
‡Published in RN © 1960;23(Mar):62. Medical Economics Publishing, Montvale, N.J. Reprinted by permission.

POETRY

Although he doesn't say so, I'm suspicious that Mark Cohen wrote this song for his school's annual follies production (see p. 8). Perhaps more students should take the plunge and try to get their work published.—H.B.

The Formulary Song*

(To be sung to the tune of Gilbert and Sullivan's "I am the Very Model of a Modern Major-General")

There's Aldomet and Atromid and Antivert and Atarax
And Dexamyl and Donnagel and Demerol and Dulcolax.
There's Tylenol and Tegretol and Riopan and Regitine
And Pertofrane and Pavabid and also Pyribenzamine.
Now if you're down there's Dexedrine and Benzedrine and Elavil,
And if you're up there's Librium and Valium and Vistaril.
There's Thorazine and Stelazine for calming schizophrenics with;
There's Seconal for sleeping and for mania there's Eskalith . . .
There's Benadryl and Gelusil and Placidyl and Peritrate
And Decadron and Parafon and Sinequan and Sorbitrate
And Miltown, Motrin, Medrol, Maalox, Myleran and Miradon
And Mycostatin, Micronor, Mandelamine and Mylicon.

There's Omnipen and Principen and Tegopen and Torecan
And Versapen and Betapen and Pyopen and Percodan.
There's Robitussin, Garamycin, also Butazolidin
And Furadantin, Coricidin, even Triaminicin.
There's Dimetane and Dimetapp and Dymelor and Dimacol
And Diuril and Dialose and Diamox and Disophrol.
There's Darvocet for headaches when you really want to stay at
    home,
But if the other end is sore, the one you need is Protofoam . . .
I know you must be weary and this song is getting pretty grim
With all these pharmaceuticals from Actifed to Zyloprim.
But just imagine what would happen if I tried to fan the flames
By starting over once again and using all generic names!

Mark L. Cohen
Pennsylvania State University
College of Medicine
Milton S. Hershey Medical Center

Hershey, PA

*Reprinted with permission from The New England Journal of Medicine, © 1977;296:520.

POETRY
111

Wise Guy*

Who knows each illness, knows each cure?
Who never doubts, is always sure?
Who gives advice to learned scholars
And shrugs aside their thanks and dollars?

Who is this learned fellow, friends?
Who is the chap who condescends
To chat with men like Mayo? Who?
It is the intern, young and new,

Who knows more than all other men.
He'll never know so much again.

Richard Armour, Ph.D.

The Surgeon†

The public views his status regal,
In our profession he's "The Eagle."
With super supple fingers slim
(Pus, blood, and guts don't bother him),
Up to his elbows, filled with glee,
With snick and slice sadistically,
Into a jar, up on a shelf
He puts a fragment of yourself.
For him no diagnostic doubt
He'll operate, and so find out.

Edgar L. Dimmick, M.D.

Off to the Yearly Convention†

Oh, we're off to the medical meeting
Where there's never a problem with seating—
Except in the bar,
Where friends from afar
Are exchanging their annual greeting.

Since the IRS didn't complain
When we held our convention in Spain,
We'll talk antibiotic
In some place exotic
And not in Dubuque or Fort Wayne.

If the papers get too soporific
We'll steal off to watch the Pacific
And we'll toss down a few—

Tax-deductible too!—
In a toast to La Vie Scientific.

And what if we do run up bills
For dinners with all of the frills?
A fine bill-of-fare
Will help us prepare
To "improve our professional skills."

So we're off to the yearly convention,
Eager to turn our attention
To the holy alliance
of Pleasure and Science
And sundries we don't need
    to mention.

Rochester, NY

David Goldblatt, M.D.
University of Rochester

*Reprinted from Postgraduate Medicine, 1962;32(8):A118. Copyright 1962 by Richard Armour; reprinted with permission of John Hawkins & Associates, Inc.
†Reprinted from JAMA, © 1967;199(6):A274, with permission from the American Medical Association.
‡Reprinted with permission from The New England Journal of Medicine, © 1974; 290:1385.

A New Personality Type*

To publish in your learned journal
One doesn't need a truth eternal.
A recent issue[1-3] made us see
Your editors like poetry.

What kind of people, you might ask,
Would spend their time on such a task
Composing lines that barely rhyme?
My goodness what a waste of time!

This group of people must be rare,
Compulsive, but with time to spare.
We've discovered they must be
Personality type, non-A non-B!

David Baer, M.D.
Debra Judelson, M.D.
Stephen Mizroch, M.D.
San Francisco, CA   Kaiser Foundation Hospital

1. Frank JB: Laments of a clinical clerk—V. N Engl J Med 298:1009, 1978.
2. Schnitzler ER: "Honeymoon cystitis." N Engl J Med 298:1035, 1978.
3. Editors: *Journal* usage under attack. N Engl J Med 298:1038, 1978.

A Referenced Poem†
by Poets Three[1]

The journal we all hold prestigious.
Whose articles both long and terse
Sport lists of authors quite prodigious,
Now gives us multi-authored verse.
Did David Baer the poem compose,
Fair Judelson his inspiration,
While Mizroch (senior author) chose
To lend his name and approbation?
How antic seem the poets of old,
Given to wry and solitary feats.
How richer *Ode to Autumn*'s gold
If writ by Shelley, Hunt *and* Keats!
A referenced poem by poets three
Is surely the best of poetry.

Frederick L. Jones, Jr., M.D.
Danville, PA   Geisinger Medical Center

*Reprinted with permission from The New England Journal of Medicine, © 1978;299:558.
†Reprinted with permission from The New England Journal of Medicine, © 1978;299:1372.

1. Baer D, Judelson D, Mizroch S: A new personality type. N Engl J Med 299:558, 1978.

POETRY
113

Additional Readings

1. Alsop RF: Let's ignore a box from Pandora (a poem about research). N Engl J Med 1977;296:887.

2. Armour, Richard: The Medical Muse.* New York: McGraw-Hill, 1963.

For those who would like more of Richard Armour, this book is a collection of poems published in *Postgraduate Medicine* from 1951 to 1963.

3. Armour R: One who needs no introduction. Postgrad Med 1951;10(8):A66.

4. Armour R: The anesthetist. Postgrad Med 1955; 17(3):A124.

5. Armour R: Growing role (a poem about computers). Postgrad Med 1965;37(6):A178.

6. Armour R: Concerning coughs (a poem about paying bills). Postgrad Med 1956;20(11):A172.

7. Bean WB: Omphalosophy: an inquiry into the inner (and outer) significance of the belly button. Arch Intern Med 134:866–870.

8. Berrett V: Ode to a flu bug. JAMA 1963;184(3): A246.

9. Butterfield WC: Know any bawdy old medical limericks? Med Economics 1973;50 (Jan 8):166.

10. Bluestone N: Who says doctors can't write? Pennsylvania Med 1983;86(11):48.

11. Caplan AN: The gout. N Engl J Med 1966;275:664.

12. Cohen JA: Lola, lowly louse. Perspect Biol Med 1981;24:502.

13. Cope, Zachary: The Diagnosis of the Acute Abdomen in Rhyme.* London: Lewis, 1962.

In this fascinating book, Dr. Cope addresses the diagnosis and treatment of the acute abdomen. Although the subject is serious, his style gives it a light touch and makes it a pleasure to read.

14. Eyerer R: Clinico-pathological exercise. J Maine Med Assoc 1965;56(12):279–281.

An otherwise serious CPC of which 50% is written in rhyme.

15. Farnum, Charles G: Medicine Could Be Verse.* New York: Exposition Press, 1949.

Dr. Farnum's poems are insightful, witty, and thoroughly enjoyable.

16. Frank JB: Laments of a clinical clerk (a poem about nephrology). N Engl J Med 1977;297:953.

17. Fruhman GJ: The superbowel (a poem about the small intestine). Perspect Biol Med 1973;17:66.

18. Green L: Requiem for an eponym. Skeletal Radiol 1989;17:589–590.

19. Hallum JV: The virologist retires or, they may be viruses to you, baby, but they're bread and butter to me. Perspect Biol Med 1989;33:106.

20. Hartley HL: Turtle trouble (a poem about salmonella). N Engl J Med 1965;273:925.

21. Kneeshaw D: The surgeon. JAMA 1966;195(1): A207.

22. Milder B: Roundsmanship. Surv Ophthalmol 1988;33:217.

23. Milder B: Ouch (a poem about acupuncture). Surv Ophthalmol 1990;36:240.

24. Milder B: The diaphragm. The Pharos 1993;56(2): 41.

25. Palmer MS: Blown out of proportion (a poem about flatus). N Engl J Med 1976;295:1204.

26. Quinn CM: The happy hypochondriac. JAMA 1961;176(12):A218.

27. Radner G: Doctors are whippersnappers. N Engl J Med 1988;319:1358.

28. Rankin HJ: Successful treatment of a compulsive limerick composer by behavioral methods. Behav Res Ther 1976;14(2):167.

29. Salit IE: Hot body, cold urine (a poem about factitious fever). N Engl J Med 1977;296:886.

30. Sanders JG: On call before Christmas. JAMA 1993;270:3054.

31. Schoen EJ: Ode to a circumcised male. Am J Dis Child 1987;141:128.

Another variation on Clement Moore's famous poem (see p. 96). In this version, St. Nick visits the ER after landing on a smoldering fire.

32. Sobin LH: Tales of the Ampulla of Vater. Berlin: Nomad Press, 1994. Distributed by the American Registry of Pathology, Washington, D.C.

The poems in this collection originally appeared in the *American Journal of Gastroenterology* and other journals. As the title suggests, the poems deal with

*These books are no longer in print, but should be available through interlibrary loan.

various maladies that afflict the GI tract. Dr. Sobin has a wonderful sense of rhythm, and his poems are very clever. They provide smiles more than belly laughs, but they're still a pleasure to read.

33. Stewart MM: Skin and bones. N Engl J Med 1968; 278:450.

34. Stewart MM: Quality control (a poem about research). JAMA 1974;230:885.

35. Stewart MM: We so move (a poem about committees). JAMA 1974;230:246.

36. Warsaw I: Inside story (a poem about the spleen). JAMA 1974;230:463.

37. Warsaw I: A little back talk (a poem about the spine). JAMA 1974;228:1137.

38. Warsaw I: The wrap-up (a poem about skin). JAMA 1974;230:1163.

39. Warsaw I: Chemo memo (a poem about the liver). JAMA 1975;231:1260.

40. Watts DG: Cholesterol lament. N Engl J Med 1969;281:113.

Oliver Wendell Holmes was an important medical and literary figure in the 19th century.[1-2] After a brief period in clinical practice, Holmes entered academic medicine becoming a professor and ultimately dean at Harvard Medical School. As a man of letters, Holmes published volumes of light verse, three novels, and wrote a column for the newly established *Atlantic Monthly*.[3] Although most of his poetry was not medical, Holmes occasionally wrote amusing medical verse. If you'd like a taste of satire from the last century, check out Holmes' *The Stethoscope Song*.[4] The poem was published approximately two decades after Laënnec invented the stethoscope. Holmes loved technical devices, and the appearance of the stethoscope was a major advance in medicine at the time. Although his poem is almost 150 years old, its message about not letting technology go to your head is just as relevant tody.—H.B.

1. Garland J: Doctors afield: Oliver Wendell Holmes. N Engl J Med 1957;256:847–850.

2. White PJ: Medical Leonardo of Boston, Oliver Wendell Holmes, MD: an evaluation of versatility. Perspect Biol Med 1981;24:411–421.

3. Martensen RL: Oliver Wendell Holmes, MD: an appreciation. JAMA 1994;272:1249.

4. Holmes OW: The Poetical Works of Oliver Wendell Holmes. Boston & New York: Houghton, Mifflin & Co. 1887 pp. 43–45.

CASE
REPORTS

Soon after they hit the wards, medical students become familiar with the language of the hospital including that all-purpose medical label: "The Interesting Case." Patients who become Interesting Cases are the ones who remain undiagnosed, presented in an unusual manner, or developed an uncommon complication of their disease. Although they are frequently the subject of much discussion, in corridors and elevators, over lunch, etc., no one should strive to become an Interesting Case. Nevertheless, medicine being what it is, there is rarely a shortage of such patients in the hospital. And what should one do with an Interesting Case? (That is, besides trying to diagnose it.) Why, write it up of course!

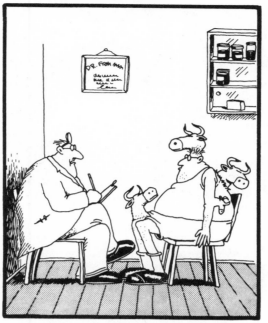

"I'm afraid you've got cows, Mr. Farnsworth."

This selection was taken from a report published in 1866. Although the piece is more whimsical than funny, I included it to show that doctors occasionally wrote humor in the 19th century.—H.B.

FRACTURED PHALLUS*

A young man who was recently married, had his wife, a day or two after the ceremony, leave him to visit a sick relative. When he woke up the next morning, the man found his penis in a vigorous state of distension. In his haste to dress (and not being patient with the natural state of things), he struck it with considerable force against the bedpost. At the instant this was done, he heard the noise of something breaking and at the same moment, a manageable condition of the member followed. Since the bedpost was noted to be sound, he concluded that his organ had suffered the damage. This was confirmed a moment later when his penis turned blue and enlarged to twice its normal size. He notified his family, and

it was soon reported that he had "fractured his penis."

The greatest possible alarm was now created in the mind of the patient and his friends. Professional aid was summoned immediately and, from the novelty and urgency of the case, further advice was sought from this physician. Among the others sent for was the newly-made bride, who, on being informed of the nature of the injury, plaintively and innocently remarked, "I'm sure this never would have happened if I had been at home."

Strict bedrest was recommended, and cold lotions were continually applied. The blood was absorbed a few days later, and the member was restored to its normal condition and usefulness.

G.C.B.

*Reprinted from the Western Journal of Surgery, Obstetrics & Gynecology, 1866;1(July):316–322. Edited from the original.

ET AL AND
THE CASE REPORT*

Theodore Kamholtz, M.D.

The urge to contribute to medical literature is motivated by more than a desire to wear the professional stole. It's as inexplicably compelling as the suicidal drive of lemmings to the sea. If the bug has really bitten you, you don't stop scribbling until, with parkinsonian hands, you caress your volume of Collected Writings.

But in order to collect your writings, you must first have something to write about. And even the most gifted clinician can't discover penicillin *and* unearth a new disease *and* find the cure for coryza *and* perfect a new operation *and* so on—for article after article.

Old hand and neophyte alike must pad. Padding comes in all sizes and shapes. In medical literature, its most familiar shape—do you recognize it?—is the case report.

By definition, a case report is proof of the precept that anything can happen and eventually does. Coincidentally, it's apt to feature the first patient you meet in the hospital after the literary fever hits you.

Having selected your case—trichinosis, let's say, in a 24-year-old white male—you must next pick your co-authors. Note the plural. Of course, it is you (singular) who will write, type, and proofread the article. But for publication purposes, the chief of service, who has never seen the case, gets top billing in the by-line.

Next comes the attending physician, who made rounds once and almost saw the case. Then the associate, who *did* see the case and contributed several grunts.

Low man on the totem pole is, of course, you—properly thankful not to be included merely as "et al" (along with "ibid" and "anon," perhaps the largest authorship fraternity in the world).

Leading off the article is your introductory review of the literature. If you are saving yourself for a solo article later, you state that a search of the literature "of the past ten years has neglected trichinosis in 24-year-old white males, though incidence of the disease in such patients is not as uncommon as the meager attention it has received would lead one to believe."

Your chief, who has gone through the same initiation, may suggest that you sweeten this up a bit. If so, you extend yourself, thus: "A search of the literature of the past *twenty* years . . ."

The question of what references you've used is a touchy one. It is not quite cricket to lift someone else's bibliography intact. Besides, you don't know where *he* got it; and you certainly don't want to fall victim to the reader who insists upon checking all references and who may then write the editor to point out that an article you've cited (presumably on trichinosis) deals actually with impotence in bald-headed men. Although a nuisance, then, it's probably best to include only those references you've validated yourself.

You've reached the peak of successful writing when your bibliography is longer than your article. This gives your work an impressive mathematical flavor: "Trichinosis[17,23,4,97] has been said[81,56,27] on several occasions[5,32,74] to be a disease[108,69,13] characterized by fever,[77,10,15] pain[11,43,91] et cetera.[16,96,103,111]"

As for the case itself, you describe it in a series of rigid clichés, following a procedure not unlike filling out a life insurance form. For example: "This was the *n*th admission of an *x*-year-old *white male* who was admitted to the *Blank* Hospital complaining of *fever and migratory joint pains*."

You go on in this vein until, in due course, "he was discharged on the *n*th day after admission, *completely relieved of his symptoms*."

It is wise not to depart from this classic form, unless you want to wind up in the Reader's Digest and out of your local society.

*Reprinted with permission from Medical Economics, © 1952; 29(June):93–97. Copyright by Medical Economics Company, Inc., Oradell, NJ 07649.

It is likewise *de rigueur* to make the patient seem as controlled as a test tube in the laboratory. You say nothing about your discovery, following a sugar tolerance test one day, that the patient had eaten breakfast beforehand. Nor do you mention the BMR that was done while the patient in the next bed delivered precipitously. Nor the sputum report that came back marked "No free acid."

In a report case, then, there are no Sunday visitors, no temperamental orderlies, no misplaced specimens, no recalcitrant patients. This requires a kind of vigorous selectivity; you must omit every detail that even smacks faintly of the human touch.

Your laboratory reports, on the other hand, must omit *nothing*. They must include every test that was performed, whether it had anything to do with the case or not. For one thing, you may as well get credit for your thoroughness. For another, someone is always ready to pounce on that lone missing test as the really important one. You're damned if you didn't perform an opsonic index; and you're damned if you did—but more faintly.

The muttered oaths directed your way from the laboratory itself are something else again. They're a tribulation to be borne during the clinical rather than the literary work-up of the case.

The next major division in the article comes under the heading of *Discussion*. Here you may—indeed, must—divulge your motive for writing the report. The medical profession does not appreciate the disease, you say. Doctors are not aware of its incidence, morbidity, mortality, curability, pathology, and so on. It has therefore occurred to you that here is a fine illustrative case to enlighten all and sundry. So runs the *stated* motive. Quite coincidental is the fact that you're going to get your name into print.

Next comes your *Summary*, a matter of delicate balance and verbal cunning. If you tell too much, the reader's interest will pall. If you tell too little, he won't be enticed either. You must show the import of your case—but tantalizingly. If in doubt, have this part of the article edited by the Coming Attractions writer at your local theatre.

Finally—the title. If you're a junior assistant, you may appropriately head your report "Trichinosis in a 24-Year-Old Male." If you're an assistant with some standing, you rate a more comprehensive title—say, "Fundoscopic Findings in Thirteen Consecutive Cases of Trichinosis."

The associate physician can take the liberty of writing about "The Psychodynamic Aspects of Trichinosis." The title of the attending's article is "Trichinosis: Its Cause and Cure." The chief of service simply asks, "Whither Trichinosis?"

Once your seniors have given the nod, the article should be mailed immediately to a medical journal. If postmarked later than midnight, it may fail to establish your priority. In fact, if you put it off for even as much as the wink of an eye, the same article may appear under a different title and a different authorship. This will not happen because of plagiarism but merely because genius these days is such a common thing.

When the nurse came to give Mrs. Johnson her heart medication, the patient looked skeptically at the pills.

"Excuse me," the patient said, "but I was just reading about a woman who checked into a hospital for heart trouble and she ended up dying because the nurse gave her the wrong medicine."

The nurse smiled. "Rest easy, Mrs. Johnson. When a patient comes in here with heart trouble, she *dies* of heart trouble."

CHICKEN SOUP REBOUND AND RELAPSE OF PNEUMONIA: REPORT OF A CASE*

Nancy L. Caroline, M.D.
Harold Schwartz, M.D.

A case is reported in which a previously healthy individual, having received an inadequate course of chicken soup in treatment of mild pneumococcal pneumonia, experienced a severe relapse, refractory to all medical treatment and eventually requiring thoractomy. The pharmacology of chicken soup is reviewed and the dangers of abrupt termination of therapy are stressed.

Chicken soup has long been recognized to possess unusual therapeutic potency against a wide variety of viral and bacterial agents. Indeed, as early as the twelfth century, the theologian, philosopher and physician, Moses Maimonides wrote, "Chicken soup . . . is recommended as an excellent food as well as medication."[1] Previous anecdotal reports regarding the therapeutic efficacy of this agent, however, have failed to provide details regarding the appropriate length of therapy. What follows is a case report in which abrupt withdrawal of chicken soup led to severe relapse of pneumonia.

Case Report

The patient is a 47-year-old male physician who had been in excellent health until 8 days prior to admission, when he experienced the sudden onset of rigors followed by fever to 105°F (40.5°C). He was seen by a physician at that time, when physical examination revealed a severely toxic man, unable to raise his head from the bed. Pertinent physical findings were limited to the chest, where rales were heard over the right middle lobe. Chicken soup was immediately begun in doses of 500 ml po q 4 hours. Defervescence occurred in 36 hours and a chest x-ray taken 5 days prior to admission was entirely normal. Because he felt symptomatically improved, the patient declined further chicken soup after this

time. He continued to feel well and remained afebrile until the night prior to admission, when he developed right upper quadrant pain, nausea and vomiting while on a visit to Vermont. His vomiting persisted through the night, and the following morning he boarded a plane for Cleveland. En route, he became severely dyspneic, and by the time he deplaned in Cleveland, he was cyanotic and in severe respiratory distress.

He was brought immediately to the hospital where physical examination revealed an acutely ill man, febrile to 104°F (40.0°C), breathing shallowly 60 times per minute, with a pulse of 140. Physical findings were again chiefly limited to the chest, where bilateral pleural friction rubs, bibasilar rales and egophony over the right middle lobe were heard. Chest x-ray examination showed consolidation of the right middle lobe, infiltrates at both bases and a questionable right pleural effusion. White cell count was 7700 without a shift to the left. Electrolytes were within normal limits. Arterial blood gases on 6 liters/min of nasal oxygen were pH=7.51, P_{CO_2}=20 torr and P_{O_2}=50 torr. Gram stain of the sputum showed swarming diplococci, and multiple cultures of sputum and blood subsequently grew out type 4 Pneumococcus.

Chicken soup being unavailable, the patient was started on one million units q 6 hours of intravenous penicillin. Failure to respond led to increases of the dose up to 30 million units daily.

*Reprinted with permission from Chest, © 1975;67:215–216.

Nonetheless, the patient remained febrile and his chest x-ray film showed progressive effusion and infiltration. On the twelfth hospital day he was taken to the operating room for a right thoracotomy. He thereafter made an uneventful recovery, maintained on 30 million units of penicillin daily during his postoperative course, and was discharged on the 25th hospital day.

Discussion

The therapeutic efficacy of chicken soup was first discovered several thousand years ago when an epidemic highly fatal to young Egyptian males seemed not to affect an ethnic minority residing in the same area. Contemporary epidemiologic inquiry revealed that the diet of the group not afflicted by the epidemic contained large amounts of a preparation made by boiling chicken with various vegetables and herbs. It is notable in this regard that the dietary injunctions given to Moses on Mount Sinai, while restricting consumption of no less than 19 types of fowl, exempted chicken from prohibition.[2] Some scholars[3] believe that the recipe for chicken soup[4] was transmitted to Moses on the same occasion, but was relegated to the oral tradition when the Scriptures were canonized. Chicken soup was widely used in Europe for many centuries, but disappeared from commercial production after the Inquisition. It remained as a popular therapy among certain Eastern European groups, however, and was introduced into the United States in the early part of this century. While chicken soup is now widely employed against a variety of organic and functional disorders, its manufacture remains largely in the hands of private individuals, and standardization has proved nearly impossible.

Preliminary investigation into the pharmacology of chicken soup (Bohbymycetin®) has shown that it is readily absorbed after oral administration, achieving peak serum levels in two hours and persisting in detectable levels for up to 24 hours. Parenteral administration is not recommended. The metabolic fate of the agent is not well understood, although varying proportions are excreted by the kidneys, and dosage should be appropriately adjusted in patients with renal failure. Chicken soup is distributed widely throughout body tissues and breakdown products having antimicrobial efficacy cross the blood-brain barrier. Untoward side effects are minimal, consisting primarily of mild euphoria which rapidly remits on discontinuation of the agent.

While chicken soup has been employed for thousands of years in the treatment of viral and bacterial illnesses, there have been no systematic investigations into the optimal course of therapy. The present case illustrates a possible hazard of abrupt chicken soup withdrawal: a previously healthy man, having received what proved to be an inadequate course of chicken soup for clinical signs of pneumonia, experienced a virulent relapse into severe bacterial pneumonia. It was not possible in this case to determine whether the relapse was caused by resistant organisms, as chicken soup was unavailable at the time treatment had to be restarted, and a synthetic product of lesser potency was used instead. Further study is needed to determine the most efficacious regimen for chicken soup. Pending such investigation, it would probably be more prudent to give a ten day course at full dosage, with gradual tapering thereafter and immediate resumption of therapy at the first sign of relapse.

References

1. Rosner F: Studies in Judaica: The Medical Aphorisms of Moses Maimonides. New York: Yeshiva University Press, 1971. Treatise 20, aphorism 67.

2. Leviticus 11:13–19.

3. Caroline Mrs Z (my mother). Personal communication.

4. Bellin MG: Jewish Cookbook. New York: Garden City Books, 1958, pp 19–20 (recipe).

THE CHICKEN SOUP CONTROVERSY*

The following letters were written in response to the article by Caroline and Schwartz. Although the three best are reprinted here, sixteen were originally published in the journal (see p. 125). These letters appeared over a five year period, which must be some kind of record in the medical literature. The article also inspired the first scientific evaluation of chicken soup (Saketkhoo K, Januszkiewicz A, et al: Effects of drinking hot water, cold water, and chicken soup on nasal mucus velocity and nasal airflow resistance. Chest 1978;74:408–410).—H.B.

To The Editor:

The report by Caroline and Schwartz is timely and alarming, for it suggests that chicken soup-resistant pneumococci may be emerging in nonhospitalized populations and that this time-honored therapeutic modality may have to be abandoned in favor of less relishable treatments. However, the authors failed to obtain *in vitro* sensitivities of the organism against chicken soup, so the presence of chicken soup-resistant pneumococci and/or the question of emerging resistance remains unanswered.

Spurred by the report by Caroline and Schwartz, our laboratories tested 100 recently isolated strains of pneumococci against chicken soup[1] serially diluted in brain-heart infusion broth (BHI). The minimal inhibitory dilution (MID) was defined as that dilution of chicken soup which visibly inhibited growth after incubation for 24 hours at 37°C. Using inocula from a 10^{-3} dilution of an overnight broth culture, 99 percent of the strains were observed to be inhibited at a dilution ≤1:64 (well within the range of levels achievable in the serum). However, one isolate was not inhibited at this dilution or, for that matter, even by undiluted chicken soup. Further examination of this putatively chicken soup-resistant Pneumococcus revealed it to contain a plasmid (labeled CS) which coded for chicken soup resistance. Not surprisingly, this CS plasmid was found to be linked directly to a plasmid coding for resistance to tea leaves (*Camellia sinensis*) and one coding for resistance to whole-wheat bread mold (*Penicillium chrysogenum?*). Regrettably, though, this multiresistant plasmid, CSTLBM, was sponta-

neously lost at such a high frequency that we could not preserve it for confirmatory studies; however, we urge others working in this field to maintain a constant vigil for the emergence of such chicken soup-resistant strains.

R. J. Duma, M.D., S. M. Markowitz, M.D.,
and M. A. Tipple, M.D.
Division of Infectious Diseases
Medical College of Virginia
Richmond, VA

Reference

1. Bellin MG: Jewish Cookbook, New York: Garden City Books, 1958, pp 19–20.

To the Editor:

As a longtime chicken-souper, I appreciated reading the article by Caroline and Schwartz.

Us chicken-soupers have long been aware of the therapeutic efficacy of chicken soup. Our data, however, have consistently been ignored by the bulk of organized medical opinion whose practitioners, as you know, are predominately affluent steak eaters.

We would like to undertake a research program to bring chicken soup into its rightful place in medical therapy. Adjunctive to this study might be the investigation of how the use of happy or unhappy chickens affects the beneficial efforts of chicken soup. In this respect, we have communicated with a contact in the chicken industry, in the hopes that he might want to finance this study with a lifelong supply of chicken legs for the researcher. We hope that

*Reprinted with permission from Chest, ©1975; 68(4):604–606.

improvement of the breed includes attitudinal programs designed to produce *happy* chickens. With the evidence presently available concerning the results of talking to flowers and plants, it is certainly reasonable to expect some degree of extra therapeutic effect from chicken soup derived from happy chickens. We must expect that even chicken brain will respond better than a weed! In any event, if chickens and plants ever take over the world, isn't it good sense to build some advanced good will for ourselves?

On behalf of the Chicken Soup Institute, we thank *Chest* for its interest in chicken soup and humanity.

Ralph Packman
Chicken Soup Institute, Philadelphia, PA

To the Editor:

I have read the interesting report of Caroline and Schwartz (*Chest* 67:215–216, 1975) on the adverse reaction to abrupt withdrawal of chicken soup in the therapy of pneumonia. While the data presented are convincing, several additional points should be made, and it need not be emphasized that we at the Mount Sinai Hospital have had extensive experience in this form of therapy.

1. Are there any data on the bioavailability of the product used? I assume, perhaps presumptuously, that Caroline produced and administered the drug to Schwartz. The question must be posed: does a girl from Presbyterian Hospital really know the laboratory methods well enough, Mrs. Z. Caroline (reference 3) notwithstanding? We have treated many patients with short-term (one to three day), parenteral, pyrogen-free chicken soup (see the following) without recrudescent disease ever being noted.

2. Was the product used in the monomeric or polymeric form? We have observed that, in the absence of mixed soup greens (Bronx Terminal Market, stall 47, Bronx, NY), only polymeric drug is produced in the fermenter vat. This tends to coalesce into oil-like droplets on the surface of the medium, and there is a tendency for some manufacturers to skim off this deposit and discard it. This, in fact, removes the major biologically active fraction from the drug.

3. Because of the growing awareness of the efficacy of chicken soup, the lack of R-factor mediated resistance, and the broad spectrum of activity, we have been faced with a severe shortage of purified drug. As indicated in the paper by Caroline and Schwartz, this is apparently a national (perhaps international) problem. We have, therefore, developed an affinity chromatography method for recovery of chicken soup from the urine. This is based on the selective adsorption of chicken soup to unleavened bread in the form of finely pulverized microspherules (Sephardex) catalytically activated with beaten eggs. The active drug may be eluted with a sodium chloride gradient using large macrocrystalline salt.

We hope this information will prove of value so that properly controlled clinical trials can be initiated.

Gerald T. Keusch, M.D.
Associate Professor of Medicine
Mount Sinai School of Medicine
of the City University of New York

The Chicken Soup Bibliography

1. Block AJ, Caroline NL: Chicken soup. Chest 1976;69:572.

2. Escher DJW, Mason D, et al: Chicken soup. Chest 1977;71:121–123.

3. Lindsey D: Chicken soup and relief of backache. Chest 1976;70:317–318.

4. Levin S: Chicken soup. Chest 1977;72:804.

5. Rosner F: Therapeutic efficacy of chicken soup. Chest 1980;78:672–674.

6. Spodick DH, Duma RJ, et al: The Chicken soup controversy. Chest 1975;68:604–606.

7. Weiss W: "And the Lord said to Moses and Aaron." Chest 1978;74:487–489.

BEEPER OBLITERANS:
CLINICAL STAGING AND NATURAL HISTORY*

To the Editor.—In this report, we describe a common but previously uncharacterized clinical entity affecting hospital staff physicians: "beeper obliterans." The essential element of this syndrome is the periodic emission of high-pitched electronic tones secondary to an ever-increasing abdominal girth that impinges on the test button located on the superior aspect of the wearer's pager-beeper.

Using a modified version of the *Disease Staging*[1] methodology, we (two staff pediatricians with 25 years of combined experience) have described this condition's inexorable march (see Table).

Advancement to stage 4 is directly correlated to a body mass index of 35 kg/m² or greater, clinical service of 10 or more years, and knowledge of the code for the patient pantry-door lock. Of interest is the notable "silent phase" seen at the level of departmental chairman (when beeper is shed and all calls are taken by the secretary, program director, or safely ignored). Further research on the natural history and treatment of this ponderous problem is suggested.

Neil Izenberg, M.D.
Steven A. Dowshen, M.D.
Albert Einstein Medical Center
Philadelphia, Pa

Clinical Staging and Natural History of Beeper Obliterans

Stage	Status and Description
0	*Condition-Free.* Beeper functions as designed. Physician alert and ready. Reaches phone within 15 s 100% of time. Body mass index (BMI) = 22.
1	*Pager Paunch.* Truncal flexion by wearer sets off beeper test button. Physician frequently confused. Answers <85% of pages. BMI = 25 kg/m².
2	*Beeper Bulge.* Abdominal overhang intermittently muffles audio tones ("soufflé effect"). Worsened by consumption of high-fiber meals. Sufferer strains at listening, ameliorated by loss of high-tone hearing. BMI = 28 kg/m².
3	*Pager Inversus.* Tone set off even by quiet respirations. Roll of pants at the belt line causes pager inversion with characteristic "echo effect." Wearer disoriented by microwave beeps in hospital snack bar; >125% of pages answered (paradoxical irritability). BMI = 31 kg/m².
4	*Beeper Obliterans.* Beeper completely enveloped by adipose tissue. Associated with increased risk of coronary artery and gallbladder diseases, as well as non-insulin-dependent diabetes; <3% of pages answered. BMI≥35 kg/m². Surgical removal or elevation to chairmanship may be indicated (see text).

1. Gonnella JF, ed. *Disease Staging.* 3rd ed. New York, NY: SysteMetrics McGraw Hill; 1986.

In a follow-up letter (JAMA 1992;267:2741), Patrice Stevenson noted that "gestational beeper obliterans" should be recognized as an accelerated variant of the above syndrome.—H.B.

*Reprinted from JAMA © 1992;267:1209, with permission from the American Medical Association.

Almost everyone in medicine knows the name of William Osler. What many people do not know, however, is that Osler's reputation is not limited to his role as physician, author, and medical educator. Throughout his long career, he was also admired for his sense of humor. Osler often expressed his less serious side with the help of an alter ego, the fictitious Army surgeon Egerton Yorrick Davis. The following letter is a perfect example of Osler's wit. According to Lawrence Altaffer, Osler sent the letter to Theophilus Parvin, a fellow editor at *Medical News* who had previously written an editorial on vaginismus in the journal. Osler disagreed with using editorial space for such an obscure topic and fabricated the case as a way of satirizing the condition. Osler did not intend for the letter to be published, but Parvin misinterpreted his hoax as a true case report. For additional articles that explore William Osler's sense of humor, see p. 135.—H.B.

VAGINISMUS*

Through the courtesy of the Editor of *The Canada Medical and Surgical Journal*, we are in receipt of the following note:

Dear Sir: The reading of an admirably written and instructive editorial in the Philadelphia *Medical News* for 24th November, on forms of vaginismus, has reminded me of a case in point which bears out, in an extraordinary way, the statements therein contained. When in practice at Pentonville, Eng., I was sent for, about 11 PM by a gentleman whom, on my arriving at his house, I found in a state of great perturbation, and the story he told me was briefly as follows:

At bedtime, when going to the back kitchen to see if the house was shut up, a noise in the coachman's room attracted his attention, and, going in, he discovered to his horror that the man was in bed with one of the maids. She screamed, he struggled, and they rolled out of bed together and made frantic efforts to get apart, but without success. He was a big, burly man, over six feet, and she was a small woman, weighing not more than ninety pounds. She was moaning and screaming, and seemed in great agony, so that, after several fruitless attempts to get them apart, he sent for me. When I arrived I found the man standing up and supporting the woman in his arms, and it was quite evident that his penis was tightly locked in her vagina, and any attempt to dislodge it was accompanied by much pain on the part of both. It was, indeed, a case "De cohesione in coitu." I applied water, and then ice, but ineffectually, and at last sent for chloroform, a few whiffs of which sent the woman to sleep, relaxed the spasm, and relieved the captive penis, which was swollen, livid, and in a state of semi-erection, which did not go down for several hours, and for days the organ was extremely sore. The woman recovered rapidly, and seemed none the worse.

I am sorry that I did not examine if the sphincter ani was contracted, but I did not think of it. In this case there must have been also spasm of the muscle at the orifice, as well as higher up, for the penis seemed nipped low down, and this contraction, I think, kept the blood retained and the organ erect. As an instance of Jago's "beast with two backs," the picture was perfect.

Yours truly,

Egerton Y. Davis,
Ex. U.S. Army

Caughnawaga, Quebec, 4th December, 1884.

*Reprinted from Medical News, 1884; 45:673. Edited from the original.

PROLONGED HAEMORRHAGE FOLLOWING NAIL CLIPPING*

J. L. Burton, B.Sc., M.D.

The popularity of the annual report of the various medical defence societies testifies to the fact that *schadenfreude*[†] is one of the more pleasurable emotions experienced by doctors. This regrettable fact prompts me to report the case of a two-year-old male who almost died from blood loss after a simple surgical procedure (nail-clipping) carried out by a surgeon with inadequate knowledge of a common anatomical variant.

Case Report

The patient was a two-year-old male green budgerigar,[‡] employed as an entertainer at a local primary school. He was the result of a normal mating between only slightly related parents, he hatched normally, and his developmental milestones, such as the ability to ring a little bell by nodding his head and stand on one leg while shelling a peanut, had been normal. He presented at the insistence of the surgeon's child's schoolteacher, who needed to find a home for him during Easter vacation. The patient had no symptoms at the time, but the surgeon's wife noticed that he had a tendency to fall off his perch because his claws were too long. Further testing revealed that he dropped his peanuts too. After due consideration of alternative therapeutic possibilities (eg, thicker perch, walnuts instead of peanuts) it was decided that claw-clipping would be the safest and quickest palliative procedure. It was felt that this operation was within the competence of the average dermatologist, and the author (who is a *very* average dermatologist) duly carried out this procedure with scissors without an anaesthetic (other than a gin and tonic) at 9 PM the same evening. It has to be noted with regret that a con-

sent form was not signed, the procedure was not fully explained to the patient, and the surgeon had never previously seen this operation performed on a budgerigar, though he had previously done a pretty good job on the school rabbit's claw, apart from lacerations of the forearm (the surgeon's forearm, not the rabbit's). Mitigating circumstances include the fact that the first assistant for the operation (the surgeon's wife) was a consultant pathologist who is not at all afraid of blood and has had considerable experience in clipping the toenails of squirmy little two-year-olds.

The immediate postoperative recovery was uneventful. The tachycardia of both surgeon and patient quickly settled, ruffled feathers were preened, and both settled comfortably on their respective perches. About 15 minutes later small beads of blood were observed at the end of each of the budgerigar's claws, and a small red stain was seen in the sawdust beneath the perch. The usual nursing observations were immediately instituted, but some difficulty was experienced because neither of the medical attendants knew how to feel a budgerigar's pulse. The carotid was not readily palpable, and attempts to locate other pulses were abandoned when the patient viciously pecked a small piece of flesh from the surgeon's finger. Palpation of the heart by the simple expedient of picking the patient up revealed that the rate was too fast to count, and it was felt that this maneuver, if repeated, was likely to excite the patient unduly and thus increase the blood loss. In retrospect a knowledge of the pulse rate would not have helped, since the preoperative rate was not recorded and neither of the medical attendants knew the normal pulse rate for a budgerigar.

The pallor proved equally difficult to assess.

---

*Reprinted with permission from the Lancet, © 1983; 2: 1484–1485.
†Enjoyment obtained from other's troubles.
‡A small Australian parrot.

Grey beaks and green feathers are a notoriously un-reliable guide to the haematocrit, and neither the conjunctiva nor the tongue were readily accessible without the risk of another painful nip.

The bleeding could scarcely be described as tor-rential, but the blood that slowly oozed from the tips of the claws did not clot, and the dark stain on the sawdust steadily increased in size. The blood vol-ume of a budgerigar is not large, and most of it seemed to be slowly accumulating as a sticky dark-red pool on the floor of the cage. By 11 PM the pa-tient's condition was causing considerable concern, since he seemed to be weakening and his head was repeatedly drooping. Whether this was due to blood loss or whether it was simply past his bedtime was not clear. At this stage cauterisation was con-sidered, but where there are capillaries there may be nerve endings, and the surgeon did not wish to add a charge of cruelty to that of negligence. Various other possibilities were discussed, such as bone-wax as used by neurosurgeons and autotransfusion as used by desperate obstetricians, but eventually it was decided that the most satisfactory solution would be to get up early the next morning before the children awoke, and if the patient had dropped off his perch during the night, a near-identical budgeri-gar would be purchased and surreptitiously substi-tuted. Experienced surgeons usually sleep soundly while patients struggle through their first postoper-ative night, but in this case the patient slept well, while the surgeon and his first assistant both spent a restless night, taking turns to tiptoe downstairs at regular intervals to check the progress of the tell-tale stain in the sawdust.

Fortunately by 6 AM the patient was considered to be out of danger, and he had completely recov-ered by breakfast-time, although the surgeon's fin-gertip continued to be painful for some days. At the end of the school vacation the budgerigar returned to full-time employment, and the teacher was so pleased with his shortened claws that the surgeon was invited to operate on the other four budgeri-gars. The offer was declined for ethical reasons.

Discussion

The human nail-plate is avascular, and haemor-rhage does not normally follow nail-clipping, even when performed by fumble-fingered dermatolo-gists. Budgerigars are different. They have a pink centre to each claw which represents the corium, equivalent to the human nail-bed. The corium is rich in blood vessels, and since birds have a longer clotting-time than mammals, careless clipping can kill. The corium is also rich in nerves, so that en-thusiastic chiropody resembles an ancient Chinese torture. The claw should be clipped about 2 mm distal to the pink corium, but this can be difficult to see if the nails are pigmented. Most veterinary sur-geons at some time or another have over-pruned the nails of various animals, including birds and tortoises. Few birds bleed to death, but the shock of handling can cause them to die from heart failure.

Dermatologists, unlike surgeons, receive very little formal instruction in common anatomical variants, which can so easily precipitate a surgical disaster. Most surgeons, as a result of their pro-longed training, would probably realise that budgerigar claw-clipping requires special skills, which they may not possess. This case illustrates the danger of allowing a nonspecialist to operate on a case that was clearly beyond his competence. It also confirms that technical incompetence does not prevent the building-up of a large private practice, providing the cage-side manner is good.

I thank Mr. A. I. Wright, BVSc, MRCVS, for technical advice after the event.

THE HAZARDS
OF DAILY LIVING

Anyone who reads *The New England Journal of Medicine* is aware of certain "Letters to the Editor" that turn up occasionally in the journal's correspondence section. These letters are different from what usually appears in the journal and range in topic from unexpected complications of outdoor activities to humorous commentaries on previously unreported ailments. Although NEJM is known for publishing these unusual letters, they appear in other journals as well. In fact, as noted in E. R. Plunkett's book, *Folk Name & Trade Diseases* (see Additional Readings), physicians have been publishing this type of clinical material for well over a hundred years. What all of these letters have in common is a catchy title and a description of an unusual and sometimes strangely entertaining malady of daily living. Although the authors frequently end their communication with a sentence or two that is humorous, the letters themselves are usually serious. The ones that follow were written with a light touch throughout. For an analysis of these letters, see the article by Kathryn Hunter in the appendix.—H.B.

PENILE FROSTBITE,
AN UNFORESEEN HAZARD
OF JOGGING*

To the Editor: A 53-year-old circumcised physician, nonsmoker, light drinker (one highball before dinner), 1.78 meters tall, weighing 70 kg, with no illnesses, performing strenuous physical exercise for many years, began a customary 30-minute jog in a local park at 7 p.m. on December 3, 1976. He wore flare-bottom double-knit polyester trousers, Dacron-cotton boxer-style, undershorts, a cotton T-shirt and cotton dress shirt, a light-wool sweater, an outer nylon shell jacket over the sweater, gloves, and low-cut Pro Ked sneakers. The nylon shell jacket extended slightly below the belt line.

Local radio weather reports gave the outside air temperature as −8°C, with a severe wind-chill factor.

From 7:00 to 7:25 p.m. the jog was routine. At 7:25 p.m. the jogger noted an unpleasant painful burning sensation at the penile tip. From 7:25 to 7:30 p.m. this discomfort became more intense, the pain increasing with each stride as the exercise

neared its end. At 7:30 p.m. the jog ended, and the patient returned home.

Physical examination at 7:40 p.m. in his apartment at comfortable room temperature revealed early frostbite of the penis. The glans was frigid, red, tender upon manipulation and anesthetic to light touch. Immediate therapy was begun. The polyester double-knit trousers and the Dacron-cotton undershorts were removed. In a straddled standing position, the patient created a cradle for rapid re-warming by covering the penile tip with one cupped palm. Response was rapid and complete. Symptoms subsided 15 minutes after onset of treatment, and physical findings returned to normal.

Side effects: at 7:50 p.m. the patient's wife returned from a local shopping trip and observed him during the treatment procedure. She saw him standing, legs apart, in the bedroom, nude below the waist, holding the tip of his penis in his right

*Reprinted with permission from The New England Journal of Medicine, © 1977;296:179.

hand, turning the pages of the *New England Journal of Medicine* with his left. Spouse's observation of therapy produced rapid onset of numerous, varied and severe side effects (personal communication).

Pathogenesis of the syndrome was assessed as tissue response to high air velocity at $-8°C$, penetrating the interstices of polyester double-knit trouser fabric and continuing through anterior opening of Dacron-cotton undershorts, impacting upon receptor site of target organ to produce the changes described.

The patient continues to jog, wearing the athletic supporter and old tight cotton warm-up pants used in college cross-country races in 1939. No recurrences are expected.

Melvin Hershkowitz, M.D.
Medical Center
Jersey City, NJ

Although he didn't know it at the time, Dr. Hershkowitz's letter would inspire someone to write a poem about his unfortunate incident (see p. 101).—H.B.

MARTINI TOOTHPICK WARNING*

To the Editor: We are writing to call attention to a new and potentially serious hazard associated with the hasty ingestion of martinis (or indeed Gibsons, as in the present case). One of us was partaking of a Gibson (gin, ice, essence of vermouth, and several cocktail onions speared on a flat wooden toothpick). As the beverage and onions were quickly consumed, the toothpick floated from the glass into the oral cavity and lodged, uncomfortably, in the posterior pharynx. An attempt to dislodge it by regurgitation resulted in transferring it up into the posterior nares, pointed end first. A trip to the emergency room brought the first author of this letter into contact with the second. Actually, this meeting occurred one hour later, after several encounters with other hospital personnel, who took the history by asking such questions as: "You have a toothpick caught where?" "Are you the man with a toothpick up his nose?" "This couldn't happen—why didn't the olive stop it?" Fortunately, the adroit second author was able to extract the offending obstruction deftly with an alligator forceps. The first author was sent home with the suggestion that he have a drink, sans toothpick. We caution imbibers to consider this potential danger at the end of a difficult day.

Daniel Malamud, Ph.D.
University of Pennsylvania
Mary Harland Murphy, M.D.
Lankenau Hospital
Philadelphia, PA

*Reprinted with permission from The New England Journal of Medicine, © 1986;315:1031–1032.

CASE REPORTS

TELEPHONE TRANSMISSION OF HEPATITIS B?*

To the Editor: The medical literature has been saturated recently with speculation about the variety of transmission mechanisms for the hepatitis B virus.[1] A recent report[2] has gone so far as to imply that even nuns, although not habit-ually important in disease dissemination, may have a greater propensity to serologic evidence of hepatitis B infection than prostitutes from the same urban area. In light of the growing complexity of the problem, we report still another potential mode of hepatitis B acquisition—telephone transmission.

During a telephone survey of transfusion recipients of a possibly contaminated commercial blood product,[3] one of us (D.B.N.), after multiple telephone calls during a single day, noted the gradual onset of lethargy, malaise, headache, otalgia, low-back pain, gluteal rash, profound anorexia, and a gnawing sensation in the upper abdomen. In an attempt to relieve those distressing symptoms, the interviewer medicated himself with a sizable quantity of ethanol. This therapeutic modality temporarily ameliorated the symptoms. By the next morning, however, new symptoms had appeared—dry mouth, nausea, and a slight darkening of the urine. A serum transaminase drawn at that time was slightly elevated. Although it was suggested that a hepatitis B antigen determination be done, the subject refused on the basis of possible medicolegal implications.[4]

Because of the nature of the telephone contacts, we have reason to believe that this case may represent the first report of telephone transmission of hepatitis B. The unusually short incubation period seen in this case may reflect the speed of sound, with the virus somehow traveling synergistically within this framework.

Although some may question the obviously theoretical nature of our conclusions, further observations in other members of the investigatory team have led to additional case-finding and possible epidemic proportions of similar illness. Unfortunately, we have as yet been unable to obtain a single blood specimen for antigen determination.

A Bell-shaped curve of the epidemic has confirmed our hypothesis, and all reputable investigators have been tapped for further ideas. We would willingly discuss our data by telephone with any interested antigen-negative person.

Phoenix, AR

Charles P. Pattison, M.D.
Center for Disease Control
David B. Nelson, M.D.
Calvin A. Klein, M.D.
Center for Disease Control

Atlanta, GA

References

1. Kew MC: Possible transmission of serum (Australia-antigen-positive) hepatitis via the conjunctiva. Infect Immun 7:823–824, 1973.

2. Adam E, Hollinger FB, Melnick JL, et al: Type B hepatitis antigen and antibody among prostitutes and nuns: a study of possible venereal transmission. J Infect Dis 129:317–321, 1974.

3. Center for Disease Control. Viral Hepatitis B Associated with Transfusion of Plasma Protein Fraction—Indiana, Morbidity and Mortality Weekly Report Vol 23, No 11. Atlanta, Georgia, The Center, March 16, 1974, pp 98–99.

4. Chalmers TC, Alter HJ: Management of the asymptomatic carrier of the hepatitis-associated (Australia) antigen. N Engl J Med 285:613–617, 1971.

For a response to this letter, see NEJM 1975;292:757–758.—H.B.

POSTER PRESENTER'S THUMB*

To the Editor: Presentations at national meetings can bring prestige and peril. The hazards of slide presentations include recalcitrant audiovisual equipment and obnoxious skeptics. Anxiety attacks and wounded egos are common. Physical injury is rare. Poster presentations decrease some pyschological and technical risks but pose a unique hazard.

A 38-year-old right-handed man used 80 Push Pins (Douglas Stewart Co., Madison, Wis.) to mount his scientific presentation on a standard, unreceptive, 1.2-by-2.4-m poster board. On completion of the task, the patient noted painful erythema on the volar aspect of his left thumb. In 15 minutes, a 6-by-7-mm blister appeared; it ruptured during the subsequent dismantling of the poster. The patient recalled similar trauma associated with his use of standard thumb tacks at previous meetings. A poll of other poster presenters revealed numerous similar unpublished cases. Prolific patients had multiple recurrences.

Considering the widespread use of poster sessions, thousands of similar cases must occur annually. Organizations that invite such sessions should provide user-friendly boards to reduce the incidence of "poster presenter's thumb."

Laurel C. Preheim, M.D.
Creighton University
School of Medicine

Omaha, NE

For three days after death, hair and fingernails continue to grow but phone calls taper off.

Johnny Carson

*Reprinted with permission from The New England Journal of Medicine, © 1986;314:1518.

SYNDROME-READER'S SCOWL*

To the Editor: Recently, I found a colleague of mine in a dark mood that I mistook for ordinary depression. Upon consultation with a specialist I was horrified to learn that he suffered from syndrome-reader's scowl.

"Note the pained curl of the brow, the wandering, fearful eyes, the cowering posture," said the specialist.

"C'mon, Brandon," I said to my friend. "You just need to have a little fun. How about some exercise?"

"Not on your life," shouted Brandon. "I might get tennis elbow, runner's knee, or frisbee finger."

I had never known Brandon to refuse exercise. "Let's catch a movie, then," I offered.

"No, no, no! Haven't you heard of popcorn-eater's grimace?"

"Intense, repetitive movements of the tongue and facial muscles in response to a morsel of popcorn lodged near the tonsils," explained the specialist. "Some victims have been known to insert a finger into the posterior pharynx and induce a gag reflex."

"Sounds beastly," I said. Brandon was agitated and weeping. "Forget the movie," I said, trying to calm him. "We'll go to the opera instead."

"Never! If I enjoy it I'll get applauder's palms."

"Painful, erythematous swelling of the hands in response to a bravura performance," said the specialist.

Brandon limped away complaining loudly that his orthotics needed adjustment.

"Your friend is very ill indeed," said the specialist, shaking his head.

"Is there nothing that will help him? What about psychotherapy?"

"He'll never submit to psychotherapy if he's heard about shrink-seer's sputter. It's an uncontrollable compulsion to speak openly about one's feelings."

The specialist was correct. We never heard from Brandon again. There were rumors that he had fled to the Bowery, where he has allowed a bad case of tipper's elbow to progress to doorway-sleeper's hip.

As for me, I sit before the pile of unopened journals on my desk, tapping my fingers, fearful of the next revelation. Finally, I can bear the pain no longer. I return to the specialist. He looks at my hands.

"Procrastinator's fingertips," he says sternly. "Be very careful."

New York, NY

David Bateman, M.D.
Harlem Hospital Center

I hate when my foot falls asleep during the day because I know it's going to be awake all night.

Steven Wright

*Reprinted with permission from The New England Journal of Medicine, © 1981;305:1595.

CASE REPORTS
134

Additional Readings

1. Doering EJ, Fitts CT, et al: Alligator bite. JAMA 1971;218:255–256.

A case report about a farmer who got free of an alligator bite by "beating it about the head with the family bible." The case prompted a field trip and bacteriologic study in which those with lesser academic rank had to capture and hold open the mouths of the alligators while the senior members obtained the cultures.

2. Ginsberg M, Green R: Manure shoveler's hip: a previously unrecognized syndrome. Arthritis Rheum 1979;22:940–941.

The authors describe a new cause of hip pain that occurs in people who shovel large quantities of manure. Individuals at risk include horse owners, stable boys, and journal editors.

3. Greengold MC: Letter from Copenhagen. JAMA 1968;204:155–156.

The author presents three case reports that show what might happen if fictional characters ever ended up in medical hands instead of literate ones. The unfortunate "patients" are: The Princess and the Pea, The Ugly Duckling, and The Emperor's New Clothes.

4. Moskow, Shirley B: Hunan Hand & Other Ailments (Letters to the New England Journal of Medicine). Boston: Little Brown and Company, 1987.

This collection brings together 20 years of letters published in the journal. The letters range from silly to serious, but together provide an interesting commentary on a way of looking at health that is unique to our profession.

5. Pedoe EJ, Lightman S: Hazards of paternity: an unreported syndrome. Lancet 1981;2:1427.

The authors describe the "Sucker-daddy Syndrome" which occurs when enthusiastic fathers attach suction toys to their foreheads. The resulting lesions progress from petechiae to purpura and are not amenable to treatment. Prevention can be achieved by using a pin to airvent the toy or, alternatively, the parent's forehead.

6. Plunkett ER: Folk Name & Trade Diseases. Stamford: Barrett Book Company, 1978.

From "Bowler's Thumb" to "Jogger's Nipples" to nearly 1500 other ailments, this book is a dictionary of conditions that have afflicted people for well over a century. Each entry is accompanied by a brief description and its original citation. Although this is not a book on medical humor, it does make for interesting reading.

The following references provide some additional examples of the type of reports presented in the "Hazards" section of this chapter.

7. Brockman MD: Voracious shredder syndrome. N Engl J Med 1993;328:359.

8. Dembert ML: Sick Santa syndrome. JAMA 1986;256:3216–3217.

9. Kamins ML: Proofreader's prostatitis. N Engl J Med 1969;280:1130.

10. Newman JO: Hula-hoop syndrome. BMJ 1958;2:1531.

11. Pinals RS. Genu amoris. Arthritis Rheum 1976;19:637–638.

12. Ragozzino MW: Stretcher's scrotum. N Engl J Med 1993;328:815.

13. Regalbuto G, Hamada P: Pseudo-enuresis recumbens. N Engl J Med 1982;306:615–616.

14. Roizen MF, Engelstad B, et al: Gaussian carditis. N Engl J Med 1982;307:448.

15. Shear NH: Snoring and calf pain. N Engl J Med 1987;317:840.

16. Sholkoff SD: Hot pants syndrome. JAMA 1976;235:2082.

17. Spitzer DE: Horseradish horrors: sushi syncope. JAMA 1988;259:218–219.

18. WB: Telephone ear. Lancet 1892;2:1369.

The following articles provide additional insight into William Osler's sense of humor.

19. Altaffer LF: Penis captivus and the mischievous Sir William Osler. South Med J 1983;76:637–641.

20. Bean WB: William Osler: The Egerton Yorrick Davis alias. In: McGovern JP, Burns CR (eds): Humanism in Medicine. Springfield, IL, Charles C Thomas, 1970, pp 49–59.

21. Blumer G: The jocular side of Osler. Arch Intern Med 1949;84:34–39.

22. Cullen TS: The gay of heart. Arch Intern Med 1949;84:41–45.

23. MacDermot HE: The lighter aspects of Osler's textbook. Can Med Assoc J 1949;61:76–78.

24. Nation EF: Osler's alter ego. Dis Chest 1969;56:531–537.

25. Tigertt WD: An annotated life of Egerton Yorrick Davis. J Hist Med 1983;38:259–297.

MEDICAL RESEARCH

Considering the amount of research that gets published every year, I did not find that much humor written on the subject. Perhaps that's because researchers are too busy writing grants to find the time to be funny. Or because no one can guarantee that a parody will get funded, and guffaws and chuckles will not feed the mice. Then again, some might argue that a lot of research is amusing anyway, especially if you read it a decade or more after it is published. One example of this type of humor can be found in an article that was published in 1879 by Dr. Allen W. Hagenback: "Masturbation as a Cause of Instanity" (J Nerv Mental Dis 1879; 6:603–612). In the conclusion to this interesting treatise, Dr. Hagenback makes a number of final remarks, the most illuminating of which is:

> That in a small percentage of masturbators, certain physical findings are present due to the vice which may prove valuable in confirming the diagnosis.

Is it possible that this is the origin of the Hairy Palm Theory? The articles that follow make some interesting claims of their own. I wonder how they'll hold up over time?

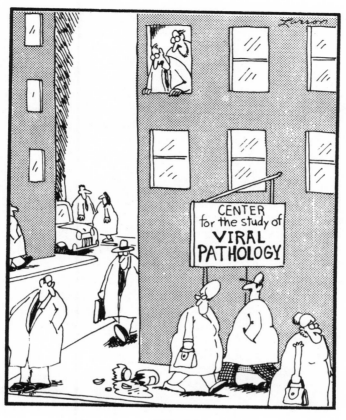

"Uh-oh."

STATISTICALLY SPEAKING*

Roger P. Smith, M.D.

Few people are aware of the significant contributions made in the early part of this century by the British statistician, William Gossett. Throughout his entire professional life, Gossett worked for the Guinness Brewery. He chose to publish his landmark studies under the pseudonym "Student."[1] These papers provided the basis for what has become known as the "Student t test." Unfortunately, few are acquainted with the true origin of the t test or how this statistical terminology has been changed from its original meaning.

Despite his employment by the Guinness Brewery, William Gossett was a devotee of the British national drink, tea. He observed that some scientific manuscripts were exceedingly boring and required more tea to stay awake than did others. This quantification led to the "tea-test" for papers and the "tea-distribution" for oral presentations. (The latter was based on the number of audience members resorting to methylxanthines to maintain consciousness.) The application of these concepts led inevitably to the "P value" and the "continence interval." A low "P value" indicated an exciting concept that required little tea to maintain a wakeful state. A shortened "continence interval" indicated that the audience wanted no more discussion on a particular point (also reflected in the "frequency" distribution, if not the urgency of some presentations).

The British preoccupation with alimentary statistics, and their sequelae, led to the concept of the "commodal value" (the most frequent place or set of observations). This has been shortened to "modal value" in the American literature.

To obtain consensus regarding a given set of statistics, Gossett would convene a group of cronies in a local pub (a "cohort study"). Assembling a group for such an uninteresting chore was sometimes a grim task. To entice participants, he had to offer both a sampling of Guinness products and the possibility of companionship with unaccompanied persons at the pub. The need to find appropriately qualified individuals who would not be distracted gave rise to both the concept of a "standard deviate" and the continuing distrust of "single observation" papers that persists today. The presentation of data around the countertops of the pub led to the idea of "tabular data" and the love of "tables" (and "bar graphs") found in modern literature. (Small fruit stains from the occasional dessert consumed during the review process are not, however, the source of the "pie chart" or "splatter-gram," though periodic announcements on the status of liquid refreshment did give rise to the "case report.")

The risk of being pinched by a bobby for excessive use of the Guinness products was recognized as potentially reducing one's "degree of freedom."

Despite the somewhat onerous job of reviewing poorly written papers night after night in a dim British pub, participation in this process was the best way for a rising mathematician to become known in the cutthroat world of statisticians. As a result, it was soon well known that you had to be "pub-ish or perish."

Reference

1. Rosner B. Fundamentals of biostatistics. Boston: Duxbury Press, 1982:147.

Now that Roger Smith has given us a "primer" on the origin of statistical terminology, I thought I'd include a couple of quotes from the last century. In addition to being an eminent surgeon and statistician, John Shaw Billings is probably the most famous bibliographer in the history of medicine (he is credited with establishing what is known today as the National Library of Medicine). Lord Moynihan was a famous British surgeon who lived from 1865-1936.—H.B.

> Statistics are like old medical journals or like revolvers in a newly opened mining district. Most men rarely use them and find it troublesome to preserve them for easy access. However, when they do want them, they want them badly.[1]
>
> John Shaw Billings

> Statistics will prove anything, even the truth.[2]
>
> Lord Moynihan

1. Medical Record. 1889;36:589.
2. Cowan L, Cowan M (eds): The Wit of Medicine. England:Leslie Frewin Pub Ltd. 1972, p. 34.

"CEPHALOMALACIA OBFUSCATE," A FOURTH GENERATION CEPHALOSPORIN*

Bruce K. Rubin, BSC, MENG, M.D.

A new fourth generation cephalosporin, cephalomalacia obfuscate, has been synthesized. Limited testing has shown this new class of antibiotic to have substantially greater bacteriopathic properties than the third generation antibiotics. The role that these properties may play in host defense is discussed.

Introduction

Since the early 1960's the cephalosporins have enjoyed great clinical success as a family of antibiotics. Laboratory manipulations have produced successive generations of this antibiotic, each more powerful than its predecessor (Fig. 1). The synthesis and testing of what we believe to be of a fourth generation of cephalosporins are reported here. We have named this antibiotic "cephalomalacia obfuscate" and hope to market it under the trade name Killacillin.

Synthesis

One of the newer third generation cephalosporins, "cephalohaematoma," was obtained from the manufacturer (Ersatz Pharmaceuticals) and a side chain was added as an offshoot to the method described by Stalin.[1] This side chain is known to both traumatize and immobilize many bacteria *in vitro.*

A phagocytic moiety was then added (Fig. 2) to produce a new class of antibiotics: the fourth generation cephalosporin.

Methods and Results

Bacteria exhibit avoidance activity in the presence of adversive stimuli. This activity has been quantified crudely in the past using the Kirby-Bauer method[2] where noxious agents in the form of antibiotic discs are placed into a colony of microorganisms, encouraging them to move away. A major difficulty with

CEPHALOSPORIN PEDIGREE

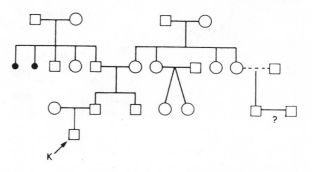

Figure 1. Cephalosporin pedigree. "Cephalomalacia" is marked with the arrow.

this method is that it does not measure the rate at which the bacteria migrate, but only the total distance travelled. Many researchers believe that this technique better reflects the stamina of the specific microorganism (B. K. Rubin, personal communication). To overcome this problem we implanted microphones into the cell walls of a fixed number of bacteria in a colony using standard microsurgical technique. When these microphones were connected to highly sensitive acoustically shielded recording and amplifying devices, we found that the rate of migration correlated well with the amplitude of the sound produced which, to our ears, sounded not unlike millions of tiny screams.

By this methodology we were able to obtain pain tolerance curves for several of the more pathogenic bacteria (B. K. Rubin, unpublished data).

A double blind experiment was then undertaken

*Reprinted from the Pediatric Infectious Disease Journal, © 1983; 2:424–425, with permission from William & Wilkins, Baltimore.

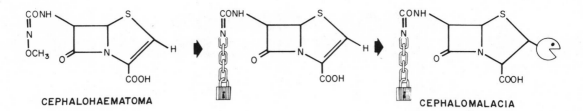

CEPHALOHAEMATOMA → → CEPHALOMALACIA

Figure 2. Synthesis of "cephalomalacia obfuscate." Funding seems to be the rate limiting step.

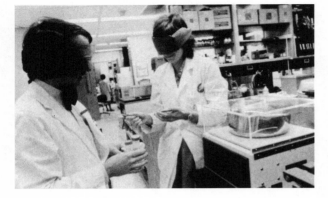

Figure 3. Behavioral bacteriology laboratory during double blind research into pain thresholds. Dr. Ford-Jones (R) is attempting to "pin the tail" on Dr. Biggar.

(Fig. 3) using alternate challenge with either "cephalomalacia" or one of the highly touted third generation cephalosporins (identified as cephalosporin "X"). The results as shown in Figure 4 show clearly that "cephalomalacia" produces more bacterial pain per unit dose in those organisms tested.

Discussion

Behavioral bacteriology is the name given to the science born of the marriage between microbiology and psychology. This field is rapidly changing our concepts of the unicellular organism. We present here both a new antibiotic and an appropriate laboratory tool for measuring an important facet of microbial socialization. This method has been used to test a new class of drug, the bacteriopathic antibiotic.

There are many factors that influence host defense. One of the most important and perhaps most overlooked is the psychologic state of the host or "will to live." Unexpected recovery from terrible disease has often been attributed to a patient's tenacious fight for life. It would be beneficial for many

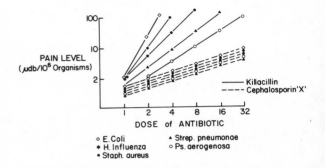

Figure 4. Bacteriopathic properties of the third and fourth generation of cephalosporin. Antibiotic dose was increased to the limit of the organisms pain tolerance.

patients to know not only that the medicine being taken is killing an infecting microorganism but also that it is making those organisms suffer. We anticipate that this sense of revenge could be valuable to the overall healing process. In this regard we feel that "cephalomalacia," the first of the bacteriopathic cephalosporins, represents a significant advance in antimicrobial therapy.

Acknowledgements

Thanks to Drs. E. L. Ford-Jones and D. Biggar of the Division of Infectious Diseases, The Hospital for Sick Children, Toronto, for performing double blind experimentation. Thanks also to Drs. A. S. Rebuck and K. Chapman of the Respiratory Division, Toronto Western Hospital, for guidance.

References

1. Stalin J: The annexation of Eastern Europe. In World War II, 1945.

2. Bauer AW, Kirby WMM, Sherris JD, et al: Antibiotic susceptibility testing by a standardized single disc method. Am J Clin Pathol 45:493–496, 1966.

RETRACTION ON
CEPHALOMALACIA OBFUSCATE*

To the Editors:

Readers of *Pediatric Infectious Disease* have been writing requesting the raw data on which my article was based. When we went to review these data we found that my research fellow, whose name was regrettably left off the preliminary publication because of an editorial oversight, had in fact "dry labbed" the entire experiment and pocketed most of the funds. The bottles of what we thought were Killacillin were in fact merely outdated tetracycline which was to be discarded. Needless to say we are all embarrassed over this incident and the research fellow has resigned his position to take a job with the government. I must therefore retract much of the data presented in the article but I am pleased to announce at this time that we are doing some exciting research into outdated tetracycline.

Regretfully our methodologist and symptomatologist both resigned their positions because of this incident, so in the future we will be forced to report on methods and symptoms rather than methodologies and symptomatologies.

Bruce K. Rubin, M.D., F.R.C.P.(C)
Queen's University
Department of Paediatrics

Kingston, Ontario, Canada

———————

Dr. Rubin isn't the only one with cephalosporin fever. A few years ago, Ludwig Lettau published a satire that described a *sixth* generation cephalosporin ("Antibiotics 1999" Ann Intern Med 1989; 110:850). Not only had Glitze Pharmaceuticals come up with an antibiotic that would kill every bacteria on the planet, but they also concocted an antifungal to deal with the superinfections caused by their new drug.—H.B.

*Reprinted from the Pediatric Infectious Disease Journal, © 1984; 3:283, with permission from Williams & Wilkins, Baltimore.

THE TEETHING VIRUS*

Howard J. Bennett, M.D.
D. Spencer Brudno, M.D.

A prospective study was carried out on 500 teething infants which demonstrated that a new infectious agent, the human teething virus, is responsible for the febrile response that accompanies the eruption of deciduous teeth. Speculations are made concerning whether or not primary care physicians will began prescribing amoxicillin instead of Jack Daniel's to treat teething infants and their parents.

Introduction

Teething has been the subject of intense interest in the medical and nonmedical community for centuries.[1] Controversy has resulted not only over the signs and symptoms associated with teething but also over the tooth fairy's impact on the family.[2,3] But perhaps the greatest controversy of all is whether or not teething causes fever. Unfortunately all of the research in this area suffers from serious methodologic flaws. McCartney et al.[4] reported that teething was responsible for fever in 20% of infants with temperatures $\geq 40°C$. That study was carried out in an emergency room setting, however, and therefore is not applicable to all infants. In addition, the authors failed to quantitate the amount of drooling that residents had to contend with and whether or not this interfered with optimal observation of the patient. More recently, Shorts[5] examined 240 teething patients in a suburban practice and concluded that teething does not cause fever. His population included school-aged children as well as infants, however, and it is well known that older children will feign illness in order to get stickers and other rewards from the doctor's office.[6]

Early in 1982 one of us was doing histopathology research on the brain cells of hairless mice that had been subjected to 36 hours "on-call." Inadvertently a sample of saliva from a teething infant (via a soggy bagel) was put under the electron microscope. To our amazement this accident uncovered a new viral particle (HJ Bennett, unpublished revelation). This discovery led to the diversion of all previously acquired grant funds into the search for the mythical teething virus. In this report we present the results of a prospective study of teething infants and young children undertaken during the Washington, DC teething outbreak of 1983 and 1984. We report our findings, which prove conclusively that the human teething virus (HT virus) is the hitherto elusive agent responsible for the fevers associated with teething.

Patients and Methods

The study included 500 infants who were followed prospectively from birth through 2½ years of age. The patients were selected from consecutive term births at our medical center. Primiparous women were interviewed by one of the authors sometime during the third trimester—usually on the way to the delivery room. The mothers-to-be were asked two questions regarding possible entry into the study: (1) If you have a baby, would you like to participate in a study of teething in infants? (2) Do you believe in Santa Claus? A positive response to either question made the infant eligible for the study.

A total of 506 mother/infant pairs were initially included in the study. The patients were matched for socioeconomic status, educational background and whether or not both parents watched "Dallas" on Friday nights. Two infants with natal teeth were subsequently excluded, though it is worth noting that in both cases the mother experienced a "warm uterine feeling" 2 weeks prior to delivery. An additional four babies dropped out of the study for unknown reasons. Their mothers reluctantly withdrew from the project as well.

*Reprinted from the Pediatric Infectious Disease Journal, © 1986; 5:399–401, with permission from Williams & Wilkins, Inc., Baltimore.

Mothers were instructed to bring their baby to the clinic at the first sign of teething. During this visit vital signs were taken and the infant was examined for physical evidence of teething using the method described by Leech.[7] Briefly, this technique involves having the infant breastfeed for 5 minutes in the office. If the mother's cry exceeds 90 dB, the baby is teething. The threshold is adjusted to 120 dB in nonnursing mothers. Infants were seen regularly during the teething period, and parents kept a diary of relevant symptoms.

Saliva was obtained on the fourth and sixth teething days by adsorption onto teething rings impregnated with human embryonic lung and human embryonic kidney. The specimens were processed using a revolutionary technique that is currently under investigation by a rival laboratory and therefore is not available for publication. Additional saliva was obtained from the subjects' mothers and in between episodes of teething such that each patient served as his or her own control. Serum specimens were not obtained due to parental squeamishness. All subjects and specimens were handled in a triple blind fashion: patients did not know why they were in the study, technicians did not know what was being studied and the authors didn't care but hoped to get published anyway.

Results

Basic research. The HT virus is a uniquely shaped viral particle with a diameter of 140 nm. The envelope surrounds a helical nucleocapsid that is covered with spherical studs (Fig. 1). Though superficially resembling a slice of white bread, the HT

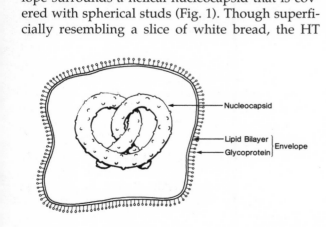

Figure 1. Schematic representation of the human teething virus.

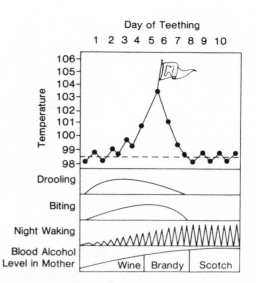

Figure 2. Schematic diagram illustrating the clinical sequence of teething.

virus is actually the first recognized member of a new family of RNA viruses to be named the masticoviridae. Details of the virus' life-style and reproductive habits will be the subject of another report.[8]

Clinical research. The 500 patients in our study experienced repeated bouts of teething during the first 2½ years of life. Teeth erupted at a rate of approximately 10 per year, which provided us with 5000 tooth-years of data. Eighty-four percent of patients became febrile during the teething process. The clinical course of these patients is shown in Figure 2. All patients recovered uneventfully from this developmental nuisance. Unfortunately, however, at least 15 divorces could be directly attributed to "irreconcilable differences" on how to manage a teething baby at three o'clock in the morning.

The HT virus was isolated by electron microscopy from well over 99% of febrile teething patients (Table 1). In fact there was only one febrile infant in whom the HT virus was not isolated, and the technician who handled that specimen admitted to misplacing the patient's teething ring and secretly testing his own saliva (J Cama, personal confession). The HT virus was not isolated from any of the nonfebrile teething patients, though it was seen in two samples taken from the mothers' group. In both cases, however, the mothers admitted to kissing their febrile babies just prior to submitting their own specimens for study.

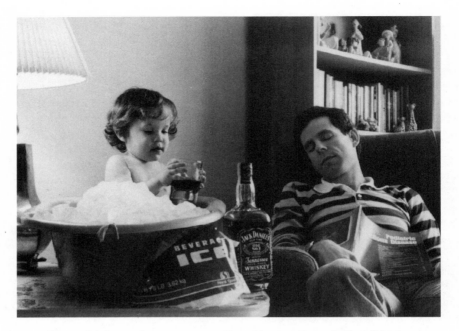

Figure 3. The modern treatment of teething: an ice and alcohol bath.

Table 1. Isolation of the human teething virus
by electron microscopy in control and teething patients.

Group	No. of Samples Tested	No. Positive for HT Virus	% Positive for HT Virus
Mothers	500	2	<1
Nonteething infants	1000	0	0
Nonfebrile teething infants	800	0	0
Febrile teething infants	4200	4199	>99[a]

[a]$P<0.000001$ by Toddler's t test and the Fisher-Price test.

Discussion

Infants acquire their primary teeth by 30 months of age. Teething occurs off and on for 24 of these months—mostly on, according to parents. We have shown that 84% of infants develop fever when teething and that it is the HT virus which causes this fever. There appears to be little doubt, therefore, that parents have been right all along. Fortunately, however, teething phobia can now be approached intelligently instead of with the irrational treatments of the past (Fig. 3).

A few questions still remain, however, concerning the pathogenesis of the HT virus. We believe that primary infections with the virus occur early in life in the majority of children. These infections are probably subclinical most of the time but undoubtedly are also responsible for many of the "idiopathic" conditions of infancy, colic and difficult temperament, to name a few. Once the primary infection subsides, the virus becomes dormant within the alveolar ridge. Then, at future points in time, the aggressive movements of erupting teeth disturb the sleeping virus who retaliates by producing local and systemic effects. The pattern of transmission is not horizontal, as one might expect, but gravitational, this of course owing to the aerodynamics of drooling babies.

As a result of this study, we have revised the anticipatory guidance given at 6 months of age. Parents are encouraged to check for teething at the first sign of fever and to quickly begin their prophylactic Valium® if the baby's Leech test is positive. Finally we recommend that practitioners approach their 2 a.m. calls as a time to educate parents about the positive aspects of teething.[9] This advice will minimize the hoarding of left-over amoxicillin until such time as a vaccine is developed to rid mankind of this pesky little virus.

Acknowledgments

This work was supported completely by a grant from the makers of Orajel® and Goldstein's Bagel Shop. Special thanks to Judith Ratner, M.D., who somehow found the time to review our manuscript in between pelvic examinations in her adolescent clinic.

References

1. Radbill SX: Teething as a medical problem: Changing viewpoints through the centuries. Clin Pediatr 4:556–559, 1965.

2. Skinner BF: The tooth ransom: Are today's children holding out for too much money? J Pediatr Bribery 86:314–316, 1980.

3. Westheimer R: Is 50¢ a tooth enough to get children to sleep in their own beds at night? J Parental Celibacy 69:123–128, 1981.

4. McCartney PL, Flintstone F, Rubble B, et al: Do teething infants need a CBC and blood culture? J Dubious Invest 59:463–468, 1977.

5. Shorts RH: Teething and fever: Another myth debunked. PMD Bull 21:459–463, 1982.

6. Munchausen BV: Factitious teething as a means to visit the pediatrician. Acta Idiotica Scand 70:212–213, 1978.

7. Leech LA: The clinical application of breastfeeding reflexes: "Let-down" means the milk is in, "Let Go!" means the teeth are coming. The Breast 36:24–34, 1982.

8. Bennett HJ, Brudno DS: The masticoviruses: Have we bitten off more than we can chew? Popular Virol, in press, 1986.

9. Weissman MI: Tootharche, menarche, and anarchy: Three developmental milestones of childhood and adolescence. Curr Prob Nightcall 12:1–7, 1983.

THE TANTRUM GENE*

(McFarland L, et al: *J Behav Genet* 83:108, 1990)

McFarland and coworkers, in collaboration with the National Time-Out Foundation, report their identification of the illusive tantrum gene. Long considered the "unicorn" of genetic research, the investigators found the gene on the short arm of chromosome 10. Sequence analysis reveals that the gene encodes for a rather sticky protein (an enzyme) that is 1284 amino acids long. The enzyme, named obstreperase by the authors, appears to regulate the suppressor activity of certain neurotransmitters in the central nervous system.

In an editorial that accompanies the article, Dr. Lars Ungstromm of the Swedish Institute of Behavioral Genetics comments that mutations have not been identified yet, but are suspected to occur in large numbers of the general population.

Comment

The fact that the tantrum gene is located on the short arm of any chromosome proves that Mother Nature does have a sense of humor. It has been suspected for years that a toddler's negativism might be the result of an autosomal dominant gene with variable penetrance. Now that McFarland et al have isolated the gene, the next step will be to figure out what factors control its suppression and activation. Determining this will not only be a godsend to thousands of exhausted parents, but it will also go a long way toward helping operating room personnel when the gene is inadvertently turned on in temperamental surgeons.

Howard J. Bennett, M.D.

SINGLE-BLIND/DOUBLE-BLIND RADIOGRAPHIC ANALYSIS: NEW VIEWING TECHNIQUES*

Michael H. Reid, M.D.
Arthur B. Dublin, M.D.

In 1982 Oestreich[1] described the cupped hand method for excluding extraneous light when viewing radiographs. Several advantages were ascribed to this simple procedure. We report two variations: 50% and 100% light exclusion.

To test the utility of these variations, we applied them to 1,000 outpatient skull films randomly selected from the discard film bin of a large university teaching hospital. These films were then viewed by two techniques on a standard radiographic viewbox independently by two radiologists as illustrated in figure 1. The results were then tabulated and compared against the original interpretation in the hospital record by a third radiologist who elected to remain anonymous. The hospital record could not be found in 55 instances.

Of the 1,000 films, 182 were normal, 58 were possibly normal, 91 were possibly abnormal, 389 were suggestive of being possibly abnormal, 82 were equivocally suggestive of pathognomonic abnormality, and 78 were uninterpretable. Of the 922 interpretable films, 318 were considered technically acceptable and should not have been discarded.

Student's t-test and Wilcoxin's paired-difference test were applied to the data. Not unexpectedly technique B (single blind) had a 50% sensitivity, while technique A (double blind) had no false positives (100% specificity).

Interpretive errors in the radiographic analysis of poor quality skull radiographs have always been a problem, and our data confirm this. While there have been many recommendations to improve viewing conditions for the radiologist, we believe our techniques are unique.

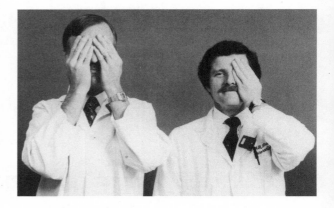

Figure 1. Anonymous radiologists demonstrating technique A (left) and technique B (right).

The contribution of technique A is the low false-positive rate (also low false-negative rate). The radiologist using technique A also complained less of eye fatigue and excessive glare. The principle disadvantage of technique A is that comparison with previous films is difficult.

We conclude that technique A (double blind) is superior when a negative interpretation is desired. Another method, technique C (no blind, not shown), has been investigated thoroughly on acceptable films but not on discarded films. Such a study, compared with techniques A and B is in progress and will be the subject of a future report.

References

1. Oestreich AE. Use of the cupped hand for improved viewing of radiographs. Radiology 1982;143:563.

*Reprinted from the American Journal of Roentgenology, © 1983;140:825, with permission from the American Roentgen Ray Society.

The *British Medical Journal* publishes a special issue each December that features, in addition to some serious articles, a number of lighter medical pieces. You can easily spot this issue because it sports an artistic cover instead of the journal's traditional blue and black. Although a lot of the material is regional, some of it does travel well. Three of the articles in the book (including the next one) and a number of "Additional Readings" were originally published in the *BMJ*'s Christmas issue. For those who do not get the journal, it may be worth a trip to your local medical library when the holiday season rolls around. Actually, considering the time it takes to cross the Atlantic, you might want to wait until mid January.—H.B.

BIOLOGY, BLIND MEN, AND ELEPHANTS*

Berril Yushomerski Yankelowitz, M.D.

Newton watched an apple fall and discovered the Law of Gravity (A). Biologists would attack such a problem more scientifically. A typical scientific approach would be as follows.

Introduction

Apples would seem to appear to fall to the ground.[1–50,52,54,57] This suggests the possibility that there is some property of apples which might result in this phenomenon. It is well known that apples falling from a height have apparent changes in tissue turgor pressure.[51,55,56–80] This might well reflect changes in intracellular water and electrolyte losses. It, therefore, appeared reasonable to determine the relationship between the apple's fall, its tissue turgor pressure, and the intracellular electrolyte content.

Materials, Methods, and Results

A total of 500 apples were randomly selected from an orchard in the State of Washington with another 500 from Wisconsin as controls. The apples were stratified by colour, number of seeds, worm content, and baseline tissue turgor pressure and intracellular electrolytes measured by methods we have previously described.[53,81–200] Each apple was num-

bered and randomly placed in brown bags (obtained through the courtesy of Cheatem Markets). The bags were then dropped from 1, 10, 20, and 100 feet (respectively 30, 300, 600, and 3000 cm) by an investigator who did not know their contents. Post-drop tissue turgor pressure and electrolyte concentrations were then remeasured by another method we have previously described.[53,201–430]

Results were analysed by the X^2, Student's test, Wilcoxon, covariant analysis, and multiple linear regression techniques with appropriate strata. There was a highly significant difference in the worm content of red apples as opposed to green ones ($P < 0.05$). Furthermore, green apples with more than 10 worms and less than five seeds showed a much greater decrease in post-fall tissue turgor if they were from Wisconsin than if they were from Washington State ($P < 0.00001$). By analysis of covariance and multiple linear regression, there was an almost linear relationship between height of drop and decrease in tissue turgor pressure (see figure). When corrected for crush artifact, no differences could be observed for pre- and post-drop intracellular electrolyte concentrations. All apples that were dropped, fell. Consequently we could not determine whether the change in turgor pressure was statistically associated with falling. Nevertheless, the inadequate number of

*Reprinted with permission from the British Medical Journal, © 1978; 2:1775. Edited from the original.

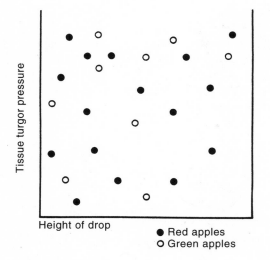

Tissue turgor pressure

Height of drop

● Red apples
○ Green apples

much criticism of our methodology—"the investigator failed to stratify by the type of apple—for example, Golden Delicious vs Beverly Hill vs Pippin, Roman." "The apples should have been allowed to drop from trees." "In our study[1-20] we found a significant correlation with temperature and season of the year—the current investigation cannot be interpreted without such data."

But once the criticism dies down, there will be a flurry of activity, investigators repeating the study with pears, prunes, pumpkins, and watermelons to show the generality of the results. The original investigators will spend six months a year on speaking tours in both the scientific and lay communities. Grant money will flow in vast rivers from both public sources and private charitable foundations. A Nobel prize should be forthcoming. In his dotage, the author should be interviewed for his political and social opinions to which he was more than entitled by virtue of his previous achievement.

While it is quite true that this type of science doesn't provide any satisfying answers, it does produce all that marvellous data that we like so much. Also, it puts bread on the table of the researcher. So, with that, I must return to my laboratory to predict elephants by examining their tails (B).

A Newton, Sir Isaac, personal communication.
B Aesop, personal communication.

drops may have led to a substantial type two error; in a more extensive trial, it is expected that a sufficient number of apples would rise to actually determine this effect.

Comment

We plan to repeat the study with a larger number of apples and also measure apple shelf life before and after dropping them. Of course, there will be

---

A drug is a substance that when injected into a guinea pig produces a scientific paper.

Anonymous

X-RAY GOGS:

Preliminary Evaluation of a "New" Imaging Modality*
David K. Edwards, III, M.D.

"X-Ray Gogs," which apparently reveal internal anatomy without radiation, ultrasound, or magnetic fields, were compared with conventional imaging modalities in evaluating a variety of pediatric conditions. Conventional techniques were preferable in terms of diagnostic accuracy and image quality, and are thus recommended in most settings. Because of low cost and lack of ionizing radiation, "X-Ray Gogs" are recommended in cases where radiography is not indicated, or where the results of radiographic study will not influence patient management, or where the diagnosis has already been established by other means.

X-RAY GOGS. You saw these advertised in comic books as a child. And you wanted them with all your heart. And your parents objected. And you yielded. And since then life has not been very happy for you, has it? We offer a second chance to buy, own and operate the famous X-ray glasses. According to the package, it is: the "scientific marvel of the century." Not sold to communist countries on the restricted list that also prohibits sales of Cray Supercomputers. $1.25 each.

Quoted with permission from *Catalog #5*[1]

In this age of rapid advances in imaging techniques, it was mildly surprising to read the above advertisement and to realize that X-Ray Gogs (XRG), which have been available to the lay public for many years, have evidently not been examined in medical context.[2] Because of parental skepticism and parsimony, the author never owned XRG, and indeed life was not riotously happy thereafter. However, a childhood friend with less frugal parents recalls that XRG permitted visualization of not only digital bones but also the lead in a wooden pencil (Bobby "Bubba" Young, personal communication).

The intent of this preliminary study was to compare XRG with conventional imaging modalities in a variety of clinical pediatric settings.

Materials and Methods

The XRG as received from the vendor (Archie McPhee & Co., Seattle, WA) consisted of plastic frames with cardboard inserts containing 5-mm openings in which a red, translucent, striated material acted as a lens (Fig. 1). The striated material proved to be part of a red feather.[3] To permit a correct interpupillary distance and to compensate for myopia, I removed the cardboard inserts and affixed them to prescription spectacles (Fig. 2).

A miscellaneous variety of pediatric sonographic ($n=30$) and radiographic ($n=97$) examinations (list available on persuasive request) were performed with simultaneous or near-simultaneous XRG observation. The bright light required by the XRG studies was intermittently turned on and off during fluoroscopic procedures.

The Human Subjects Committee responded to routine petition in an uncouth, jocular manner that was interpreted as approval. Because of the benign nature of XRG studies, informed consent was considered implicit. Pediatric patients (age, 1 day to 10 years) were employed both because of the author's area of specialization and because adults, encountered in hallways, responded adversely to the examiner's appearance (Fig. 2), whereas children

*Reprinted from the American Journal of Roentgenology, © 1988;150:731–734; with permission from the American Roentgen Ray Society.

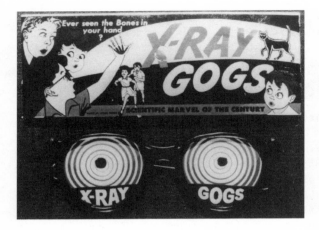

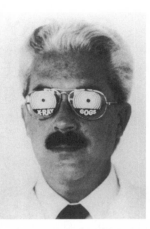

Figure 1. Obverse of X-Ray Gogs and package label, photographed on corduroy (5.5 ridges/cm). Reverse of package label (not shown) contains instructions and faintly distasteful insinuations about seeing through clothing.

Figure 2. X-Ray Gogs modified for use with prescription lenses.

seemed intrigued, and infants oblivious. The passive voice was used where possible in this report.

The obviously harmless character of XRG allowed bypassing tedious laboratory investigation involving rodents and other vermin. Following the model of the similarly seminal early communications of Wilhelm Roentgen,[4] this study was not cluttered with annoying gibberish about line-pairs, ROC curves, sensitivity/specificity, and similar incomprehensibilities.

Results

Preliminary Evaluations

When used as instructed (i.e., viewing structures against a strong light), the XRG displayed the soft tissues of the fingers in a pleasing pink, with darker central regions that were surely either bones or something else (Fig. 3). Similarly, a wooden pencil thus viewed revealed pink edges and a dark central line that suggested the pencil's graphite core. The potential, hinted by the manufacturer, of seeing through clothing was explored with selected female staff members to the point of eyestrain, without success. Continual wearing of the XRG offered the advantage that the eyes remained dark-adapted; however, it was difficult to find one's way about the department in what seemed a dense red fog, hounded by the jeers of one's colleagues.

Comparative Study

The results comparing XRG and conventional studies are presented in Table 1. Conventional studies were notably superior in furnishing the correct di-

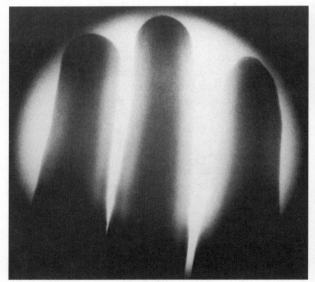

Figure 3. Three of the author's fingers viewed through X-Ray Gogs.

agnosis. The XRG studies provided the correct diagnosis only in those instances when the conventional study also revealed no abnormality. An important reason for this disparity appeared to be image quality, which was invariably inferior with XRG. Indeed, on no occasions were axial skeletal structures, soft tissue-gas interfaces, or administered contrast materials discernible with XRG; all that was seen was a pink, patient-shaped blur.

On the other hand, XRG was superior in terms of ease of examination (one had only to look at the patient with a bright light in the background), cost (negligible), and radiation dose (nil). With these advantages in mind, the cases were reviewed retro-

Table 1. Comparison of X-Ray Gogs and Conventional Radiographic Techniques (127 Examinations)

	Correct Diagnosis[a]	The preferred study in terms of:			
		Image Quality	Ease of Examination	Cost of Examination	Radiation Dose[b]
Conventional techniques	112 (88%)	127	0	0	0
X-Ray Gogs	60[c] (47%)	0	127	127	97
Significance of difference	$p \ll$ tiny[d]	$p <$ SC[e]	$p <$ SC	$p <$ SC	$p <$ SC

[a]Pathological, surgical, or clinical confirmation.

[b]30 sonograms not included.

[c]Where the correct diagnosis was "no abnormality seen," or thereabouts.

[d]Conventional techniques were correct and X-Ray Gogs wrong in 61 cases, while X-Ray Gogs were correct and conventional techniques wrong in 9 cases.

[e]SC = smoking computer: the clone, using the sign test and attempting to compute the infinitestimal "p" values of chi-square in the megaton (100+) range, began to smoke: heavily, indoors, and in defiance of local ordinance and several clearly visible signs.

spectively to define the actual benefit afforded the patient by the imaging study; 13 cases (10%) were found in which the benefit of the XRG study was at least the same as that of the conventional study. These were cases in which at least one of the following pertained: (1) the radiographic study was not indicated; (2) no change in patient management would occur whatever the results of the radiographic study; or (3) the diagnosis was already firmly established by other means. Examples of such cases follow.

Exemplary Case Reports

Case 1.—A 4-year-old girl presented to the Emergency Room with a hurt finger. The intern, swamped with patients, injudiciously ordered radiographs before examining the child. The finger proved to have been hurt by a bee sting.

X-Ray Gog Examination: Soft tissue swelling dorsal to distal phalanx. No bony injury seen.

Radiographic Examination: Ditto.

Comment: No imaging examination was indicated.

Case 2.—A 3-year-old boy was evaluated for unexplained fever. Examination revealed otitis media, purulent nasal discharge, and tenderness over the left maxilla. The discharge was sent for culture, and the patient was begun on antibiotics and decongestants. As the child was leaving the clinic, a Waters view of the paranasal sinuses was requested and obtained.

X-Ray Gog Examination: No abnormality seen.

Radiographic Examination: Radiopacity of the left maxillary antrum.

Comment: The XRG diagnosis was clearly wrong. However, the clinicians proposed to treat the child the same whatever the radiographic study showed.

The film added nothing except a nebulous entity called "baseline."

Case 3.—A 1-month-old boy presented with projectile vomiting. Examination revealed mild dehydration, peristaltic waves across the upper abdomen, and a palpable mass ("olive") in the right abdomen. Sonography demonstrated a lengthened pylorus with a wall thickness of 5.5 mm; pyloric stenosis was diagnosed. However, an upper gastrointestinal series (UGI) was demanded and, after unseemly shouting and flexings of ego on the part of the clinicians and radiologists, grudgingly performed.

X-Ray Gog Examination: Barium sulfate suspension, administered by bottle and nipple, was not seen to flow freely through a normal esophagus. The filled stomach was not observed in several projections. Pyloric lengthening and marked narrowing ("string sign") were not noted. Distal to the narrowing, a normal duodenal sweep and ligament of Trietz were not appreciated. Hypertrophic pyloric stenosis was not diagnosed.

Fluoroscopic Examination: Ditto, deleting the word "not."

Comment: The diagnosis of pyloric stenosis was established prior to further study, if not clinically then certainly by sonography. The unnecessary UGI cost $203 and inflicted an active marrow radiation dose of perhaps 0.1 rad (0.001 Gy).

Discussion

Red goggles, long a radiologic mainstay until the development of image intensifiers, are now useless save possibly for staring at the superficial veins of breasts.[5] Indeed, if tinted goggles are to be worn, they probably should be yellow, to enhance depth perception.[6] Breasts were not visualized in the current study (although not for want of trying), and any potential advantage of XRG in maintaining dark-adaptation was vastly outweighed by several painful collisions with both fixed and animate objects.

The imaging ability of XRG, when judged by the limited, picayune standards of diagnostic accuracy and image quality, is admittedly abysmal. Nonetheless, this study suggests a definite role for XRG in the diagnostic imager's armamentarium. The modality is invaluable in the following common settings: (1) where radiography is not indicated but someone badly wants it anyhow; (2) where the results of radiographic study will not influence patient management; and (3) where the diagnosis has already been established by other means (i.e., "The more times you run over a dead cat, the flatter it gets."[7]).

It is recommended that every radiologist purchase XRG and modify them to his or her ocular needs. Then, when one of these settings is encountered, the radiologist should vigorously recommend to the clinician an XRG examination in lieu of whatever conventional radiation-laden and/or costly study is requested. This recommendation may be enhanced by slowly and portentiously donning the XRG, gazing solemnly about, and finally stumbling off in the general direction of the patient. Then, having performed the XRG examination, only one diagnosis need be pronounced: "*No abnormality seen.*" The advantages to the radiologist, and especially to the patient, are obvious. However, further investigation supported by substantial and tax-exempt grants is needed (and isn't it always?).

Acknowledgments

Gratitude is expressed to the unknown founder(s) of April Fool's Day; to the *AJR* editorial staff for helping commemorate it;* and to Carol A. Edwards and Marcia L. Earnshaw for their photographic assistance.

References

1. Anonymous. Catalog #5. Archie McPhee & Company, Box 30852, Seattle, WA 98103, 1987:20.

2. In other words, if X-Ray Gogs *were* previously tested, the report is buried somewhere beyond reach of the author's bibliographic search service and (one hopes) beyond reach of the reader's memory as well.

3. Yes, a feather. I know little of matters avian, but my parents did provide a childhood toy microscope, and I do know feathers. X-Ray Gog barbicels and hamuli were clearly discernible at 30X.

4. See any comprehensive medical history text. Direct citation of Dr. Roentgen might imply that I read German, or have read translations, which I don't and haven't. Give me a break.

5. Dunn FH. Red goggles and the mammographic physical examination. Radiology 1970;95:618.

6. Kinney JA, Luria SM, Schlichting CI, Neri DF. The perception of depth contours with yellow goggles. Perception 1983;12:363–366.

7. Schreiber MH. Wilson's law of diminishing returns. AJR 1982;138:786–788.

*Since 1983, *AJR* has published a humorous article in most of its April issues.—*H.B.*

Additional Readings

1. Foraker AG: The temptation of Dr. Faust. Perspect Biol Med 1970;14:473–476.

Dr. Faust loses his funding from two institutions that had accepted his grants for years: The Geltmore Foundation and The National Omphalological Institute. While he is frantically preparing a new application, he is visited by that well known subspecialist from below.

2. Fraser AG, Rees A, et al: The haggis tolerance test in Scots and Sassenachs. Br Med J 1988;297:1632–1634.

This study examined the lipemic effect of haggis, the national dish of Scotland, on two groups of subjects. Haggis is made from lamb's heart and lung, pig's liver, beef perinephric fat and oatmeal that are seasoned and boiled in a sheep's stomach. Although one probably needs to be British to actually eat haggis, the article itself is quite palatable. To quote the authors, "This study was ill conceived and badly designed, but brilliantly executed."

3. Greenberg DS: Grant Swinger's innovations. N Engl J Med 1977;297:459–460.

A dialogue with Grant Swinger, the Director of the Center for the Absorption of Federal Funds. He suggests two innovations that would improve the climate for scientific research: (1) The Fund for Dubious Projects (2) The Journal of Rejected Manuscripts.

4. Greenstein JS: Studies on a new, peerless contraceptive agent: a preliminary report. Can Med Assoc J 1965;93:1351–1355.

A new contraceptive is inadvertently discovered while the author is working to control the odor problem in his animal research lab. The agent is 100% effective and, except for increasing the libido, is totally free of side effects.

5. Iverson OH: Volvolon: a recently discovered peptide hormone from the pineal body. Can Med Assoc J 1982;126:787–790.

A new hormone is discovered that regulates body movements during sleep (Lat. volvo: I roll). A number of isomers exist which explains why people turn in both directions at night. The effect of volvolon stops after death, which puts to rest the old belief that the actions of young people make their fathers turn in their graves.

6. Kline NS: Factifuging. Lancet 1962;1:1396–1399.

This is a clever article that describes how to deflect all arguments against your findings—even in the face of overwhelming evidence. (See also, Dillon PF: Data manipulation: Dr. Factifuge meets the three stooges. Perspect Biol Med 1990;33:231–236.)

7. Lieu T, Fleisher G: The brownie study. Med Decision Making 1986;6:207.

This is a brief report about brownies—the chocolate kind, not junior girl scouts. Using doctors, nurses, and one *bottomless stomach*, the authors determined that Betty Crocker Brownie Supreme is the best tasting mix. In a follow-up letter, "Some Fudge About Brownies" (1987;7:133–134), the authors were criticized for their "half-baked" analysis.

8. Onestone AP: Further studies on the antirhabdomyelic effect of iso-2-pallallic acid. Obstet Gynecol 1956;7:361–362.

This article satirizes some of the complexities of scientific research, including the propensity for different researchers to refute each other's work.

9. Perkins RP: How to live with statistics (without having to marry them). Obstet Gynecol 1988;72:422–424.

This article is similar to the one by Roger Smith (p. 139), but the author goes in a different direction. In this case, he describes the "Chi-Line Test," "Digression Analysis," and other statistical tools.

10. Umpierre SA, Hill JA, et al: Effect of coke on sperm motility. N Engl J Med 1985;313:1351.

The authors compared the spermacidal effects of four different types of Coca-Cola. Diet Coke was best, but in comparing New to Classic Coke, the authors found that Classic Coke "is it."

11. Warburton FE: The lab coat as a status symbol. Science 1960;131:895.

This article provides some insight into the evolution of the scientist's lab coat: "When work is unavoidable, he will be found in his shirt sleeves, in a coarse brown smock, or in plastic. His lab coat, clean, pressed, possibly even starched, hangs safely behind the door, to be worn only when he is lecturing or greeting official visitors."

12. Weiss RA: Dorian Gray mice. Nature 1993;362: 411.

This article appeared in the April 1 issue of a usually sedate journal. The author describes the genetic engineering of mice that do not age.

13. Yankelowitz BY: How to create a data base. BMJ 1979;2:596.

As an international authority in umbilical research, the author uses his own example to show how, by following a few simple rules, you can turn out 2000 or more studies in your own chosen field.

———✦———

Mr. Chase was having terrible headaches, so he called his doctor for an appointment.

"I can squeeze you in next week," the receptionist said.

"Next week? Lady, I could be dead by then."

"In that case," she said, "please have someone call and cancel the appointment."

THE DOCTOR AT WORK

There are a number of safeguards built into medical practice that are designed to prevent boredom. Besides having to deal with lab personnel, answering services, hospital administrators, and upset families (our patients'), we also have to contend with specialists, partners, busy schedules, and upset families (our own). With so much to do, it's a wonder more of us don't quit and go into law.

Although I did not actively look for jokes during my research, I did run into a number of funny ones along the way. Therefore, to kick off the chapter, I am including the following joke from Patricia Thomas' article, "The Anatomy of Coping: Medicine's Funny Bone" (see Appendix).

A doctor dies and goes to heaven, where he finds a long line at St. Peter's gate. As is his custom, the doctor rushes to the front, but St. Peter tells him to go wait in line like everyone else. Muttering and looking at his watch, the doctor stands at the end of the line.

Moments later, a white-haired man wearing a white coat and carrying a stethoscope and black bag rushes to the front of the line, waves to St. Peter, and is immediately admitted through the pearly gates.

"Hey!" the doctor says angrily. "How come you let him through without waiting?"

"Oh," says St. Peter, "that's God. Sometimes he likes to play doctor."

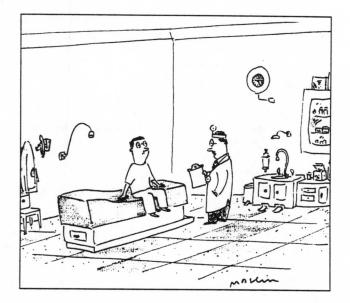

"You'll be coughing up big bucks for quite some time, Mr. Vanihorn. Don't be alarmed—it's perfectly normal."

READERS OF THE LOST CHART

AN ARCHAEOLOGIC APPROACH
TO THE MEDICAL RECORD*

Frederick L. Brancati, M.D.

The first 2 years of medical school are spent in class memorizing biochemical details such as the Krebs cycle, visualizing the anatomy of the pterygopalatine fossa and making up lewd mnemonics for the cranial nerves—facts that instructors insist will be crucial to becoming a successful clinician. Why, then, once finally arriving on the wards, do students feel as clueless and misinformed as Dan Quayle at a cabinet meeting?

Think. While students perform excruciatingly complete histories and physical exams and continuously review pocket notes on inborn errors of metabolism, the resident is focused on the ever-expanding document of patient knowledge—the medical record.

The medical record is regarded as an object of awe, much as historians revere the Dead Sea Scrolls or Harvard graduates worship their diplomas. Although it contains the distilled wisdom of past physicians and the resulting truths of prior studies, these revelations are obscured by strange idioms and are buried in an avalanche of bureaucratic landfill. Like Indiana Jones, the astute physician must take an archaeologic approach to becoming a reader of the lost chart.

The Nursing Note. Exploration of nursing notes is risky. They have the potential to contain buried clinical treasures—perhaps the first mention of delirium or a critical summary of important psychosocial

*Reprinted from JAMA © 1992;267:1860–1861, with permission from the American Medical Association. Edited from the original. Drawing by Michael Maslin; ©1993 The New Yorker Magazine, Inc.

factors. On the other hand, they may contain no data at all. An "alteration in comfort" may signify anything from nasal congestion to a ruptured aortic aneurysm. An "alteration in bowel habits," although more specific, is hardly news in a hospitalized patient. Especially worrisome, however, is a flat-line flow sheet, in which the same values (most commonly respiration 20, pulse 80, blood pressure 120/80 mm Hg, and temperature 37°C) are recorded for 3 consecutive days. The status of patients during the flat-line interval is uncertain; they may be gravely ill, dead, or vacationing in the Caribbean.

Adventitious Markings. Food stains related to note writing in the hospital cafeteria are easily identified by color and aroma. A clear stain is pathognomonic for the drool of an exhausted intern who has fallen asleep while writing. The finding of a long, straight pen line trailing off the side of the page confirms the impression of sudden somnolence. Such markings often precede a collection of medical mumbo-jumbo that reflects neuronal activity emitted solely from deep in the midbrain and should prompt skepticism of the chart's reliability.

The Surgical Note. The beauty of the surgical note is its simplicity. For example: "Post-op day #2, afebrile, vital signs stable, exam unchanged, continue post-op care." It's refreshingly clear, free of the detail, insight, and deliberation that so often mars the notes of internists. Do not, however, underestimate the significance of even small deviations in the content of the note from day to day. For example: "Post-op #3, temp 37.5, vital signs now stable, exam improved, continue current management" means that the previous night, the patient developed septic shock, was pancultured and started on a third-generation cephalosporin, and will possibly require transfer to the surgical intensive care unit later in the morning.

The Consultant Note. To the untrained eye, this note appears to be divine scripture written with the authority born of specialization. Textual analysis, however, reveals that it is actually the work of several all-too-human authors writing at different times. The "M Source," or medical student, composes the bulk of the treatise, usually one and a half pages of transcribed text that avoids providing any opinion or recommendation. The "R Source," or resident, generally edits the work of the M Source and provides commentary. The written tone of the R Source is one of righteous indignation, heaping judgments on medical student, patient, and referring physician alike.

Squeezed on the bottom edge of the second page are the cryptic markings of the "A Source" or attending physician. The A Source is best recognized by its constant repetition of two phrases: "Agree with above plan" and "Will follow with you." Since neither the M nor the R Source ever really describes a plan of action, and since it is unusual for the A Source to inscribe even one follow-up note, experts believe that these phrases are to be understood in purely mystical terms.

The Medical Student Note. Warning: these notes are dangerous. Many physicians have been missing for hours or even days sifting through the seething miasma of verbiage spewed out by earnest medical students. Moreover, because of their prodigious length, these notes are hard to avoid. Scientists estimate that medical student notes account for more than 60% of the chart's weight. Fortunately, several features make medical student notes easily recognizable: (1) compulsively neat penmanship, (2) unusual ink colors (including the popular lavender and green), (3) diagrams of family pedigree so extensive as to include deceased in-laws and close childhood friends, (4) stencils of neck and abdominal anatomy, and (5) liberal use of stick figures. These notes should be explored only by teams of experienced, well-rested professionals in brightly lit rooms using modern excavating equipment.

FORMPHOBIA *

To the Editor.—We report the first case of formphobia. The index patient, a physician, was cared for in our offices recently. He appeared to be mumbling numbers: "414.0, 715.9, 162.9, 250.0, or what is 250.4 (see also 581.81)?" After a consent form had been signed, a cup of hot tea was administered orally and a cool compress was placed on the physician-patient's forehead. When he was calm and rational, his history was obtained.

He was a 52-year-old internist who graduated from medical school in 1963, completed an approved internship and residency in internal medicine, and served in the military; he had been in private practice (with a university affiliation) since 1969. He was board certified in internal medicine and in a subspecialty. Sensitive to his patient's needs, he always filled out insurance forms carefully and promptly to ensure payment and reimbursement. Despite the profusion and confusion of the forms, whether from Blue Cross/Blue Shield, Group Health Insurance, Medicare, or one of the many health maintenance organizations, he had mastered them all. He had memorized procedure codes for Medicare. Now, with the new requirements for *International Classification of Diseases—Ninth Revision—CM* codes instead of narrative diagnoses, he had spent the first 3 months of the calendar year poring over the two large volumes that embrace the proper numbers. On April 1 he was ready; however, as he bent to fill out his first Medicare form his eyes glazed, his hand started to shake uncontrollably, and he began to recite code numbers as if they were his mantra. Always self-aware, he now sought immediate help: he received none.

We call this syndrome *formphobia*. We recognize that this coinage is etymologically inept, constructed of a Latin prefix and a Greek suffix, but it has the advantage of euphony. We believe that many cases of this syndrome will be seen as soon as physicians fail to fill out the forms with facility. There is no known treatment.

The syndrome should have an *International Classification of Diseases—Ninth Revision—CM* code; we propose 300.29.

#079-30-1199[†]
#130-28-40789[†]
Bronx, NY

A doctor made a brief house call to one of his patients. As he left the house, he told the man's wife, "There's nothing wrong with your husband. He just thinks he's sick."

A few days later, the doctor stopped by to see how his patient was doing.

"How's you husband today?" the doctor said.

"He's worse," said the wife. "Now he thinks he's dead."

*Reprinted from JAMA © 1989; 262:500, with permission from the American Medical Association.
[†]Formerly Leonard G. Dauber, MD, and Gerald M. Fleischner, MD.

PERMISSION FORMS MAY BE HAZARDOUS TO YOUR HEALTH*

Howard J. Bennett, M.D.

I was sitting in my office the other day, minding my own business, when one of my nurses came in with a pained expression on her face. As she approached my desk, I put down my tunafish sandwich and braced myself for the worst.

"It's the Bluebird Nursery School," she said. "They need a note authorizing them to give Tylenol to Daniel Krauss in case he hurts himself at school."

"Didn't we send that last week?"

"No, last week you gave permission to use sunscreen if Daniel went outside on a day with less than 50% cloud cover."

"Isn't Tylenol included on our form allowing them to take children outside where they can get poison ivy, tick bites, or fall down a hundred times a day?"

"No, I'm afraid the Outdoor Activities Form doesn't cover medication."

"What about our Standard School Form?"

"Sorry, it doesn't include medications either. It simply gives the nursery school permission to feed the children, wash their hands, take them to the bathroom, read them books, and let them play with the school's pet hamsters and baby chicks. It also contains a rider letting the teachers explain where babies come from, in case anyone is curious enough to ask. Of course, the form also stipulates that parents must promise not to sue if their children embarrass them in the future."

"What about our Emergency Authorization Form? Certainly that covers Tylenol."

"I wish it did. Unfortunately, I just read it, and it only gives the teachers permission to perform cutdowns, intubations, and arterial line placements in children over 12 months of age. Since the students all know CPR and the Heimlich maneuver by now, the teachers don't need authorization for those procedures."

"I'm almost afraid to ask, but don't we have a Medication Form?"

"Actually we do, but it only covers prescription items. Your attorney said it would be better if you had a separate Nonprescription Medication Form since he's not sure you can authorize giving over-the-counter medicine in the first place."

At this point, I was beginning to tremble and wondered why I had not listened to my parents and gone into neurosurgery like they suggested. Fortunately, my intrepid RN had already dashed off a nonprescription form, filled in the blanks, and stuck it in front of me for my John Hancock.

After I signed the form, I returned to my tuna sandwich, which now looked soggy and limp and was no longer fit for human consumption. However, no sooner had I taken a bite of my apple than I was jolted upright by the office intercom.

"Dr. B., it's Bluebird on line 8. They want to know if it's OK to change Rachel Cama's diaper?"

There are two kinds of adhesive tape: that which won't stay on and that which won't come off.

Maria Telesco

*Reprinted with permission from Contemporary Pediatrics © 1993; 10(2):135–136. Edited from the original.

WHAT IF MEDICAL ADS READ LIKE THE PERSONALS?*

Howard J. Bennett, M.D.

Anyone who's ever had to replace a nurse on short notice or fill a residency position in August knows how tough it can be to attract medical staff through the classifieds. But long hours and low pay notwithstanding, one of the obvious problems with medical ads is that they are so boring. Just think what an improvement it would be if we borrowed the language and style used by singles in search of a mate.

DIVORCED FAMILY PHYSICIAN—45, into double booking, working through lunch, and late nights at the office. Seeking residency graduate to join lucrative practice. Kill yourself for a few years and perhaps you'll make partner. Send CV and recent stress test to Box 438.

CLINICAL RESEARCHER—43, seeks position as Director of Research at a prestigious medical center. I enjoy creative statistics, large-scale, multicenter trials that bring big bucks to the university, and multiple authorship (the more names on a paper the better). Also, any rumors you've heard about me related to ethical misconduct are totally untrue. Box 711.

CHRONIC CARE HOSPITAL—138 (beds), is looking for an RN, age 22 to 82, who likes bedpans, foleys, NG tubes, and central lines, for long-term relationship. Box 802.

PRACTICE FOR SALE—Solo practice located in remote wilderness setting. Rugged townsfolk rarely get sick, though you will need to attend to livestock on occasion. Only 1200 miles from a major city, and no lawyers in the area. Box 892.

LET'S MAKE A DEAL—Suburban HMO is seeking a physician who is secure, sensitive, and saucy to join its network of primary care centers. Are you ready for excitement (overbooked schedules), travel (between our six clinics), adventure (taking call three times a week), good food (5-minute lunches), witty conversation (nitpicking over cost containment) and traditional values (no profit sharing)? If so, reply with photo and note to Box 891.

TEACH A LITTLE/PRACTICE A LITTLE—This is the position you all talk about during your residency interviews. University Dept. seeks primary care physician who is into research, teaching, and more. Must be turned on by the thought of going to endless meetings, serving on countless committees, lecturing to comatose students at 7:30 AM, and padding your CV. Box 141.

IS NIGHT CALL A DRAG?—If so, why not try this new, elegant answering service. Our operators are into accurate spelling, reciting numbers in the proper sequence, and following your instructions to the letter. We promise no 2 AM calls for someone else's patients, and we'll always wake you with a smile. Box 123.

ARE YOU CHIEF RESIDENT MATERIAL?—Residency Director, 78, is seeking that special someone who will tread where others fear to go. Are you into making schedules, revising schedules, and arguing over schedules? Are you ready to share life's adventures with bleary-eyed residents who will complain about everything from too much night call to having to work with outdated PMDs? If so, this could be a match made in HEAVEN! Box 666.

LOOKING FOR DR. RIGHT—Here's the scenario: We're a big, sprawling teaching hospital in a seedy part of town. We haven't matched in three years and our Physician-in-Chief just quit to go to law school. Are you an academic doc who is ready to deal with motivational atrophy, turf battles, cost overruns, sneering, pimping, and an occasional food fight? If so, this could be the chance of a lifetime. Send CV and three references (preferably in English) to Box 489.

WE KNOW YOU'RE OUT THERE—Busy group practice seeks an RN who enjoys telephones that never stop ringing, doctors that never stop running, and babies that never stop peeing. If this sounds like fun (and it is), send note and photo to Box 327.

CLIA? PHOOEY!!—Are you a savvy MD who is tired of regulations telling you how you can and cannot practice medicine? Would you like to qualify for a Level 1 or Level 2 lab in the blink of an eye? Well, for a limited time only, pathology residencies are available through a two-week mail order program sponsored by The University of Hubris School of Medicine. Send your application and $500 to Box 903.

*Reprinted from The Journal of Family Practice, 1992; 35:216, with permission from Appleton & Lange, Inc.

WHAT IF DOCTORS ADVERTISED?*

Howard J. Bennett, M.D.

Here's what the Yellow Pages may look like if the squeeze on health-care dollars continues and doctors have to work a little harder to attract patients

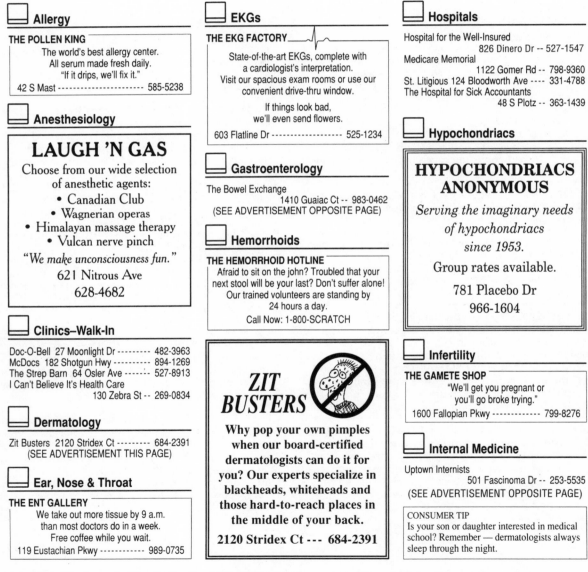

Allergy

THE POLLEN KING
The world's best allergy center.
All serum made fresh daily.
"If it drips, we'll fix it."
42 S Mast ---------------------- 585-5238

Anesthesiology

LAUGH 'N GAS
Choose from our wide selection
of anesthetic agents:
- Canadian Club
- Wagnerian operas
- Himalayan massage therapy
- Vulcan nerve pinch

"We make unconsciousness fun."
621 Nitrous Ave
628-4682

Clinics–Walk-In

Doc-O-Bell 27 Moonlight Dr --------- 482-3963
McDocs 182 Shotgun Hwy ---------- 894-1269
The Strep Barn 64 Osler Ave ------- 527-8913
I Can't Believe It's Health Care
130 Zebra St -- 269-0834

Dermatology

Zit Busters 2120 Stridex Ct --------- 684-2391
(SEE ADVERTISEMENT THIS PAGE)

Ear, Nose & Throat

THE ENT GALLERY
We take out more tissue by 9 a.m.
than most doctors do in a week.
Free coffee while you wait.
119 Eustachian Pkwy ----------- 989-0735

EKGs

THE EKG FACTORY
State-of-the-art EKGs, complete with
a cardiologist's interpretation.
Visit our spacious exam rooms or use our
convenient drive-thru window.

If things look bad,
we'll even send flowers.
603 Flatline Dr ------------------ 525-1234

Gastroenterology

The Bowel Exchange
1410 Guaiac Ct -- 983-0462
(SEE ADVERTISEMENT OPPOSITE PAGE)

Hemorrhoids

THE HEMORRHOID HOTLINE
Afraid to sit on the john? Troubled that your
next stool will be your last? Don't suffer alone!
Our trained volunteers are standing by
24 hours a day.
Call Now: 1-800-SCRATCH

ZIT BUSTERS
**Why pop your own pimples
when our board-certified
dermatologists can do it for
you? Our experts specialize in
blackheads, whiteheads and
those hard-to-reach places in
the middle of your back.**

2120 Stridex Ct --- 684-2391

Hospitals

Hospital for the Well-Insured
826 Dinero Dr -- 527-1547
Medicare Memorial
1122 Gomer Rd -- 798-9360
St. Litigious 124 Bloodworth Ave ---- 331-4788
The Hospital for Sick Accountants
48 S Plotz -- 363-1439

Hypochondriacs

HYPOCHONDRIACS ANONYMOUS

*Serving the imaginary needs
of hypochondriacs
since 1953.*

Group rates available.

781 Placebo Dr
966-1604

Infertility

THE GAMETE SHOP
"We'll get you pregnant or
you'll go broke trying."
1600 Fallopian Pkwy ------------- 799-8276

Internal Medicine

Uptown Internists
501 Fascinoma Dr -- 253-5535
(SEE ADVERTISEMENT OPPOSITE PAGE)

CONSUMER TIP
Is your son or daughter interested in medical
school? Remember — dermatologists always
sleep through the night.

*Reprinted from The Journal of Family Practice, 1994; 39:89–90, with permission from Appleton & Lange, Inc.

THE TROUBLE WITH TREATING YOUR RELATIVES*

Ralph T. Streeter, M.D.

You probably owe your relatives a lot for the way they helped you get started in practice. But do you owe them the care of their pets and other oddities?

Every movie fan knows that a small boy with an injured puppy is every young doctor's first patient. Every experienced physician knows that this boy is a relative of the young doctor he goes to. And in *my* experience, the aunt who sent her boy and his dog over to me thought treatment of an injured paw was about the limit of my ability.

Doting aunts are quick to spread the word of your skill as a physician. But they themselves won't follow your advice, even if you simply suggest that they take two aspirins for a headache.

While still in medical school, I was often asked my medical opinion by members of the family. I realized that this was in the nature of chaffing a young fellow who had graduated from high school eight years ago and had yet to earn his first dollar. It was later, while I was serving my internship, that I became seriously initiated into that vast subspecialty of every doctor: *relative* practice.

Father-in-Law's Rx

My father-in-law developed a mild case of conjunctivitis during the course of a week-end visit to my home. I was delighted to be of some help to him. I presented myself at the corner drugstore, borrowed a prescription pad, and wrote a beautiful prescription for benzalkonium chloride (refined) 1:5,000 in normal saline with gtt i epinephrine hydrochloride 1:1,000 to the ounce.

My father-in-law thanked me. My mother-in-law thanked me. But after they left, I found the unopened bottle on the top shelf of a bookcase.

A few days later, my mother-in-law phoned.

"We're so proud of you," she said. "The Lincoln Life nurse said it was conjunctivitis, just as you did. She gave Walter some eye drops, and they're clearing his eyes nicely."

There's no way to avoid this segment of practice. Even if, you're an orphan, there are always plenty of friends to fill your kinless vacuum.

I don't mean casual acquaintances, whose questions can usually be stopped by suggesting an appointment. The friends I speak of are those old and dear ones who consider themselves part of the family.

All such friends and relatives can be divided into three categories. There are the ones with pets, the ones with absurd ailments, and the ones who belong to *other* physicians. (As a matter of fact, *all* of them are regular patients of other doctors. But we'll go into that later.)

To begin with, let's look at category #1:

Their Pets Are Sick

There was the friend who called me at 2 AM one winter morning to assist in the delivery of a litter of pups. A week before, the dog had defecated in the room we call my study. This apparently gave my friend the idea that he ought to call *me* rather than disturb the veterinarian.

That tops anything my relatives have ever done. In fact, it tops anything I've ever heard, except for the colleague who was called out of a staff meeting to prescribe an abortifacient for a neighbor's cat. At least *I* wasn't asked to do anything questionable.

Relatives with pets have to be handled with just as much tact as the old maid in your private prac-

*Reprinted with permission from Medical Economics, © 1957;34 (Dec):141–147; Medical Economics Company, Inc., Oradell, N.J. 07649.

tice with a positive serology. A faltering diagnosis on a helpless animal can ruin you.

I almost lost an old and trusted friend when I failed to recognize an advanced case of Bumblefoot in an owl he'd acquired. It's doubtful if his wife's obstetrician would have recognized it either. Still, I came off better than another of his M.D. friends who prescribed streptomycin for the owl. As soon as the needle was withdrawn, the bird fell over dead.

It took a lot of persuasion and the better part of a bottle of brandy to re-establish my friend's faith in medicine. He seriously questioned whether doctors who couldn't treat an owl were any better equipped to treat humans.

It's just such a challenge that made a competent orthopedist of my acquaintance put a modification of a Peterson nail in a parrot's femur. Or that pushed a certain psychiatrist into an attempt to resolve the frank homosexuality of a French poodle. Or that caused a full professor of pathology whom I know to section a piece of steak, in order to convince his mother that the butcher wasn't selling horse meat.

The Queer-Ailment Ones

Category #2 consists of relations who ask you to treat vague complaints of bizarre etiology, without recognizable pathology. These ailments, you've probably noticed, occur only on those portions of the body that can be shown without taking off anything (except, rarely, a shoe). And the suffering relative always points out that the problem is too trifling to bother his regular doctor—the difference between you and a "regular doctor" being that he sends a statement.

You Know the Type

I have a light-headed second cousin with recurring ganglia on her wrist. With each occurrence, she admits that the lump appears only when she wears her wrist watch. My recurring answer is that the cause might be pressure from the band. She smiles vaguely and says something like: "It's a very good watch, Ralph dear." And so she goes on thinking of me as Betsy's boy, the one who took so long to get through school.

There is in every family a brother-in-law with athlete's foot. My brother-in-law's last athletic experience was touch football at Yale ten years ago; but his dermatomycosis pedis is refractory to all the sample medications that pile up in the mailbox. Every time I see him, he says: "I've still got that itch on the bottom of my foot."

He says it in an injured way. He's indicating that a better, more responsible doctor would have cleared it up by now.

The easy way out would be to suggest that such individuals see their own physician. But only a narrow, begrudging doctor would refuse a few words of advice to an uncle or an old friend—especially if he's a hydraulics engineer and only last week advised you on the best way to drain your new patio. The main difference is that *you* followed *his* advice.

Cured—by Someone Else

Some of these relative ills can be helped, of course—but never by you.

The tic in my older brother's left eye failed to respond to all the ophthalmology, psychiatry, and neurology I knew. But it has been completely cured at the neighborhood health bar with a daily pint of carrot juice and eight ounces of sunflower seeds. Naturally, he tells me about it every chance he gets.

Our cook acts the same way. Long ago, I urged treatment for her goiter, and I made appointments for her with qualified men. She didn't keep them, but the goiter disappeared. She says a practitioner of black magic conjured it away by laying on the hand of a recently demised seventh son of a seventh son.

The only person in our household who doesn't chuckle when she tells the story is me.

They Have Other Doctors

Finally, we come to category #3: the friends and relatives who are already being treated by their own physicians. If you can handle them, you're probably qualified to get Hungary back from Khrushchev. They present their signs and symptoms in detail, and all they want is for you to tell them what the doctor's doing wrong.

Naturally, you take a firm stand. "I think yours is a very interesting case, and Dr. Blank is doing exactly the right thing," you say firmly.

But this doesn't help, since everybody's aware of medical ethics. "But what do you *really* think?" asks the persistent sister-in-law (females outnumber males about four to one on this). "Don't you think it's taking too long to get results? Don't all those X-rays show that Dr. Blank doesn't know what's wrong?"

You repeat your first statement with increased firmness. The following day, she calls your wife and asks *her* opinion of your opinion. She explains that the serious expression on your face the evening before suggested that hers is a far advanced and hopeless case. (A smile, however, would have convinced her that Dr. Blank is an utter incompetent. And on her next appointment she'd probably have implied as much to him.)

'Check Me, Daddy'

In the relative practice of medicine, nobody can cause you more self-doubt, nobody can frustrate and harass you more, than your own wife and children. The only time the married physician really envies his bachelor colleagues is when he's nursing a bruised ego as the result of making an effort to play the role of family doctor (as opposed to doctor in the family).

My 4-year-old son has never awakened me at dawn with a cheery "Good morning," as I'm told lawyers' children do. Mine comes stumbling in with the demand: "Check me, Daddy." Only a hand on his forehead, with assurance that he's in excellent health, gives him the strength to continue through the day.

So far he's too young to doubt my word. But he'll learn. The doctor's immediate family are never silly enough to believe Daddy really knows medicine.

During my senior obstetrical clerkship days, I expressed the opinion that my wife and I were shortly to become parents of twins. She expressed the opinion that I needed more practice on the maneuvers of Leopold. Six weeks later the obstetrician and X-ray confirmed my diagnosis. She was as surprised as if she were hearing it for the first time.

Doctor's Best Friend

Occasionally, though, you *will* find gratitude in the immediate family. One of the most grateful patients I've ever had was our dog, Genevieve. During my residency, she kept giving birth to litters of tremendous size and variety. All canine preventive measures failed; so we decided to make a permanent change. Since the veterinarian's fee was almost the same as my monthly salary, my wife took the familiar attitude that anyone who can treat people can certainly treat cocker spaniels.

A fellow gynecology resident, an anesthesia resident, and I planned the operative procedure. We were a little handicapped because none of us could read German, and the only appropriate book in the medical library was entitled "Der Hund." But all things considered, the operation went very well.

During the immediate postoperative period, I carefully examined the incision and probed the abdomen morning and night. That was four years ago. For four years now, every time I come home Genevieve lolls foolishly on her back with all four legs extended. I say, "Nice incision, Genny." And she gets up and romps gratefully away.

I should like something of the same brand of respect from my children. But their mother is teaching *them* to be brighter than Genevieve.

And now I see my nephew and his dog coming up the walk. Browny has the mange. I must get back to my subspecialty again. How's it with yours?

YOUR MOST MYSTERIOUS COLLEAGUE*

Theodore Kamholtz, M.D.

You've never met him, yet you hear about him all the time. He's the least rational, most inscrutable physician you know of.

He's your patient's Former Doctor.

Let's say you're taking a history on a new patient. She's fair, fat, and forty. She has cholelithiasis. She sticks to a diet ninety-nine days out of a hundred. Every hundredth day, she just can't resist potato pancakes with gravy, and she's rewarded with a 3 AM seizure of biliary colic.

So far, no surprises. But suddenly the cogs slip. "My former physician"—says the patient—"gave me some medicine and then massaged the stone right out."

"Massaged?" you asked warily.

"Oh, yes." And she shows you some calculi removed in just that way. As a matter of fact, the Former Doctor had a way with renal calculi, too. He had a medicine that dissolved them.

One characteristic, then, of the Former Doctor is that his medicine appears to be entirely different from yours. It's not that he's a charlatan. It's just that a few details get garbled when the patient relays them from doctor to doctor.

You recall one of your own patients who thanked you profusely for curing his cough and palpitations during fluoroscopy. That form of therapy really impressed him. You shudder to think how it will sound when he describes it to the next doctor who sees him.

Meanwhile, you still have a sneaking suspicion that your colleague's psychotherapy is more flamboyant than yours. This is particularly true after a patient tells you that his previous physician uses gold and silver hypodermic needles.

Another thing that impresses you about the Former Doctor is that he has a pharmacopoeia substantially different from yours. One day, a patient asks if the medication his last doctor prescribed could cause numbness in the ears. You've never head of the drug in question, so you look it up. Two hours in the medical library produce only one small reference to it—and that in an untranslated Swedish journal published more than twenty years ago.

Shot Therapy

Another patient wants an injection of the stuff his former physician gave him. It cured his psoriasis overnight. He went to bed in misery and awoke the next morning unblemished. The scales are beginning to come back now, and . . .

Sometimes you wish that his Former Doctor would just hang onto his patients. (It probably comes to you as a second thought that he wishes the same thing.)

A woman with a kidney condition tells you her previous physician put her on a diet of almond, celery, potatoes, and apricot brandy. Should she continue it? You can't detect one iota of logic in it. Yet can you unhesitatingly condemn? After all, they laughed at Pasteur . . .

You suggest that she return to the other fellow for management of her case. But she can't. She never paid his bills.

Most of the time, you're grateful that you don't actually know your predecessor on the case. Occasionally, however, you do get to know him. Then you discover that the irrational Former Doctor doesn't really exist.

"I saw a patient of yours the other day—Egbert Blank," you may say to your colleague in the hospital staff room. Then you add hesitantly:"He says you cured his tuberculosis with shoe supports."

Your colleague laughs. Then he tells the story:

*Reprinted with permission from Medical Economics, © 1958;35 (Apr 14):122–128; Medical Economics Company, Inc., Oradell, N.J. 07649.

Egbert had been coming home tired and aching all over. Even his feet had hurt him. When his great aunt died of tuberculosis, he became convinced he had it, too. He began to lose weight and to have night sweats. No amount of X-rays, examinations, or assurances helped.

Your colleague found a local foot condition, prescribed supports, and told him that as long as he was going to die of tuberculosis (which the patient believed and the doctor doubted), he might as well die with happy feet.

"I gather it worked," your colleague says. "What's his trouble now?"

"Nothing much," you reply. "Just syphilophobia."

For each case handled by the mysterious Former Doctor that finally is clarified, a dozen cases remain tantalizingly unbelievable. His office, seen through your patients' eyes, varies from alchemist shop to temple; his prescriptions are incantations.

They'll Talk About You

But, aware of your own patient's misunderstandings, you hesitate to criticize, no matter how wild the story. After all, a patient of yours may tell *his* next doctor that his wife's menses became regular after *he* took a tonic—forgetting all about the intensive course of estrogen therapy she was given. If so, your only hope is that he also forgets your name.

Top Ten Reasons to Work for an HMO*

10. You've always wondered what it would be like to see 80 patients a day.
 9. The thought of running streptokinase drips at home sounds like fun.
 8. Your accountant thinks you should be in a lower tax bracket.
 7. You get a free tote bag with the plan's logo on it.
 6. It's a good transition job before you make the jump to professional wrestling.
 5. You can star in a TV commercial.
 4. It gives you something to brag about at college reunions.
 3. It's a challenge to manage patients without any lab work.
 2. Big bonuses are earned for reusing tongue depressors.
 1. Lawyers rarely belong to HMOs.

*Reprinted from The Journal of Family Practice © 1996;43:110, with permission from Appleton & Lange, Inc.

SHORT COURSE IN EUPHEMISM*

Philip A. Kilbourne, M.D.

After a few years of practice, most of us get pretty slick at interpreting "patientese." We soon learn, for example, that "Spare no expense" or "Money is no object" can mean "I have no intention of paying you anyway."

All well and good. But how about the other side of the coin? The list that follows is a mere neophyte's armamentarium of some reliable clichés of consulting-room technique. The column on the left represents the actual spoken words; the column on the right, the thought behind them.

If some of you younger men in the front row still haven't caught the knack of it, maybe you'd better see me after class for further coaching. But perhaps it will help if you simply keep this point in mind: Your diploma only starts you in practice; it's your diplomacy that keeps you there.

When you say:	You may mean:
"Just get this prescription filled and come back in about two days."	"Darned if I know what you've got. I'll need a couple of days to read up on the symptoms."
"Who's your regular physician?"	"How many doctors did you shop before you got down to me?"
"When a child like yours presents a behavior problem, it often helps to look for environmental causes."	"There's nothing wrong with your kid that a new set of parents wouldn't cure."
"Let me just check the current cost of this drug."	"I'm looking up the dose in the PDR."
"I'm sure that if Dr. Smith had not been so terribly overworked he'd have arrived at the same diagnosis as I did."	"That cloth-head couldn't diagnose his way out of a wet paper bag."
"Yes, you went to the only man in the country who could have performed that operation."	"Old Krankheit's the only man in the country who still *does* that operation."
"I happen to have limited stock of that drug right here, so we can get you started on it now."	"The detail man just left."
"Your baby certainly looks like his father."	"No teeth, no hair, and the same pot belly."

*Reprinted with permission from Medical Economics, © 1963; 40(Feb 25):90–91; Medical Ecomonics Company, Inc., Oradell, N.J. 07649.

THE INDEX OF ARRIVAL*

Theodore Kamholtz, M.D.

In medicine, doctors start at the bottom of the ladder and climb up rung by tedious rung. The pursuit of the apex is so demanding that they rarely survey their position. Will you get the appropriate signal once you've reached the top? Or will you overshoot your mark like the comic hero in a cartoon movie? Perhaps you should take stock of your position and determine your own index of arrival.

There is a little old lady who can tell when you've arrived. She works behind the counter in the hospital cafeteria. She looks gossamer frail, but has the soul of a meat grinder. When you first enter the hospital, she serves your soup half in the bowl and half on the tray. One day when you order chicken salad, she indicates that she recognizes you. She knows you are up and coming so she gives you sliced corned beef instead. But when you reach the top, she no longer tries to please you but to do good by you. She casts an appraising look at your belt size, ladles out a 32 calorie portion of cottage cheese and says, "Here you are, Curly." You've arrived!

The elevator operator is an expert at rating the status of doctors. When you first come to the hospital, your capital epiphyses have just fused. He takes one look at you and says, "Where's your pass, Sonny?" He begins to think you're a regular guy when he lets you see the photograph of him kissing a starlet good-bye after her 12th suicide attempt. You're promoted when he starts to plumb your professional judgment. "Say Doc, are you going to operate on the guy in Three North whose wife tried to knit him to death?" But when he stops the elevator between floors to show you the largest scrotal hernia in the hospital—You've arrived!

The x-ray technician has a keen sense about the relative status of doctors. If he takes your requisition slip, asks blandly what idiot filled that out, and tosses it in the waste basket—you are gauche. When he acquiesces to your request for taking the skull and foot on the same film, he believes you are headed in the right direction. But when he tells you the radiologist has read the GI series as negative, but that if he were you he'd look twice at that ulcer niche high on the lesser curvature—You've arrived!

The operating room squad has great facility in recognizing which side of the bread is buttered. When you first arrive you not only get little time in the O.R., but are also assigned scrub nurses with PMS and interns who have lost the toss of the coin. As your prestige mounts, they give you 15 minutes prime time, the chief resident, and all the instruments you need. But when you've been working all morning over a hot belly and the circulating nurse goes out of her way to scratch your back and give you a soggy paper cup filled with hot, undrinkable coffee—You've arrived!

Hospital administrators indicate the status of doctors by the quality of their introductions. At your first staff meeting, he introduces you as Dr. David Clown when your name is really Dr. Robert Brown. You have moved up a notch when he introduces you to the ladies auxiliary as Dr. Brown, our eminent neurosurgeon, even though you're board certified in hematology. But when he introduces you at an annual dinner as "Dr. Robert Brown, a man who needs no introduction" and then launches into a 15 minute one—You've arrived!

In the final analysis, however, it is your colleagues who determine your true status as a doctor. If they refer you patients who live out of town and require home visits at night, your meteor has not yet left the ground. If they refer only their headache patients, but at least the ones who will pay, your star is in its ascendancy. If they refer all their cases to you, the dull and the interesting, the penniless and the wealthy, your star is bright. But if they refer only relatives (not the paying kind) they are indicating that you possess not only the highest medical skill, but the highest ethical standards as well—You've arrived!

*Reprinted from JAMA, © 1963; 186(6):A206–207, with permission from the American Medical Association. Edited from the original.

Additional Readings

1. Bennett HJ: How to keep your practice in the pink. Postgrad Med 1992;92(3):49–52.

In order to stay competitive in the future, the author provides a number of interesting suggestions. For example, "Schedule only one patient per hour, post your home phone number in the waiting room, and offer to baby-sit for patients on weekends."

2. Bluestone N: Professional courtesy. New Physician 1979;28(11):6,26,28.

After the author refers her mother to a group of colleagues for a minor ailment, a lively bit of correspondence ensues regarding the etiquette of professional courtesy.

3. Cohn A: See this tic? I owe it to "Alternative Therapists." Med Economics 1988;65(Nov 21):205–214.

In this amusing satire, the author relates some of his experiences with chiropractors, homeopathists, foot reflexologists and other practitioners from the opposite side of the tracks. Dr. Cohn also writes under the pseudonym Oscar London (see below).

4. DePaolis M: Festive answers to holiday medical questions. Postgrad Med 1991;90(7):18–20.

While it's relatively safe to go to hardware stores, at parties you're never more than an hors d'oeuvre away from a free consultation. According to the author, primary care docs get bugged more than specialists. For example, could you imagine someone going up to a gastroenterologist and saying, "Hey doc, I think I'm having a little ascending cholangitis. Could you take a look?"

5. Egerton JR: Please get my patient off the referral merry-go-round. Med Economics 1983;60(Nov 14):313–315.

This article pokes fun at the way specialists refer patients to each other without consulting a patient's primary care physician.

6. Felson B: My most unforgettable patient. Seminar Roentgen 1976;11:77–79.

A radiologist tells the story of how he ended up x-raying a cow in his hospital. Getting the films done was a little tricky, and the cow retaliated with some emissions of her own.

7. Greengold M: I'm 100% publicly owned! Med Economics 1964;45(May 18):94–99.

This is an amusing story about a doctor who incorporated his practice and then "went public" by selling shares of himself to his patients.

8. Guttman D: Things they never warned me about in medical school. Med Economics 1985;62(Dec 23):59.

In this brief article, the author presents 15 bits of wisdom he has learned as a practicing pediatrician. For example, "Never trust a naked baby," and "The only way to keep a child from ingesting a drug is to prescribe it for him."

9. Lettau LA: From the Centers for Fatigue Control (CFC) weekly report. Ann Intern Med 1991;114:602.

In this mock report from the CDC, the author describes the incidence of *Lime disease* in the U.S. Risk factors include attendance at cocktail parties and exposure to media stories about Lyme disease. (Some positive and negative correspondence followed this article. See, AIM 1991;115:157–158 and 1991;115:500.)

10. London, Oscar: Kill as Few Patients as Possible (and fifty-six other essays on how to be the world's best doctor). Berkeley: Ten Speed Press, 1987.

A collection of essays on medical practice that are witty, amusing, and provocative.

11. London, Oscar: Take One As Needed. Berkley: Ten Speed Press, 1989.

This is a second book of amusing essays by Dr. London. Although many of the pieces are general, with titles like "A Hospital Bill to Die Over" and "God Bless Your Chiropractor," this collection certainly qualifies as medical humor.

12. Matz R: Principles of medicine. NY State J Med 1977;77:99–101.

13. Matz R: More principles of medicine. NY State J Med 1977;77:1984–1985.

The author presents 144 rules and laws of medicine. Most ring true and some are funny. For example, the Principles of Intensive Care: (1) air goes in and out (2) blood goes round and round (3) oxygen is good.

14. Matz R: Still more principles of medicine. NY State J Med 1980;80:113–116.

After a three year hiatus, Dr. Matz returns with an additional 113 rules. For example, "Confidence is the feeling you have before you understand the situation," and "If you can't be brilliant, be careful."

15. Meador CK: The last well person. N Engl J Med 1994;330:440–441.

This article satirizes man's preoccupation with wellness and medicine's preoccupation with disease: "A well person is a patient who has not been completely worked up."

16. Robertson RG: Lights, camera, prevention. J Fam Pract 1995;40:542.

The author pokes fun at Hollywood's penchant for exaggerated medical drama by showing how a scene in primary care could be just as dramatic as a full code.

17. Rose I: Robert's rules of parliamentary procedure: III. the phenomenon of records. Can Med Assoc J 1963;89:308–309.

This article satirizes a physician's least favorite task—dealing with medical records.

18. Schiedermayer DL: The Hippocratic oath—corporate version. N Engl J Med 1986;314:62.

A brief satire that updates the original. For example, "I will not use the knife unless I am a surgeon, but I will try to learn some form of endoscopy."

19. Shaw BA: If doctors bargained like car dealers. Med Economics 1987;64(Sept 7):139–143.

The shoe is on the other foot!

20. Vainder M: Certified circumcision. Med Economics 1966;43(Sept):20.

Having to deal with protocols is an inevitable part of a doctor's job. When a baby is born outside the ER, an amusing administrative tangle results.

21. Wolf JA: Phone calls that are shortening my career. Med Economics 1981;58(Feb 16):165–171.

The author presents a handful of "off-the-wall" phone calls he's received over the years. Remember, what drives you crazy at 2 AM is often funny by the light of day.

KEEPING UP WITH MEDICINE

When I finished my residency in 1980, keeping up with medicine was a manageable affair. I got three or four journals per month and, while I did not read them cover to cover, they could at least be stacked in such a way that I rarely tripped over them. Now, however, with many more subscriptions and with "throwaways" arriving almost every day, my monthly journals have taken on menacing proportions. They not only threaten to knock me down if I make a wrong turn, but I'm sure they snicker at me when I sit at my desk trying to ignore them.

Of course, reading the literature is only one of the ways that doctors try to keep up with medicine. Informational indigestion is also available through grand rounds, local lectures, and national meetings. And finally, for the overworked and bleary-eyed, there is always the 6 o'clock news.

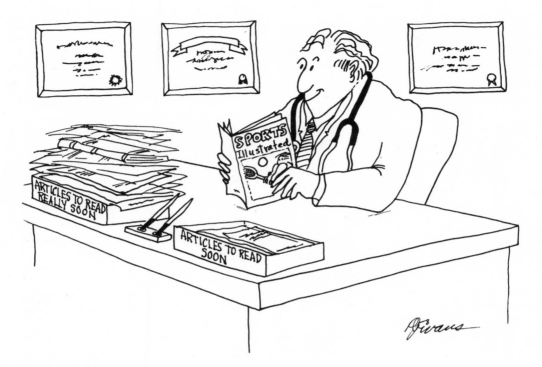

KEEPING UP WITH THE LITERATURE*

Howard J. Bennett, M.D.

When I began my medical education almost 20 years ago, I had no idea what a medical article was. In those days I was a textbook man—a rather plodding fellow who liked his information organized, summarized, and neatly packaged between the covers of a book. The first time I actually saw an article I was sitting in pathology lab looking at a slide of my own blood. In between glances at neutrophils and lymphocytes, my lab partner handed me a copy of an article from a pediatric journal. "What's this?" I asked, glad for the chance to talk to a multicellular organism. "It's an article on CBCs," he said. "Did you know there's a shift to the right with viral infections?" "No," I said rather sheepishly. The only shifting I knew about was shifting dullness, and I had only learned about that the week before. Nevertheless, since ignorance is something medical students learn to live with, I leaned forward with my best I'M REALLY INTERESTED IN THIS face. "What else does it say?" I queried. "A lot," he said. "I'll copy it for you after class." At which point we went back to looking at doughnut-shaped RBCs, platelets, and the like.

*Reprinted from JAMA ©1992;267:920, with permission of the American Medical Association.

I still remember how excited I was after class. Wow! I thought. So this is what the medical literature is all about. Copying articles and reading stuff that's so new it hasn't made it into the textbooks yet. When we got the library, I actually felt taller, as though I had traversed some major evolutionary step in an instant. Little did I know, however, that one day I would look back on this afternoon with a somewhat different perspective.

The problem, I learned, is that it's impossible to keep up with the medical literature. This is not the fault of the literature itself, but rather of those individuals who keep adding to it as though it were an endangered species. Unfortunately, while most of us cannot keep up with our reading, we all know people who say they can. But is this really true? Are there people out there who do not need to eat or sleep? People who never need to change diapers, attend ballet recitals, or plant azaleas? People who take their journals with them wherever they go?

To settle this issue, I spent the last few years examining the reading habits of all the physicians I know. What I found out is that few physicians actually go to bed with their journals at night (this was a comforting observation). I also discovered that physicians go through stages in their reading just like other areas of development. And, as we all know, the important thing about developmental stages is finding out whether you are reaching your milestones. Therefore, I have compiled the information I collected into a Table for your review. If your reading habits are in sync with the listed categories, you can relax and should no longer feel guilty when you pick up a beer instead of a medical journal. (Remember, older golfers don't hit in the 70s anymore, so why should you?) On the other hand, if you don't "fit" anywhere in the Table, perhaps now is the time to take a sabbatical or open up that restaurant you've been talking about all these years.

Bennett's Classification for Reading Medical Articles

Medical Student	Reads entire article but does not understand what any of it means.
Intern	Uses journal as a pillow during nights on call.
Resident	Would like to read entire article but eats dinner instead.
Chief Resident	Skips articles entirely and reads the classifieds.
Junior Attending	Reads and analyzes entire article in order to pimp medical students.
Senior Attending	Reads abstracts and quotes the literature liberally.
Research Attending	Reads entire article, reanalyzes statistics, and looks up all references, usually in lieu of sex.
Chief of Service	Reads references to see if he was cited anywhere.
Private Attending	Doesn't buy journals in the first place but keeps an eye open for medical articles that make it into *Time* or *Newsweek*.
Emeritus Attending	Reads entire article but does not understand what any of it means.

In 1978, David Durack published an amusing article called "The Weight of Medical Knowledge" (N Engl J Med 1978;298:773–775). The author was intrigued with the explosion of medical information and set out to determine when doctors would be buried in the medical literature. Assuming that the weight of *Index Medicus* bears a rough relationship to the number of articles published each year, the author recorded its weight from 1875 to 1977. Although the *Index* only weighed 32 kg in 1977, he discovered an exponential curve which suggested that by 1985 the *Index Medicus* would weigh in at a hefty 1000 kg. Fortunately, a follow-up study done in 1989,[1] revealed that Dr. Durack's prediction was premature. According to the new figures, the *Index Medicus* won't reach 1000 kg until the year 2027. Happily, most of us will be in nursing homes by then.—H.B.

1. Madlon-Kay DJ: The weight of medical knowledge: still gaining. N Engl J Med 1989;321:908.

The New England Kernel of Medicine*

Established in 1612 as The NEW ENGLAND KERNEL OF MEDICINE AND SORCERY

VOLUME 642   OCTOBER 20, 1993   NUMBER 4

Howard J. Bennett M.D.

*Reprinted from The Journal of Family Practice 1994; 38:427, with permission from Appleton & Lange.

PRIMARY CARE UPDATE 1999*

Howard J. Bennett, M.D.

■ **Sunday**

7:00 PM   Registration and nude swim

■ **Monday**

DERMATOLOGY

8:00 AM   **The Diagnosis of Rashes that Resolved Last Week**

9:00 AM   **Antioxidants and the Prevention of Male Pattern Baldness**

9:30 AM   **Itchy Trigger Finger**—Pitfalls in management

10:00 AM Break—10K run

SURGERY

10:15 AM **Flatus in the OR**—Old problem, new rules

10:45 AM **Colonoscopy of the Rich and Famous**

11:30 AM **Irritable Jowel Syndrome**—Surgical management of patients who talk too much

12:00 PM Lunch

INTERNAL MEDICINE

1:30 PM   **Medical Treatment of Diseases Contracted in Past Lives**

2:30 PM   **Drug Rep Inhibitors**

3:00 PM   **Congestive Chart Failure**—Pathophysiology and management

3:30 PM   Break—Massage and sauna

4:00 PM   **Acute and Chronic Death**—Management options in primary care

5:00 PM   **Diseases of the Xiphoid Process**

■ **Tuesday**

INFECTIOUS DISEASES

8:00 AM   **A New Look at Infections Picked Up During UFO Abductions**

8:30 AM   **Diseases Acquired from Postage Stamps**

9:15 AM   **The Child with Too Few Infections**

10:00 AM Break—Lox and bagels

EMERGENCY MEDICINE

10:30 AM **Pinworm Emergencies in Primary Care**

11:00 AM **Advances in Turfing Patients**

11:45 AM **Carbohydrate Emergencies**—How to avoid raiding the refrigerator when you're on call

12:15 PM Lunch

MISCELLANEOUS TOPICS

1:30 PM   **What to Do When Specialists Use Abbreviations You Don't Understand**

2:00 PM   **Imaging the Big Toe**

2:30 PM   **Excessive Nose Hair**—Common problems in management

3:00 PM   **Nocturnal Emissions**—Screening, detection, therapy

3:30 PM   Break—Dunk the professors

4:00 PM   Workshops (choose one)

    A. State-of-the-Art Rectal Exams

    B. Renal Biopsies for Non-Nephrologists

    C. Slide Seminar: Prostates I Have Known

■ **Wednesday**

SPORTS MEDICINE

8:00 AM   **Failure to Drive**—New trends for avoiding sandtraps

9:00 AM   **Reactive Fairway Disease**—Preventing tantrums on the back nine

9:30 AM   **Iron Deficiency**—A practical approach to chip shots

10:00 AM Break—Mud wrestling

OPHTHALMOLOGY

11:00 AM **Red Eye/Pink Eye/Blue Eye/Green Eye**—2nd annual Dr Seuss memorial lecture

12:00 PM Lunch

OBSTETRICS

1:30 PM   **Ultrasound Diagnosis of Attention Deficit Disorder**

2:00 PM   **Intrauterine Circumcision**—An idea whose time has come

2:45 PM   **Controversies in Cord Clamping**—Catch the baby or catch the dad?

3:30 PM   Break—Pin the tail on the lawyer

MANAGED CARE

4:00 PM   **Advances in Billing Republicans**

4:30 PM   **Admission Channel Blockers**

5:00 PM   **Interventional Stonewalling**

5:30 PM   **Adjourn**

    (For hotel information, call 1-800-EASY CME)

*Reprinted from The Journal of Family Practice, ©1994; 39:523, with permission from Appleton & Lange, Inc.

THAT'S FUNNY—SOMETHING IS GAINED IN THE TRANSLATION*

L. A. Healey, M.D.

At international medical meetings where papers are presented in several different languages, simultaneous translation enables the audience to understand the speakers. Yet it hasn't been widely recognized that translation can also offer much in local meetings where it's assumed that everyone speaks the same language. Here's a list of statements commonly heard at the latter sort of meeting. Following each, in parentheses, I've given the actual meaning. Take this with you to the next meeting you attend and see if it doesn't add quite a bit to your comprehension of the presentations.

1. I do not have to relate in detail for this audience the history of this condition. (*I didn't look it up in the literature.*)

2. For purposes of the present discussion, let us assume that . . . (*This is the key to my argument but I can't quite prove it.*)

3. This slide depicts the results of a representative study in one dog. (*This is the only one that came out right.*)

4. Careful clinical observations show . . . (*If I'd had controls, I'd be presenting this at the A.M.A. clinical convention.*)

5. Omphalograms were not performed at this time. (*I forgot to do that.*)

6. Probst reports a recurrence rate of 20 per cent, but in our experience, this has not been the case. (*Neither of my patients had one.*)

7. Time does not permit us to describe fully the enzymatic pathways that are involved in this type of reaction. (*I never was very good in biochemistry.*)

8. That's a good question. (*I don't know.*)

9. Please repeat the question. (*I don't know that either.*)

10. That's a very interesting question. (*That I know.*)

11. The cases are potentially complicated, and consultation with a specialist should be obtained early. (*I need referrals.*)

12. For the most part, such cases are readily managed by the primary physician. (*I have a busy practice, thank you.*)

In 1993, Mark DePaolis published a satire about going to medical meetings (Conference Call. Postgraduate Medicine 1993;93(5):57–58.) Here are two pearls from that article.—H.B.

1. Medical conferences are always held at nice locations. (This is based on the educational principle that to learn anything important, you must be able to swim or ski afterward.)

2. There's no need to ask questions after a conference because everything the speaker said is in the syllabus. (In fact, everything *anybody* has ever said is in the syllabus: It's a little known fact that the word "syllabus" is taken from the Greek "syl" meaning outline and "labus" meaning lumbar disk injury.)

*Reprinted with permission from Medical Economics, © 1971;48 (Aug 30):137. Copyright by Medical Economics Company, Inc., Oradell, NJ 07649.

CLINICAL ALGORITHMS*

R.G. Neville, MRCGP, DRCOG

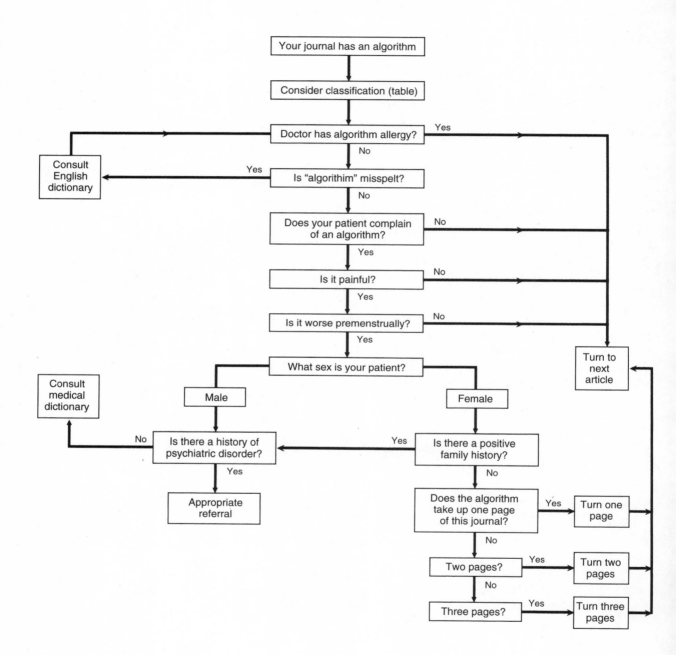

*Reprinted with permission from the British Medical Journal, ©
1985; 29:1819.

Additional Readings

1. Augsburger JJ, Gamel JW, et al: The risk of major audiovisual problems during ophthalmic presentations. Surv Ophthalmol 1992;36:390–392.

The authors analyzed over 4000 presentations to determine the best combination of variables for predicting a person's risk for experiencing an AV problem during a lecture. They accomplished this using the SWAG method of data analysis (stupid wild ass guess).

2. Bennett HJ: Do articles have wings? J Emerg Med 1995;13:253–254.

The author muses about getting older and how difficult it is to remember not only what we read, but where we read it.

3. Dorfman W: How to prepare a medical talk. JAMA 1964;190:A227.

The author provides some helpful hints about what's expected when doctors go to medical conferences. If you're in the audience, you're supposed to stay awake. If you're on the podium, you're supposed to have something to talk about (staying awake is optional).

4. Goldwyn RM: Meeting mania. Plastic Reconst Surg 1993;91:144–145.

This article is about a prominent surgeon who practices with a slide projector instead of a scalpel.

5. Harvey RF, Schullinger MB, et al: Dreaming during scientific papers: effects of added extrinsic material. BMJ 1983;287:1916–1919.

The authors investigated the prevalence of sleeping and dreaming at medical meetings. In addition to creating a "stupor index," they studied how extraneous material (i.e., provocative slides) affect the retention of clinical information.

6. LaCombe M: The spouse's programme. JAMA 1990;263:2099.

This is an amusing tale about what happens when the author escorts his wife, an orthopedic surgeon, to a medical conference.

A malpractice lawyer, and HMO administrator, and a Medicare auditor jump off the Empire State Building at the same time. Which one hits the ground first?
Who cares?

INFORMED CONSENT & OTHER COMPLICATIONS OF HEALTH CARE

The articles in this chapter and the one that follows poke fun at some of the frustrations endemic in medicine. Although the division of articles is somewhat arbitrary, the ones in this chapter seemed to fit better under the subtitle, "Complications of Health Care." It also made sense to group them with the two parodies on Informed Consent. Considering the range of subject matter and the dates of publication, it is surprising how up-to-date the articles appear. George King's article, the "Human Nature Chart," is particularly revealing in the durability of its satire. Although it is listed as a 1965 publication, the article originally appeared in *Medical Economics* in the early 1930's. I used the 1965 citation because that issue is more likely to be available for anyone who wants to review the journal itself.

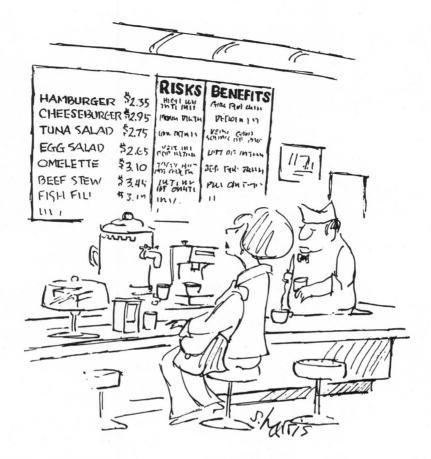

The menu board reads:

		RISKS	BENEFITS
HAMBURGER	$2.35		
CHEESEBURGER	$2.95		
TUNA SALAD	$2.75		
EGG SALAD	$2.65		
OMELETTE	$3.10		
BEEF STEW	$3.45		
FISH FIL	$3.19		

FRENETIC PHARMACEUTICALS*

Paul L. Fine, M.D.

"Good morning, Dr. Fine. Would you like some Psychocort playing cards?"

I turned around. I couldn't help myself. I was on my way to the cafeteria after a particularly grueling call night, one in which refractory hypotension seemed to be as contagious as the common cold. Perhaps my dilapidated condition left me unable to resist the bait.

Dave, a drug rep who looked suspiciously like Bob Costas, felt the tug on his opening line and be-

gan to reel me in. "Psychocort," he explained, "is a true breakthrough, a combination of prednisone and Haldol for patients who experience unwanted and embarrassing psychotic effects from steroid therapy." I glanced down at the slogan that decorated the cards: *Play the prednisone game with a full deck.*

"That's certainly a unique blend of medications," I admitted. "And I've never seen a deck of cards in which the King and Queen were quite so cushingoid."

*Reprinted from The Journal of Family Practice, 1994;38:627–628, with permission from Appleton & Lange, Inc. Edited from the original.
Drawing by S. Harris; © 1979 The New Yorker Magazine, Inc.

"Well, here at Frenetic Pharmaceuticals we believe in offering our clients convenient products that combine two or more medications. Our company motto is *Compliance instead of complaints.*"

I must have looked skeptical, because he continued as if answering an unspoken objection. "Conclusive studies have demonstrated the efficacy of such combinations. For example, let me give you this monograph on our Panaceabid formulation. Panaceabid is a combination of ciprofloxacin, trimethoprim-sulfamethoxazole, and doxycycline—definitive twice-a-day therapy for patients whose doctors are concerned about infection but can't find a source. As you can see here, 88% of the doctors prescribing Panaceabid in this series reported 'significant relief' of their anxiety. The *P* value was less than .01."

"But what about the patients? Did they—"

"Here, doctor, have a doughnut. The cinnamon glaze is conveniently combined with a tart lemon filling. You know, we're very excited about another new product, Impactocard. It combines quinidine and Imodium for patients who find that retaining a normal sinus rhythm is not sufficiently rewarding to offset the frequent trips to the bathroom. I was just chatting with your chief of cardiology, and he thinks Impactocard will be of great value."

"What does it cost?"

"Let me pour you a cup of coffee, doctor. No, you don't need to add cream. We mix it in as part of the recipe. Over here, we have samples of Omnipatch, which contains transdermal preparations of estrogen, clonidine, nitroglycerine, nicotine, and scopolamine. It's the only patch approved by the FDA for postmenopausal women with hypertension and angina who plan to quit smoking while on a cruise."

"I really have to go now," I said quickly. "I think I feel my pager vibrating."

"Sure, doctor. Thanks for your time. Let me quickly remind you that Prilopril, a combination of captropril, enalapril, lisinopril and quinapril, is now available for hypertensive patients whose doctors can't decide which advertisements to believe. We also throw in some dextromethorphan for cough suppression."

What could one say in response? I started to suggest that his company promote Prilopril by distributing decks of play cards from which all of the aces had been removed, but Dave appeared so earnest that I changed my mind. Instead, I mumbled some thanks for the doughnut and coffee, and slumped into a chair.

The next day was Saturday, and I slipped out of the hospital in time to do some shopping at the local Discount Drugstore.

"Hello, Dr. Fine. How nice to see you." It was Dave. He had exchanged his three-piece suit for the full regalia of a drugstore employee, including a badge that read *I'm Dave. Ask me about our contraceptives.* With an abrupt motion he grabbed my hand and forced a can of soup into it. "Did you know that Frenetic Pharmaceuticals is a leader in the pharmacologic supplementation of common household products? We're working very closely with a number of retail stores," he bragged. "That, for example, is a can of our innovative Chicken Noodle 'n' Lasix Soup, a tasty treat for patients with congestive heart failure who would like a bowl of soup without committing themselves to a week in intensive care. There's also a chunky variety, with K-Dur tablets."

Dave led me a little farther down the aisle and handed me what appeared to be a candy bar. "Over here," he continued, "let me show you Hershey's Euglycemia Bar, made with creamy milk chocolate, nougat, caramel, and delicious morsels of glyburide. For only $5, patients with type II diabetes can relish a tasty chocolate treat and still control their glucose levels. In fact, our study showed that an incredible 50% of the patients in a group consuming two Euglycemia Bars each day fell below the group's median level of glycosylated hemoglobin."

"But 50% always fall below *any* median, by defin—"

"And the packaging is so convenient! See how the paper wrapper can be detached and used as a urinary glucose test strip?"

There was clearly no point in debating a man who responded to a statistical challenge by advocating the desecration of candy wrappers, so I murmured something vaguely congratulatory and attempted to escape into the personal hygiene area. Unfortunately, Dave followed me, and I noticed that his speech was beginning to sound pressured. "We have several products in this section that are doing exceptionally well. First, there's Amoxifloss, a dental floss with an amoxicillin coating, for patients with rheumatic heart disease. It lets them care for their teeth and gums without having to worry about endocarditis. And speaking of dental hygiene, we also have a toothpaste that is really—"

"I know, I know," I interjected. "It has fluoride in it. They all do."

"Sure it has fluoride," he snapped. "But it also has a potent sublingual nitroglycerine formulation, for patients with coronary artery disease. When angina demands urgent medical attention, Nitrodent relieves the chest pain *and* keeps your breath fresh and minty for the trip to the emergency room. Wouldn't you say that it fights plaque in a more effective manner than other toothpastes?" Before I could answer, he emitted a nervous giggle and began to hop up and down in an agitated manner, glancing repeatedly at my receding hairline. "You should also be interested in our latest product for the, uh, follicularly challenged. It's a hair-styling gel with minoxidil called 'Groom & Grow.' Not only will your hair look great at the end of a busy day, *but there will be more of it!*"

Dave's eyes were becoming glazed, and I detected a slight intention tremor. In desperation, I grabbed the largest container of laundry detergent I could find and made a run for the checkout aisle.

Dave seemed confused and upset. "On your way out," he yelled after me, "be sure to notice the E-Z Breathe Cigarettes behind the counter. They have special heat-labile formulations of Proventil and Vanceril for patients with COPD who can't stop smoking long enough to use their inhalers."

Don't look back, I thought to myself. *Just get out as quickly as possible and never go near the hospital cafeteria again.*

I paid for my detergent and was putting my wallet back in my pocket when a small projectile hit me squarely on the back of the head. "That's a package of Addictochew," Dave called out as he ducked behind the deodorant display, "a snappy spearmint gum supplemented with Antabuse, nicotine, and methadone. It's ideal for the man who used to have everything!"

Dave was clearly out of control and he knew it. After he managed to calm himself, he jogged up to the checkout counter to apologize. "I'm very sorry, doctor, but sometimes my manic disorder gets the better of me when I have forgotten to take my Litho-cells." He was just reaching over the counter for a package of lithium batteries when I hurried out of the store.

The CEO of a managed care company dies and goes to heaven, where he meets St. Peter at the Pearly Gates.

"I want to be admitted to heaven," the CEO demands. "I've lived a good life, and I've made health care more affordable."

"You can come in," St. Peter answers. "But you're only authorized for two days."

"NOW, MRS. BLARE, ABOUT THE COMPLICATIONS . . ."*

William P. Irvin, M.D.

After his lawyer left, Dr. Jones sat at his desk, staring moodily out the window. He was thinking of what he'd just heard about informed consent: "I guess you have to warn patients about almost everything that might go wrong," he told himself. "I sure wouldn't like to get hit with a $100,000 verdict, like that radiologist who gave local X-ray treatments without telling the patient about possible burns."

His reverie was cut short by the entrance of his nurse. "Mrs. Blare is here, Doctor."

"Oh yes, she's to be admitted to the hospital tomorrow for surgery, isn't she? Send her in."

Mrs. Blare entered, sat down, and lit a cigarette. "Well, here I am, Doctor. My husband was a little upset until I told him you said it was just a fibroid tumor, just a simple hysterectomy, and there really wasn't much to it."

Dr. Jones winced. What his lawyer had told him made him sorry he'd used those words. "Now, Mrs. Blare, I didn't exactly mean it that way. You see . . ."

"Doctor, what is it? Do I have cancer?"

"No, still fibroids, Mrs. Blare. But a hysterectomy—well, frankly, there are some things that can go wrong. Not often, of course. But I should tell you of the possibilities."

"Oh, I'm not worried, Doctor. But if it'll make you feel better, go ahead and tell me."

"Well, after you're admitted to the hospital, they'll shave you. And occasionally they may nick the skin a little. . . . No, I realize that's not so bad. . . . Yes, I realize you're not the type to get upset over little things. . . . Well, then they'll draw your water. Sometimes this can cause a little inflammation of the bladder. . . . That's right—like you had with your last pregnancy. . . . Well, I know it took four months, but usually we can cure it much faster. We'd use some of the new drugs because they don't

cause as many reactions. . . . A reaction? Well, you break out in a rash and itch and . . . That's right—like your cousin, John, after he got penicillin. . . . He died? Oh, I didn't know. Mrs. Blare, you're shaking ashes all over my rug.

"Next they'll draw some blood from your arm for tests. . . . Yes, I know you've had it done before. But sometimes you can get a virus infection that causes a little liver reaction. . . . Your friend's husband died, too? Well, most people get better. Of course, it takes years sometimes, and—well, anyway, it doesn't happen often. Mrs. Blare, you look pale. Here, take this pill. That's better.

"Now at bedtime, they'll give you some drugs to help you sleep. . . . Yes, I guess you could get a drug reaction from them, but usually . . . No, I don't mean that would be your second drug reaction, I mean you probably wouldn't have any reaction. . . . Yes, I know what I said about the bladder.

"You'll also get a little enema at bedtime. . . . Mrs. Blare, what happened to your cousin in Omaha has nothing to do with this case. They won't push a hole in your intestine. . . . Of course, I don't guarantee it. . . . Peritonitis? Well, yes a hole in the intestine can cause it, but nobody will punch a hole in your intestine. . . . No, I was not aware that your brother is a lawyer.

"Well, let's see. Early the next day they'll take you to the operating room, which brings us to the anesthetic. Occasionally, it can cause a little problem. . . . Well, the heart might stop working. . . . Oh, yes, we can start it again. Usually. If we can get it going, it usually keeps on working O.K. Of course, if the brain has been damaged, the patient might not be too bright after surgery. . . . Yes, an idiot, you might say—but really, that doesn't happen often.

"Next we open the abdomen and remove the uterus. Of course, once in a while—not very often,

*Reprinted with permission from Medical Economics, © 1971; 48(Apr 12):183–190, Medical Economics Company, Inc., Oradell, N.J. 07649.

you understand—but just sometimes . . . Mrs. Blare, just because your grandmother said you were born under an unlucky star . . . Now stop shaking. Here, take another pill. . . . No, it won't cause a drug reaction—I don't think. You mustn't worry so, Mrs. Blare.

"Now, in removing the uterus, we might—on very rare occasions, you understand—get into the bowel. . . . I mean, we might cut a small hole in the bowel. Sort of like the enema thing, yes. . . . Well, we just sew it up. . . . Yes, peritonitis is possible.

"If all goes well, and we haven't nicked the ureter . . . Oh, the tube that goes to the bladder. . . . Well, it might cause a fistula and—let's talk about that later. . . . Yes, your insurance would cover it if it should happen.

"Now, the uterus is out, and the incision is closed. . . . No, we won't sew the bowel up too tight. I mean, we won't touch the bowel. . . . Yes, I know what I said before. . . . No, I'm not contradicting my-self. Now, now, please relax. . . . After the surgery you'll be given some fluids through a needle in your vein. . . . Well, yes, I guess so. That old virus and the liver again. . . . Yes, you mentioned that he died.

"If the wound doesn't break open we'll . . . Well, all your intestines could spill out. . . . Oh, we'd put them back. . . . No, that wouldn't cause idiocy.

"There's only one more thing. Of course, it doesn't happen often. We call it a Staph infection. . . . Oh, you've read about it in the papers? . . . They all died? But that was in a nursery. . . . Well, yes, grown-ups can die from it, but we have drugs, and . . . Well, a drug reaction isn't usually as bad as a Staph infection.

"To sum it all up, Mrs. Blare, a hysterectomy really isn't so simple. Now if you'll just sign this paper that says I've informed you of these little complica—Mrs. Blare! We're not through! Where are you going? *Come back, Mrs. Blare!*"

Top Ten Rejected Names for Managed Care Plans*

10. McHealth Care

9. Suboptimum Choice

8. Sri Lanka Health Plan

7. Equivocare

6. Premiums Plus

5. You'll Get That Procedure Over Our Dead Body Health Plan

4. Cut-Rate Health Care

3. Gatekeepers USA

2. Chapter 11 Health Plan

1. Kevorkian Plus

*Reprinted from The Journal of Family Practice © 1996;43:110, with permission from Appleton & Lange, Inc.

PROPOSED INFORMED-CONSENT FORM FOR HERNIA PATIENT*

Preston J. Burnham, M.D.

I, ..., being about to be subjected to a surgical operation said to be for repair of what my doctor thinks is a hernia (rupture or loss of belly stuff—intestines—out of the belly through a hole in the muscles), do hereby give said doctor permission to cut into me and do duly swear that I am giving my informed consent, based upon the following information:

Operative procedure is as follows: The doctor first cuts through the skin by a four-inch gash in the lower abdomen. He then slashes through the other things—fascia (a tough layer over the muscles) and layers of muscle—until he sees the cord (tube that brings the sperm from testicle to outside) with all its arteries and veins. The doctor then tears the hernia (thin sac of bowels and things) from the cord and ties off the sac with a string. He then pushes the testicle back into the scrotum and sews everything together trying not to sew up the big arteries and veins that nourish the leg.

Possible complications are as follows:

1. Large artery may be cut and I may bleed to death.

2. Large vein may be cut and I may bleed to death.

3. Tube from testicle may be cut. I will then be sterile on that side.

4. Artery or veins to testicles may be cut—same result.

5. Opening around cord in muscles may be made too tight.

6. Clot may develop in these veins which will loosen when I get out of bed and hit my lungs, killing me.

7. Clot may develop in one or both legs which may cripple me, lead to loss of one or both legs, go to my lungs, or make my veins no good for life.

8. I may develop a horrible infection that may kill me.

9. The hernia may come back again after it has been operated on.

10. I may die from general anesthesia.

11. I may be paralyzed if spinal anesthesia is used.

12. If ether is used, it could explode inside me.

13. I may slip in hospital bathroom.

14. I may be run over going to the hospital.

15. The hospital may burn down.

I understand: the anatomy of the body, the pathology of the development of hernias, the surgical technique that will be used to repair the hernia, the physiology of wound healing, the dietetic chemistry of the foods that I must eat to cause healing, the chemistry of body repair, and the course which my physician will take in treating any of the complications that can occur as a sequela of repairing an otherwise simple hernia.

_____
Patient

_____
Lawyer for Patient

_____
Lawyer for Doctor

_____
Lawyer for Hospital

_____
Lawyer for Anesthesiologist

_____
Mother-in-Law

_____
Notary Public

_____
Date

_____
Place

*Reprinted from Science, © 1966;152:448–449, with permission from the American Association for the Advancement of Science. Edited from the original.

THE PROFESSIONAL PATIENT*

Ian Rose, M.B., B.S.

The concept of the professional patient is new to most people. Therefore, it must be understood at the outset that professionalism is essentially a state of mind. The patient must realize at all times that he is the essence of medicine. Where would the physician or surgeon be without him? Harvey, Lister, Pasteur and all the other greats of medicine would have lived in vain, if not for the patient.

He must also remember that the patient-doctor relationship is a constant battle. The patient must learn not to give an inch, yet his approach must be subtle. As we shall see later, it is always possible to thwart the doctor without open revolt. Thus, when the patient is told to go into the examining room and take his clothes off, he should not object, but merely enter the room and hang his hat upon the peg. This has been classified as Phase I of the examination revolt.

Phase II occurs when the physician returns, finds the patient still fully dressed, instructs him in peremptory tones to strip, and then leaves again. The patient should then remove his jacket and open his shirt. The original description of this revolt contains 16 phases through which the patient moves before he has reduced his physician to a state of servile impotence; and only then does he allow himself to be examined in the nude.

The History

Once the initial greeting is over, the lead should be passed to the doctor. Rule IV clearly states that the history should never be given; the physician must be made to extract it.

When the physician is ready to take the history, the professional patient falls silent and waits with a pleasant and confident look on his face.

The first response to the doctor is of utmost importance. It must undermine his confidence and make him realize that he is dealing with a nimble mind. As the doctor has certain standard openings, the patient should use standard replies or counters. A selection of these follows:

Doctor: Well what seems to be trouble?

Patient: That's what I'm here to find out.

Doctor: And how are you today?

Patient: I'm hoping you'll be able to tell me at the end of the examination.

The really experienced physician will often open with: "What are you complaining of?" and sit back with a complacent smile on his face because he feels that there is no effective counter to this approach. Segway Mathieson disproved this on many occasions and in his paper, "The Conquest of Dr. Tinglefoot," concludes that the best counter-move was to reply quietly: "I am not complaining of anything except, perhaps, your phraseology, which is ugly, unworthy of your noble profession, and ends in a preposition!"

Contrary to what many people expect, the professional patient will lead the doctor through the chief complaint without confusion, because this lulls the physician into a false sense of security and he is less wary of the pitfalls that lie before him. However, exceptions can be made to this general rule in special circumstances; for instance, when a doctor is insistent on the exact time of origin of a symptom the special process of "time derouting" is appropriate. This process is best explained by an illustration. The following example is taken from Fanny Timberflossetts' book, "Thoughts of a Picaresque Patient—The Naked Truth."

On being pressed for the date of origin of a symptom such as diarrhea, constipation or anything else, she would hesitate and appear to think for a moment.

"It was just after Fred had his accident," she would say, smiling sweetly at the physician. When he did not look satisfied, she would hurriedly add,

*Reprinted with permission from the Canadian Medical Association Journal, © 1965;92:923–926. Edited from the original.

INFORMED CONSENT & OTHER COMPLICATIONS OF HEALTH CARE

"Yes, I'm sure it was about two months after his accident."

"And when did your husband have his accident?" "Oh my husband hasn't had any accident."

"Then who is Fred?"

"Fred, he's my eldest boy."

"All right" (the doctor is now controlling himself with difficulty), "when did Fred have his accident?"

"Which accident?" Then, noticing the flushed face of the doctor, she would add, "He's had two bad ones, and was on Compensation for a long time with them."

Fanny says that this is generally a turning point in the conversation. More excitable doctors will have an explosion of temper at this point, while in the more phlegmatic such an outburst may be delayed further. The latter will say that they are interested in the accident that occurred just before onset of diarrhea. Fanny would then continue: "Oh, that one. That was when he twisted his back on the uneven path leading to the restroom at the construction site where he was working. He was in hospital for two months and had to have traction and . . ."

Fanny says that she has never yet been able to finish her account of Fred's second accident, although she committed a 200-word description of it to memory. It may be thought by many that, at this point, the doctor would give up and pursue a different symptom, but doctors usually show a remarkable perseverance and will return to the direct attack after an interval in which they either light a cigarette or attempt to tear the phone book in half, depending on their temperament.

The questioning by the doctor is now very direct. He says: "When did the diarrhea begin?" Or alternatively, "When was the last time you felt perfectly well and had no diarrhea?"

In either case Fanny's response to renewed questioning had no reference to Fred's illness but she would start out on a completely new tack.

"Oh, you want to know when the diarrhea started?"

"Yes."

"Oh well, that's easy. It started about five or six days before the headache."

"And when did the headache begin?"

"I've just told you. About five or six days after the diarrhea."

Owing to limitations of space we cannot quote this dialogue at greater length. However, the gen- eral tenor of time derouting can be easily discerned from the foregoing. As long as the doctor returns to the same questions, they can be easily evaded by associating the temporal origin of a symptom with something in the patient's private life rather than with a calendar. Eventually the doctor will give up if no other reason than that set out in Rule V: *The doctor has less time than you do.*

Past and Family History

A great deal of time can be wasted with the past history and the family history. The patient should carefully prepare beforehand and memorize all the illnesses he's ever had, together with their complications, their dates of origin, and their duration. These must include all childhood illnesses, all attacks of flu, colds and accidents, however trivial. These should be given to the doctor at dictation speed. If there is one important illness among them, such as rheumatic fever, tuberculosis, typhoid, and so on, this provides a good opportunity to practise time derouting.

Similarly, the family history should be learned and include all brothers, sisters, aunts, uncles and first cousins. It's likely that the doctor will interrupt the process, but such preparation is the first sign of professionalism in the patient.

The Physical Examination

We have already alluded to the possibilities that open up for the patient when he is told to disrobe for the examination. This matter will not be discussed further at this point.

Head and Neck. The tactics to be used during this examination are sufficiently obvious that they need not be described in detail. Such measures as choking on the tongue depressor and coughing in the doctor's face; turning the head to the left when the left ear is being examined and to the right for the right ear, causing the eyes to wander and the eyelids to close for a funduscopic examination—are all parts of the rather obvious gambits of this phase.

In a similar way we may dispense with a detailed description of examination of the limbs and lymphatic system. A high degree of ticklishness underlies an elementary but highly effective technique.

The Chest. When the doctor places his stethoscope anywhere near the sternum or underneath the fifth rib, the patient should breathe in and out deeply and noisily. When the doctor attempts to listen to any other part of the chest, the breath should be held. Breaths should be taken hurriedly while the doctor is moving the bell of his stethoscope from one place to another.

Occasionally the doctor will notice the absence of breath sounds and will instruct the patient to breathe. When this occurs the patient should inspired as slowly as possible, hold his breath for at least 30 seconds, and then exhale equally slowly.

Rarely, a persistent physician may not instruct the patient to breathe but will wait patiently for cyanosis and the inevitable breath. When it's impossible to hold the breath any longer, victory may still be obtained by covering a few quick gasps of life-giving oxygen by a fit of paroxysmal coughing.

It should be noticed that we have not advised the ploy of talking while the doctor is trying to listen. This is too obvious and we feel that it raises the doctor's suspicions. The processes we have described are sufficiently subtle to be effective with most physicians.

The Abdominal Examination. The abdominal examination can be made frustrating and almost impossible by three simple maneuvers. (1) By complaining of the coldness of the doctor's hands; this causes delay while he tries to warm them. (2) By squirming and laughing because he is tickling. (3) By raising the head each time his hand touches the skin of the abdomen—this effectively tenses the abdominal muscles, making it impossible for him to feel any of the internal organs.

C.N.S. The examination of the central nervous system is a highly specialized subject and will not be referred to in this elementary text. Those interested are referred to the paper "Physicians, Jerks, and Neurosurgeons", by Stetler and Merryweather, published in the April 1964 issue of the *Journal of the Canadian Professional Patient.*

Conclusion

In conclusion, certain general rules may be advanced for the guidance of practising or would-be professional patients.

1. Never go to the doctor's office if a house call will do.

2. Never call the doctor during the day if a night call will do.

3. Never openly oppose the doctor; the art of professionalism must be more subtle.

4. Make the doctor extract the history. Remember, you're paying him.

5. Take your time. The doctor is probably in more of a hurry than you are.

6. The doctor needs you more than you need him.

The foregoing article is intended to be of an introductory nature only, and the serious student is urged to join the local chapter of the Society of Professional Patients of Canada where group classes and practical demonstrations are arranged monthly. For those unable to attend, the Society has a correspondence course entitled, "New Horizons for the Patient in Six Easy Lessons." Please enclose 50 cents for handling and the top of any unpaid doctor's bill.

A male gynecologist is like an auto mechanic who never owned a car.

Carrie Snow

ALCOHOL PERMITTED *"It certainly is great to be alive."* ★

OUT OF BED *"I'm in luck. What a doctor!"*

BATHROOM PRIVILEGES *"Ain't nature grand?"*

SITTING UP *"That doctor is a wizard!"*

VISITORS *"So I said to him . . ."*   ALLOWED TO GO HOME *"I guess I wasn't as sick as I thought."*

STITCHES REMOVED *"Not so bad."*

FIRST SMOKE *"What a relief!"*   WEEK AFTER *"I certainly got trimmed for that."*

FIRST REAL MEAL *"Um-mm, that was good."*

PASSED GAS AFTER ENEMA *"Thank Heaven for that!"*

ORANGE JUICE RETAINED *"I'm going to make the grade after all."*   MONTH AFTER *"Let him wait. He has plenty."*

LINE OF NORMAL GRATITUDE

RECOVERY FROM ANESTHESIA *"So far, so good."*

DAY OF ENTRY TO HOSPITAL ☆
"I'm the sickest man in the world."

THREE MONTHS AFTER *"I don't think I needed that operation."*

DAY OF OPERATION *"Hope I live through it!"*   KINDLY REMIT *"Rushing me, huh? I'll show him!"*

PAYMENT DEMANDED *"Who the devil does he think he is?"*

☆ **PROPER TIME TO MAKE FINANCIAL ARRANGEMENTS**   LEGAL ACTION *"Swindler! Faker!"*

★ **PSYCHOLOGICAL MOMENT TO RENDER BILL**   FORCED COLLECTION *"I'll tell the world what a crook he is."*

HUMAN NATURE CHART:
THAT'S GRATITUDE!*

George S. King, M.D.

Above is a chart that shows how a patient feels, at each stage of his sickness and convalescence, about his doctor and the doctor's fee. The chart first appeared in the May, 1934, issue of *Medical Economics*. We published it again in 1956. And we still get requests for copies.

So does the chart's creator, Dr. George S. King, a still-active 86-year-old G.P. from Bay Shore, N.Y. Over the years, he estimates, nearly 1,000 doctors have asked him for copies. He has sent reprints all over the world. Twice his own framed copy has been stolen from his office wall.

The chart has been reprinted in consumer magazines, newspapers and a textbook on business procedures. A medical school handed out copies of the chart along with diplomas. It has been distributed by the New York County medical society and the Australian Medical Association to all their members.

Why such widespread and continuing interest in a chart that was first published more than 31 years ago? "The world changes, and medicine changes," answers Dr. King, "but human nature remains the same."

*Reprinted with permission from Medical Economics, © 1965;42 (Nov).:102–103, Medical Economics Company, Inc., Oradell, N.J. 07649.

DIAL-A-LAWYER*

Dale Orton, M.D.

On first thought, a 24-hour-a-day legal question answering service seems a great idea. On second thought. . .

DOCTOR: Hello? Is this 1-800-LAWYERS?

LAWYER: Yes, it is. Please give me your Visa number and expiration date or your Federal DEA number if you are a physician, osteopath, or veterinarian.

Thank you. How may we help you paddle up life's legal rivers?

DOCTOR: First of all, I think this 24-hour-a-day legal question answering service is a great idea. We doctors are always being second-guessed, but now we can have that legal advice right from the beginning.

You see, I'm the doctor on call tonight in the emergency room, and I've got this drunk here who was punched in the nose. He won't let me examine him.

LAWYER: Was he the fighter or the fightee?

DOCTOR: He's not sure.

LAWYER: What?

DOCTOR: He drank a fifth of Old Grand Dad before arriving.

LAWYER: Did he sign a permission-to-treat form?

DOCTOR: Yes, he did.

LAWYER: Then I see no problem. You'll just have to treat him.

DOCTOR: He did sign the chart permission form, but I doubt that Screw You is his legal name.

LAWYER: So do I. This could be a problem. Why don't you ask him if he wants to be treated? A verbal permission is better than nothing.

DOCTOR: I did, but he wanted to talk about my mother's nationality and sexual preferences instead.

LAWYER: Your patient has come to your emergency room, and you have an obligation to treat him.

DOCTOR: Easy enough for you to say, but this fellow wants to tear my head off. By the way, let's say this guy punches me, too. Can I sue him?

LAWYER: Well, we lawyers are an argumentative lot, and that question could go either way, especially if a 40-percent contingency fee were at stake. I think the real question here involves that venerable legal tenet called The Law of the Deep Pockets. Are you familiar with it?

DOCTOR: No, but I'm afraid to ask.

LAWYER: To put it in a nutshell—at our dollar-a-minute telephone charge, I'm sure that's what you want—if you have insurance, you can and you will be sued.

DOCTOR: Even if not guilty?

LAWYER: Yes.

DOCTOR: How about the patient?

LAWYER: Does he have insurance?

DOCTOR: Not unless it's on the Harley-Davidson sitting out in the parking lot.

LAWYER: That brings us to the other cornerstone of modern legal thought, which is, by the way, the converse of The Law of the Deep Pockets. Plainly stated: A Bum is Judgment Proof.

DOCTOR: So if I don't treat him, I get sued, but if he beats me up, that's too bad.

LAWYER: So to speak.

DOCTOR: Wait a minute. I think my problems are over. The patient just took a swing at the investigating police officer. His nightstick accidentally struck the patient on the head, and he's out cold. I'll call the neurosurgeon in. Besides, the city must have an excellent liability policy.

LAWYER: Isn't that called "turfing" in medical parlance?

DOCTOR: Yes, it is. But I'm asking the questions here. While you're on the line, how about a quickie?

LAWYER: Lawyers don't do quickies, not at $75 an hour.

DOCTOR: I have another patient here, a cute lit-

*Reprinted with permission from MD, © 1986;30(1):37–44.

tle four-year-old named Sally. She fell off her Hot Wheels and bumped her forehead. She didn't lose consciousness and looks entirely normal to me right now.

LAWYER: What's the problem?

DOCTOR: Her mother watched "Half-Hour Magazine" last week. Some guy said that the only way to really diagnose head injury is with a CT scan. If I order the test, the girl would receive an unneeded dose of radiation, and it would be expensive.

LAWYER: What are the chances that there could be something wrong on the scan?

DOCTOR: Oh, I'd guess about one in 500.

LAWYER: Are you a betting man?

DOCTOR: Not usually.

LAWYER: Do you want to see your whole medical career go down the drain in case you're wrong?

DOCTOR: No, but . . .

LAWYER: Tell you what, go back and explain to the mother what you've just told me. I'll do some quick research on the issue and put you on hold. Besides, there's a wife-beater on the other line who's frantic and needs my advice.

DOCTOR: Hello? I talked with the mother and she said no go. She wants the CT scan and mumbled something about paying all those insurance premiums, but when you need the coverage, they always try pinching pennies.

LAWYER: Let's see. *Roe vs Wade . . . Miranda . . . Escobedo.* Ah, here it is. An interesting case on the West Coast. Just last year a teenager fell down and hit her head. She also didn't lose consciousness. The physician who first saw her didn't find any physical signs of closed head injury and refused any further tests. The girl complained of headaches for the next week and finally she managed to convince another doctor to perform a CT scan on her.

DOCTOR: What did they find?

LAWYER: Nothing. Unfortunately, they sued the first doctor anyway and collected ipso facto because he caused her the pain and suffering of *not* knowing that there was anything wrong. What did your four-year-old's mother say?

DOCTOR: First of all, she took out a note pad and copied my name off my name tag. Then she asked me if that was my legal name. Right now she's calling her lawyer.

LAWYER: Did you inform her of our service?

DOCTOR: No.

LAWYER: Just kidding. I rest my case. Look on the bright side. This country already spends $30 billion a year on preventive medicine. So what's another $600? Fire up the CT scanner.

DOCTOR: I will. First I need to get permission. I'll have to call 1-800-BUREAUCRAT, the clearinghouse for hospital admissions and tests not covered under 1-800-FEDERAL, the clearinghouse for Medicare and Medicaid patients.

LAWYER: Just mention our discussion. If they refuse, inform the mother that she can sue them, too.

DOCTOR: Well, it's been interesting.

LAWYER: And your bill is only $24.95. Now isn't that a small price to pay to sleep well at night?

DOCTOR: It certainly is.

LAWYER: Don't forget to tell your colleagues about our new program—Rent-A-Lawyer. For the next month, you can take advantage of our introductory offer. We'll give you an attorney who will follow you on rounds and advise you on any legal pitfalls right on the spot. He even brings his own lab coat. At just $495 a day, this is really a bargain.

Have a nice day.

"THIS IS CORPORATE MEDICINE. PLEASE HOLD . . . PLEASE HOLD . . ." *

Kenneth L. Toppell, M.D.

A physician imagines what might happen if corporate medicine were carried to its logical extreme. You can laugh . . . for now.

Woolworth J. Smith, M.D., reached for the phone as soon as Mrs. Way nodded. Tired, short of breath, and in pain, she'd given in and agreed to enter the hospital. Her physician was concerned, but confident that a few days of inpatient care would relieve her symptoms and allow her to resume her active life. Now all he had to do was get her admission approved.

Smith was pleasantly surprised to hear the phone ring only once. Usually his secretary, Pat Wordwhiz, handled details such as these, but today she had jury duty, so the doctor was on his own.

"CorpuCare Practitioner Services and Support," a Voice answered. "Your well-being is our problem; your problems are our well-being."

"Yes, um, I'm Dr. Smith, and I'd like to admit Mrs. C. N. Way. She's. . ."

The Voice broke in: "Is Mrs. Way a member of our Plan?"

"Yes, of course. Her number is 11-426-72." Smith smiled with satisfaction, thinking, "They never expect physicians to have that information."

The Voice responded: "Is that her authorization number?"

"No. That's her membership number. I'm trying to admit her to the hospital," Smith said.

"She must have an active authorization before she can be admitted." The Voice continued, "I'll transfer you to Authorization."

The phone clicked a few times, and an electronic message intoned: "Please wait. All of our operators are busy, but you will be serviced in a moment."

"Serviced?" Smith thought.

The sound of music, as if transmitted through cloth wrapped in plastic, drifted through the phone. It was a full orchestral treatment of "Yellow Submarine."

Abruptly a higher-pitched, nasal Voice cut in. "Authorization."

Smith identified himself and repeated his goal, "I'm trying to admit Mrs. C. N. Way, member No. 11-426-72."

"What is your patient's name?" the Voice asked.

Puzzled, Smith tried again. "She is Mrs. C. N. Way. Her membership number is 11-426-72."

"Thank you. Please hold." The muffled holding music was now playing "Don't Fence Me In," full orchestra. Smith smiled benignly at Mrs. Way, who was now leaning a bit to the right in her chair. The telephone symphony had swung into "Muskrat Ramble" before the new Voice cut back in. "The beneficiary's authorization number is 74-A-Arnold-B-Box-26."

Mildly annoyed, Smith hung up the phone, and hurried around his desk to straighten up the tilting Mrs. Way. She had chronic forniculation. This was her first full-blown attack since Smith had made the diagnosis some months earlier.

Regatta Lovely, Smith's laboratory assistant, came to take Mrs. Way to the hospital. The patient was calm, relieved to know that her discomfort would soon be ended.

As Regatta and her charge were leaving, Pat returned, released from the jury box once the plaintiff's lawyer learned she worked for a physician. She was the most efficient secretary Smith had ever employed, and until today she'd shielded him from CorpuCare's admissions process. He told her of his phone call, and she smiled knowingly.

*Reprinted with permission from Medical Economics, © 1987;64 (June 8):171–175, Medical Economics Company, Inc., Oradell, N.J. 17649.

INFORMED CONSENT & OTHER COMPLICATIONS OF HEALTH CARE

Smith returned to the preparation of his evening lecture, "The Role of Body Language in the Treatment of Chronic Forniculation." He was a fornicular specialist, renowned in his field. It seemed that only a few moments has passed when he heard a knock on his door. "Come in," he called, and Pat and Regatta entered his office. Smith was surprised to see Mrs. Way, propped up against the wall.

"Dr. Smith, the hospital won't admit Mrs. Way," Regatta announced. "The business office said she hasn't received preadmission clearance."

"I spoke to CorpuCare myself," Smith said, indignant. "What are they talking about?" He reached for the phone again.

"CorpuCare Practitioner Services and Support. Your well-being is our problem; your problems are our well-being." It was the same Voice, at least.

"This is Dr. Woolworth Smith again. I just called to arrange to admit Mrs. C. N. Way, member No. 11-426-72. The hospital says she hasn't been cleared. What's going on?"

"Is that her authorization number?" said the Voice.

"No, that's her membership number. Her authoriz. . . ."

"I'll transfer you to Authorization, Doctor."

"Wait!" Smith sputtered helplessly as the phone clicked and the syrupy sounds of "Girls Just Want to Have Fun," full symphonic arrangement, came through. As the orchestra swung into "On the Road Again," he was tapping his fingers impatiently on his desk.

"Authorization." It was the same nasal Voice. "How may we help you?"

"You can't," Smith began to explain. "I have an authorization number for my patient. I am trying to get her admitted."

"You need to speak to Someone Else, Doctor. This is Authorization. I'll transfer your call."

The lush notes of "Monster Mash" made Smith's eyes cross. He looked out to see Pat lifting Mrs. Way's head from a tub of ivy as Regatta wiped the potting soil from her once-smart coiffure.

Someone Else came on the line. "Practitioner-Provider Relations. How may we help you?"

"This is Dr. Woolworth Smith. I have been trying to admit a patient to the hospital." Hearing the angry edge to his voice, Pat was worried.

"Is the patient a beneficiary?" Someone Else asked.

"Beneficiary, hell! She's a member of the plan. She has been authorized. And she is sick."

"There is no need for profanity, Doctor." Someone Else sounded a bit prissy. "What is her membership number?"

"11-426-72."

"What is her authorization number?"

"74-AB-26."

"Is that B-box or V-vehicle?"

Smith paused and forced himself to swallow before he answered, "B-box."

"Thank you. Please hold." Before Smith could react, the phone had clicked and the telephone orchestra was playing "Itsy Bitsy Teenie Weenie Yellow Polkadot Bikini."

Pat could feel the tension in the room. Smith was holding the phone by the mouthpiece, leaning forward at his desk. His knuckles were white, and there was a line of sweat glistening on his upper lip. In the waiting room, Regatta was trying to keep Mrs. Way from forniculating in the wheelchair.

Someone Else came back on the line, saying, "Now then, how may I help you?"

"First, do not put me on hold. Next, tell me how to get my patient into the hospital." Smith was trying to regain his composure; surely he could reason with the Voices.

"Certainly. All the beneficiary needs is a preadmission clearance."

"But I was given an authorization number to admit Mrs. Way," Smith's voice was rising slightly.

"An authorization doesn't mean anything," Someone Else chuckled. "That's just the number you use when you call for preadmission clearance. What is the nature of your patient's problem?"

"Acute exacerbation of chronic forniculation," Smith answered smoothly, back on his own turf at last.

"And who gave the second opinion?" Someone Else was obviously filling in blanks on the preadmission clearance form.

"I didn't get a second option. There's not time. Mrs. Way is acutely ill," Smith's voice was much louder. Through the door, he could see Regatta and Pat lifting the twitching Mrs. Way back into the wheelchair.

"We have found that many admissions can be avoided if another physician sees the patient. Often these problems can be handled on an outpatient basis," Someone Else was reciting. "We recommend that Dr. Woolworth Smith review all forniculation cases. Why don't you call him?"

As Smith screamed, "I *am* Woolworth Smith!" Someone Else hung up.

Pat heard the scream and sensed what was needed. She grabbed the damp washcloth off the now comatose Mrs. Way's forehead and forced it into Smith's mouth. She gently guided him onto his couch. Then she went for decaffeinated coffee.

When she returned, Smith was back at his desk. "Who's the medical director of that damned plan?" he was back in control—angry, but controlled.

"R.I.P. King," Pat replied immediately, and provided the telephone number from memory. She'd run this maze often.

Smith dialed King's office.

"CorpuCare, Medical Director King's office." It was a recording. "Dr. King will return your call after 11 PM if you leave your name, number, and a brief message after you hear the tone. . . ."

Smith didn't hang up the telephone. He dropped it on his desktop as he rose with enormous dignity, removed his white coat, slipped calmly into his sports jacket, straightened his necktie, and stepped over to open the window of his 12th-floor office.

Pat dived for his ankles as he got the window fully open. Regatta helped her to wrap the struggling, howling Smith in the straightjacket he kept on hand for the most acute fornicular episodes. Then Pat picked up the phone and dialed. It rang just once.

"CorpuCare Practitioner Services and Support," the Voice answered. "Your well-being is our problem; your problems are our well-being."

<hr />

For additional satires on managed care, see the following:

1. Parker DS: With HMOs—well, who really knows. JAMA 1996;276:1006u.
2. Savinese SJ: What an HMO really is. Med Economics 1992;69(Mar 16):79–83.
3. Weinberg RB: The once and future physician. Ann Intern Med 1989;110:753.
4. Williams BJ: The train is leaving the station. N Engl J Med 1994;331:1316–1317.

QUAC: A MODEST PROPOSAL FOR OPTIMAL USE OF CT SCANNING EQUIPMENT*

Michael H. Reid, M.D.
Arthur B. Dublin, M.D.

Many articles have addressed the issue of cost containment in medical care, and the high cost of computed tomography (CT) has been used to illustrate this problem.[1-3] The impact of diagnostic-related groups (DRGs), preferred-provider organizations (PPOs), cost-conscious hospital administrations, and increased governmental controls is certain to affect the practice of radiology.[4] We describe a new technique that will enable increased diagnostic examination output in the face of limited resources and funds.

Current estimates suggest 1500–2000 body CT examinations per CT scanner per year as an appropriate patient load, but it is likely that budget limitations and the rising costs of CT facilities will necessitate heavier use. However, it is unlikely that CT efficiency can be increased with current operating techniques. We propose multiple simultaneous patient examinations—quantity uniaxial compositomography (QUAC)—as an alternative.

Technique

Figure 1A illustrates this new multiformat examination technique with four children in prone, supine, and right and left lateral decubitus positions symmetrically placed about the central CT axis. Occasionally, five children and rarely, only three might be accommodated. Figure 1B illustrates two adult patients and Figure 1C, the resulting image. Using the format shown in Figure 1B, 4000 examinations per year could be performed with a single scanner. In a children's hospital with smaller patients, this figure would be 6000–8000 or even higher. For neuroradiologic studies, the number of examinations possible with the QUAC technique rises precipitously, particularly in practices restricted to patients with small heads.

Manufacturers should be encouraged to develop CT scanners with large padded apertures with low-friction Teflon coating for ease in patient positioning. Water-soluble sonographic jelly could be used as a nonstaining aperture lubricant to aid in patient packing by hydraulic ram, if necessary. Small wiggling children might require a multinippled pacifier suspended in the gantry to reduce anxiety and motion artifacts.

Discussion

Anticipated savings in the cost of medical care are significant. Special "batch" rates could be offered to groups of patients with the same disease and/or same insurance carrier. For areas with certificate-of-need limitations on CT scanner purchases, this method provides an obvious solution. Multiinstitutional sharing of a CT scanning facility with the various patient slots (positions) assigned to different hospitals (e.g., hospital A patients at 3 o'clock position, hospital B patients at 9 o'clock position) is another possibility.

Among the advantages of the QUAC technique, air-tissue artifacts due to incomplete filling of the gantry aperture will be eliminated. Ideally, studies should be restricted to all male or female subjects,

*Reprinted from the American Journal of Roentgenology, © 1984;142:845–846, with permission from the American Roentgen Ray Society.

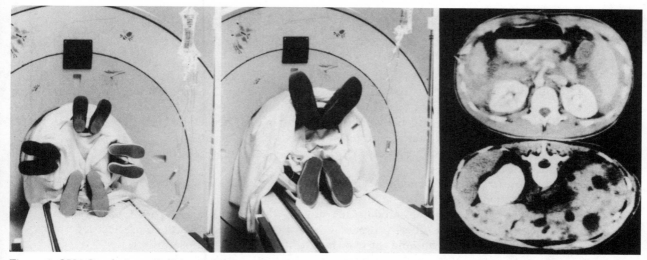

Figure 1. QUAC technique. A, Four pediatric patients positioned in CT gantry aperture. B, Two adult patients positioned for simultaneous examination and (C) resulting image (*bottom*, liver cysts; *top*, ruptured spleen [unrelated to patient positioning within gantry]).

radially oriented with anterior surfaces outward, for patients' comfort and privacy. In view of the cost savings and other benefits, it is unlikely that patients will complain of used x-ray photons. Multiple simultaneous patient examinations recorded on the same film will provide some normal anatomic control, thus making abnormalities more apparent. Some examinations may be difficult to combine, for example, pelvic CT with cranial CT. Otherwise, QUAC has much to offer the future practice of diagnostic radiology.

References

1. Evens RG, Jost RG. Computed tomography utilization and charges in 1981. Radiology 1982;145:427–429.

2. Schoppe WD, Hessel SJ, Adams DF. Time requirements in performing body CT studies. J Comput Assist Tomogr 1981;5:513–515.

3. Hughes GMK. National survey of computed tomography unit capacity. Radiology 1980;135:699–703.

4. American College of Radiology. TEFRA and DRG's: section 108 revisited. ACR Bull 1983; Sep 7.

The above article reminds me of another radiologist with a great sense of humor. Benjamin Felson was the editor of *Seminars in Roentgenology* from 1966 to 1988. Throughout his career, Dr. Felson had a penchant for collecting unusual radiographs which he occasionally published in the journal. Most of them fell under the heading, "Foreign Bodies I Have Known." The others consisted of amusing interpretations of the shadows and artifacts that turn up on x-rays from time to time. For the uninitiated, see the following references in *Seminars*.—H.B.

1981;16:159–161.   1986;21:1–2.
1983;18:167–168.   1988;23:235–237.

QUAC PROPOSAL*

In perusing the April 1984 issue of *AJR*, I was chagrined to see that our more aggressive West Coast friends[1] once again have "scooped" their more conservative East Coast colleagues, who are still collecting cases. We agree that packing children in groups of four with their heels together and toes pointing outward (as shown in the authors' Fig. 1A) is the only sensible way to perform computed tomographic (CT) scanning in a pediatric practice.

However, I do not think that Figures 1B and 1C illustrate the optimal scanning position for adults. We have found that in selected cases, it is preferable to place one patient prone and the other supine, with the toes of each patient toward the toes of the other. This makes the examination considerably more enjoyable for the patients and can even lead to lasting relationships. I am surprised that the California-based authors did not think of this possibility.

It is reassuring to see that *AJR* is devoting some much-needed time and effort to improving the efficiency of medical care and lowering its cost.

Robert H. Freiberger, MD
Hospital for Special Surgery

New York, NY

Reference

1. Reid MH, Dublin AB: QUAC: a modest proposal for optimal use of CT scanning equipment. AJR 1984;142:845–846.

Reply

The Pauli exclusion principle prevents two electrons of a pair from facing in the same direction (i.e., spins must be opposite); the Reid-Dublin exclusion principle prevents two persons in a magnetic resonance scanner or computed tomographic scanner from facing in the same direction—except perhaps in San Francisco.

Michael H. Reid, MD
University of California, Davis School of Medicine

Sacramento, CA

*Reprinted from the American Journal of Roentgenology, © 1984;143:433, with permission from the American Roentgen Ray Society.

WHAT IF THE PATIENTS BILLED US?*

Howard J. Bennett, M.D.

After many years in practice, I've become accustomed to a certain amount of give and take with patients. Compromising about which lab tests are necessary or when to seek a second opinion are part of day-to-day medical care. I've even mellowed in those situations when patients need to exercise some control in their lives—even if the research they quote comes from the Journal of Community Advice or from Grandparent's Quarterly.

But I never thought I'd see the day when I might have to compromise on the most fundamental aspect of the doctor-patient relationship—namely, who bills whom. Given the current climate of patients' attitudes toward health care (not to mention its practitioners), I can now imagine certain scenarios in which that, too, comes into question.

Case 1: Be Late, Be Billed

It's 1 PM on a Friday. Following a rough night on call, Dr. Daniel Krauss has just worked through his fifth lunchtime this week. He's finishing up with his last patient when the child's mother hands him a bill for $165.

"This is my fee for Jacob's visit today," Mrs. Wright says.

"Pardon me?" asks a bewildered Dr. Krauss.

"It's a late fee."

"A what?"

"A late fee. You know, for being late."

"But you never objected to my being late before," says Dr. Krauss.

"Well, no, but I was never a member of P.A.I.D. before."

"What's P.A.I.D.?"

"Patients Against Inconsiderate Doctors. It's a new consumer group."

"Catchy name," says Dr. Krauss.

"Our motto is 'A doctor's time is just like mine.'"

"I see," Dr. Krauss says. "So you're billing me for the 50 minutes I kept you cooped up in the waiting room."

"Exactly," Mrs. Wright says. "And, as you'll recall from that rather long social history I provided at Jacob's first visit, I work as a lobbyist for a prestigious firm downtown."

"I remember," Dr. Krauss says.

"My consulting fee is $200 an hour," Mrs. Wright adds.

Not bad, Dr. Krauss thinks to himself, wondering if it's too late in life for a career change. If not as a lobbyist, then perhaps as a professional patient. "Will a check suffice?" he asks.

"That will be fine," Mrs. Wright says. "Just remember to put your Social Security number on the back."

Case 2: The Costly Pinworm

It's 8 AM on a dreary Thursday, and Dr. Joseph Cama has just finished his morning telephone hour. He leans back to relax with his second cup of coffee when the phone rings.

"This is Dr. Cama."

"Yes, this is Roberta Barnes. I'm Chester Barnes' mother."

"Hello, Mrs. Barnes, how can I help you?"

"I wanted to talk to you about Chester's last visit. If you check his chart, you'll notice that we were in about a month ago."

"Well, ummm, I don't actually have his chart in front of me at the moment."

"Oh, that's okay. I realize that you're busy, and I want to let you know that I didn't mind having to wait an hour to see you last month."

*Reprinted with permission from Medical Economics, © 1990;67 (July 9):83–87. Copyright by Medical Economics Company, Inc., Oradell, N.J. 07649.

"Thank you for being so understanding, Mrs. Barnes."

"After all, Chester is a resourceful child. He busied himself with your toys, while I spent the time writing a letter to my ex-husband."

"It's always good to keep busy."

"Dr. Cama, have you ever seen what some children actually do with the toys they find in your waiting room?"

"I try not to."

"Well, about three days after the visit, Chester came down with a terrible case of pinworms. And I am certain that he picked up the infection at your office."

"I see," says Dr. Cama. "Is he still having trouble?"

"No, he's okay now. But the night he got sick was awful. He began scratching at 3 AM and had the whole house up by 4."

"I'm sorry to hear that."

"I knew you would be, Dr. Cama, since you've always been a sensitive doctor."

"Thank you, Mrs. Barnes. I try my best."

"I want you to know that I have discussed this issue extensively with Chester's therapist. Although she reassured me that pinworms will not cause an anal personality disorder, I've come to the conclusion that the only way we can put this episode behind us is to have you pay the emergency room fee. Including X-rays, the bill came to $287. I will be glad to do my share and pick up the cost of the medication."

A loud thud is heard from the upper end of Mrs. Barnes' receiver.

"Hello? Dr. Cama? Are you there?"

Case 3: Paying for Pox

It's 5 PM on a Friday, and Dr. Agnes Ryan is getting ready to leave for a well-deserved vacation. After she finishes with her last patient, she stops to read the mail before heading out to meet her husband. The first thing she picks up is a registered letter that her receptionist signed for earlier in the day.

Dear Dr. Ryan:

This is to inform you that your patient, Emily Stone, returned to nursery school before all of her 463 chicken pox lesions had completely crusted over. Based on interviews with the girl's parents, it is apparent that this breach in the school's health policy was a direct result of improper patient education on your part.

The consequences of this omission can hardly be overstated: Every child in our school and three staff members (one of whom was about to get married) came down with chicken pox over the past six weeks.

Enclosed you will find an itemized bill for all of the physician, lab, and hospital fees that accrued as a result of this epidemic. Also included is the cost of cleaning calamine lotion out of the school's two Oriental rugs, and the cost of replacing our pet hamsters (Ying and Yang) who died mysteriously during this time. The total bill comes to $28,417.

We accept all major credit cards.

Sincerely,

Bernice Johnson, Director
The Get Ahead Nursery School

Of course, it's doubtful that any of these cases would *really* take place. But if they did, would we be ready to face the challenge?

Would existing malpractice insurance pay these new costs? Or would we need a new breed of coverage? In addition to Blue Cross insurance for patients, would there be Double Cross coverage for doctors? And finally, would competition among carriers lead to the development of prepaid patient payment organizations (PPPOs)?

I can hardly wait to find out.

Additional Readings

1. Anonymous: The doctor-witness who didn't keep his cool. Med Economics 1979;56(Jan 22):81.

Since lawyers usually have the upper hand in the courtroom, this article is fun to read. It contains a brief excerpt from an actual court transcript. After a doctor is grilled about his credentials and experience, he snaps back with the last word: **Q.** Do you recall the time that you examined the body of Mr. Edgington? **A.** The autopsy started around 8:30 PM. **Q.** And Mr. Edgington was dead at that time? **A.** No, you dumb ass! He was sitting on the table wondering why I was doing the autopsy.

2. Bennett HJ, Weissman M: Agenesis of the corporate callosum: a new clinical entity. N Engl J Med 1987; 316:1220.

This is a satirical case report about a new corporate malady. It involved a health maintenance organization, Moneycare Corporation of America, and a community hospital (St. Avarice).

3. Bennett HJ: Health care reform or bust. J Fam Pract 1994;39:393–394.

This article satirizes the current debate over health care reform. Assuming that change is inevitable, the author ends on this note: "No longer will obstetricians be allowed to admit patients for routine deliveries. No longer will brain stapling be an acceptable treatment for obesity. And finally, *primum non nocere* will no longer be taught to medical students. From now on the first rule of medicine will be *primum no dinero*."

4. Bennett HJ: Who's suing and who's sick. Med World News 1991;32(9):61.

This is a satire about a doctor who sues one of his patients for noncompliance.

5. Fred HL: On being politically correct. South Med J 1992;85:865.

Given the current preoccupation with not offending anyone, the author presents both a traditional and a politically correct case report. For example, an 80-year-old patient is "chronologically gifted," and someone who's dead is "terminally inconvenienced."

6. Kamholtz T: When you're the patient. Med Economics 1957;34(Oct):148–149.

The author presents some amusing thoughts about what happens when doctors are on the other side of the stethoscope.

7. Markle GB: What if everybody had to get informed consent? Med Economics 1976;53(Apr 5):148–152.

The author ponders what might happen if nonprofessionals were required to tell customers about the risks associated with their services.

8. Morgan KR: What to tell third parties who use and abuse you. Med Economics 1974;51(Aug 5):130–135.

The author, who is tired of dealing with myopic insurance companies, presents some of the pungent letters he has written over the years on his patients' behalf.

9. Reemtsma K, Maloney JV: The economics of instant medical news. N Engl J Med 1974;290:439–442.

The reporting of medical "breakthroughs" in the lay press has been a problem for many years. After studying this phenomenon, the authors came up with a new law of medical economics: "The public impact of instant medical reporting is inversely related to the intrinsic merit of the observation."

10. Rochelson B, Stone ML: The designated defendant. Obstet Gynecol 1987;70:662–663.

The authors propose that elderly physicians (85+ years of age) be used as the attendings of record at teaching hospitals. That way, in the ten or more years it would take for a malpractice case to get to court, that should be the worst of their problems.

11. Schrifrin BS: The biblical basis for the rising Cesarian section rate. J Perinatal 1986;6:99–100.

This article demonstrates how humor and satire can be used to address a serious topic in health care.

12. Venuti FJ: If Medicare ran baseball. Med Economics 1993;70(March 22):94–100.

Games would be held in the snow, some home runs wouldn't count, and new rules would come out every other week. Sound familiar?

13. Vosk A: New stratagems for dealing with Medicare's prospective payment system and other cost-containment measures. JAMA 1991;266:121–122.

This clever article spears Medicare and DRGs with the following conceit: the best way to keep hospitals in the black is by admitting and providing care to dead patients—i.e., low overhead but good reimbursement.

SURGEONS &
OTHER SPECIALISTS

More than half of the articles in this chapter were written by or about surgeons. Whether this implies that surgeons are more revered than other specialists or less, I'm not sure. In any event, the chapter does offer a revealing look at the consulting process and some of the specialties. The reason each organ system is not fully represented is that a lot of humor never makes it out of the cath lab. It's clear from the following excerpt, however, that no one in medicine gets off scot-free.

> "Humor is quite common when house officers refer to specific rotations and hospitals to which they are assigned . . . No specialty is spared. Radiology becomes radioholiday, while nuclear medicine is known as unclear medicine. Gastroenterology is referred to as scoping for dollars and anesthesiology is known as doping for dollars. Urology probably has the most nicknames, such as stream-team and whiz-kids, to name a few. Orthopedic surgeons have to be strong as an ox and only twice as smart, and think that the sole function of the heart is to pump antibiotics to the bones."
>
> From "Humor and the Physician" by Fred D. Cushner, M.D. and Richard J. Friedman, M.D. (see Appendix).

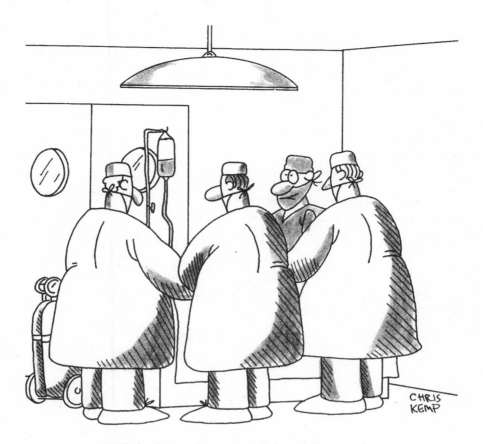

With the chest cavity open and the heart fully exposed,
Dr. Robbyn suddenly regretted cutting class to go pub crawling
that crisp fall day four years ago.

COMMUNICATING WITH SURGEONS, ONCE YOU LEARN THE LANGUAGE, IS POSSIBLE MOST OF THE TIME*

Patty Swenson, R.N.

An area close to my heart (and quite possibly my ulcer) is "Communicating in the O.R." The reason there are difficulties in this area can be directly traced to the fact that most O.R. nurses sign on with only their mother tongue as a means of communication. Although the job descriptions never mention it, fluency in "Surgeon Speak" and its several dialects—one for each surgeon—is easily the key to on-the-job success or failure.

For example, the manufacturer's catalog will refer to a certain instrument as a Mayo clamp, but only a fool will ever expect to hear it called by that name. Instead surgeons will ask for heavy curves, curved sixes, fat Kellys, and in moments of intense concentration, "that one over there." Kitners, kuntners, peanuts, and occasionally, cherries, all refer to the same blunt dissector. Schnitz, snits, and tonsils are the same stroke to different folk.

One surgeon will call an instrument by many pet names, depending upon how it will be used. Alone it's a right angle; feed a piece of suture into its little beak and you have a tie on a mixter. The list is endless, and I will bet there are some regional variations that would bring tears to my eyes.

But conversation in the O.R. is less than stimulating, despite the occasional burst of confusion from instrument names. Most of the exchanges are hardly enough to keep the mind alive. I quote:

"Give me a tie."
"What kind?"
"Any kind."
"Here's 3-0 silk."
"Terrific!"
"You're welcome."
"I didn't ask for a rope. I asked for a tie."
"You have it."
"Then what is THIS?"
"Three-0 silk."
"Man oh man. This sure doesn't FEEL like 3-0."
"What DOES it feel like?"
"It feels like 2-0."
"Trust me."
"I TRUST you. But next time I want thin 3-0."
"Ooookay."

Surgeon Signal

Next we have "Surgeon Signal." This is a series of hand signals substituted for the spoken word, used to request objects with perfectly good given names. They are used instead because the surgeon in question (a) doesn't know the real name, (b) is saving his voice for bigger and better things, (c) assumes the scrub nurse is deaf, or (d) all of the above.

Among the more common signals are

- The forefinger and middle finger moving up and down against each other in a scissors-like fashion meaning "I wish to cut."
- The thumb and forefinger meeting one another in a rapid pinching motion usually indicating the desire for a pickup.
- The hand formed into a semi-fist and whipped rapidly in a partially clockwise direction, quaintly requesting a needle and thread on a needle holder. Now really, wouldn't the simple use of the word suture be a lost less wearing on everyone?

One of my favorite surgeons has a habit of simply holding out his hand, as if to make a left-hand turn, giving you the option of placing in it whatever you think will strike his fancy.

Surgeon Snag

To me, the average surgeon's concept of time is the eighth wonder of the world and something for which there is no rational explanation. "Surgeon time" is not necessarily "clock time" as we know it. There is no established rule for converting one to the other, but a safe guideline is if your surgeon says, "This will only take 45 minutes," DOUBLE it! In many cases—and these you quickly become familiar with or go mad—TRIPLING it is a more realistic approach to estimating when the room will be available for someone else. No matter what *they* say, *you* know better. And *they* know *you* know. And *you* know *they* know *you* know. Which explains the half-crazed expressions worn by surgery supervisors during working hours and why they are so often observed babbling pathetically to no one in particular.

The final thing that contributes to the downfall of even the brightest and best O.R. supervisor is directly traceable to the "Supply and Demand Equation." This boils down to something like, "The number of supplies and instruments a surgeon says he will need is inversely proportionate to the amount he will ultimately require." This law is most effective after 3 PM and on weekends.

All in all, after years of research, observation, and personal experience, I can safely say that communicating with surgeons, once you learn the language, is possible most of the time.

A GUIDE FOR INTERPRETING WHAT SPECIALISTS REALLY MEAN*

Howard J. Bennett, M.D.

Communicating with specialists can be a tricky business. This is especially true for those of us who refer patients to academic medical centers. Interactions with our learned colleagues generally fall into three categories: the consultation letter, getting put on hold by their receptionists, and actual conversations if we are lucky enough to catch up with them when we're rounding at the hospital. Of course, once we do connect, it takes experience and cunning to figure out what the specialist is actually trying to say. Therefore, I offer the following guide to help bridge the gap between what our colleagues say and what they really mean.

What the Specialist Says	What the Specialist Really Means
Thank you for the letter you sent detailing the patient's history.	I didn't actually read it, but I'm sure it was interesting.
I'd like to do a full diagnostic workup to ensure that we've ruled out all organic possibilities.	This guy looks like he'd sue his mother.
Thank you for allowing me to assist with the care of your patient.	Send me all the cases you can. My kid just got into Harvard.
The patient made an uneventful recovery after surgery.	If you call respiratory arrest, septic shock, and a week in the ICU uneventful.
I'm sorry it took so long for this letter to arrive, but the typing pool has been backed up lately.	I misplaced your patient's chart under a pile of grant applications.
The physical examination was unremarkable.	I'm only interested in procedures anyway.
Thank you for giving me the opportunity to see this pleasant family in consultation.	Boy, am I glad I didn't go into primary care.
I think we'll need to admit your patient for additional diagnostic studies.	The hospital census is low.
I think we can complete the diagnostic workup on an outpatient basis.	I don't have a fellow on the wards this month.

*Reprinted from The Journal of Family Practice 1992;34:505–507, with permission from Appleton & Lange, Inc.

What the Specialist Says	What the Specialist Really Means
Thank you for referring this most interesting patient.	It was pretty boring, actually, but I'm always glad to help out.
After an exhaustive workup, a review of the literature, and a discussion with my colleagues, we have not yet arrived at a definitive diagnosis for your patient.	Damned if I know what's going on.
I don't need to see your patient again unless unexpected complications develop.	I'm busy writing up a research proposal.
This letter was dictated but not read.	I'm on service this month and actually had to take call last night.
I agree with your excellent diagnosis.	Even a third-year medical student could have picked this one up.
Don't hesitate to call if you have any questions concerning your patient.	I'll be on vacation for the next 2 weeks, so call as much as you'd like.
The following studies have been done, but the results are pending at the time of this dictation.	So you better check them yourself.
I recommend that your patient get a PET scan.	We just bought our own PET scanner.
As you know, we just published this treatment protocol in the *Journal of Definitive Research*.	You *did* read our article, didn't you?
I recommend that you send your patient to one of my colleagues who is a leader in this field.	I don't see HMO patients.

This is obviously just a sampling of the many verbal maneuvers available to the seasoned consultant. Considerable variations are possible for those with creative imaginations.

COME BACK DR. CURMUDGEON*

Kenneth R. Morgan, M.D.

The old-time practitioner was a fiery autocrat compared to today's colorless counterpart, says this Connecticut OBG man. If the trend towards docility continues, these ghastly scenes may occur.

In the days between World Wars I and II, no surgeon worth his salt ever left an operating room unless the scrub nurse was in tears, the anesthetist cowering in a corner, and the assistants nursing their bruised knuckles in ashen dismay. When he stomped down the corridor, glowering left and right, the orderlies ran for cover, and the medical students took to the hills like frightened deer. It's a pity this splendid prima donna has disappeared from our midst.

An occasional pallid imitation still wields his knife in the amphitheatre, but the spirit has seeped out of him. He knows in his heart that the scrub nurse will tolerate his ferocity only so long as it amuses her; that the intern, if he is lucky enough to have one, will break scrub and find more congenial company unless the old bomber remembers to be polite; and that the anesthetist will treat him with a lordly disdain at the first sign of pique.

I won't be at all surprised if a few years hence the typical operating room scene will be played out something like this:

SURGEON: Suture!

SCRUB NURSE: Say please.

SURGEON: Suture, *please!*

SCRUB NURSE: Once more. And no sarcasm this time.

SURGEON: Please?

SCRUB NURSE: That's better. (*She forks it over.*)

SURGEON (*to assistant*): Would you mind sponging the wound so I can see?

ASSISTANT (*bursting into tears*): I can't stand it! Orders, orders, all day long! Never a kind word!

SURGEON: There, there. After the operation we'll have a little chat about a raise in salary, and I'll try to be a little more understanding in the future.

ASSISTANT: All right—as long as you promise.

SURGEON (*to anesthetist*): The patient seems to be getting a little light. Muscles are kind of rigid.

ANESTHETIST: It's not necessary to reflect on my ability. You'll notice that I refrain from criticizing *you.*

SURGEON: No criticism intended. I simply meant that because of my own ineptitude I need more muscle relaxation for exposure than most surgeons do.

ANESTHETIST: In that case I accept your apology.

SURGEON (*concluding operation and beaming at everybody*): Thank you, thank you, one and all! You've been most tolerant this morning. . . .

In the old days, the atmosphere was as tense outside the operating room as in. For example, what floor nurse would have dared remain seated when old Tyrannosaurus rex stormed into the ward trailed by his house staff? At the first sound of approaching thunder she tossed her copy of Elinor Glyn into the wastebasket and leaped to attention, reciting a catechism of temperature readings, pulse fluctuations, and bowel movements as if entranced.

Nowadays, the doctor making rounds goes through a sort of ritual courtship of the head nurse before extracting the requisite information. It won't be long before you can expect the nurses' station to be the setting for this short drama:

DOCTOR: I hate to disturb you, Miss Imperious, but how is Mrs. Brown doing?

NURSE (*busy manipulating six ball-point pens of different colors to make an artistic time sheet showing who will be on night duty next week*): I wish I could tell you, Doctor, but as you well know—or should— Miss Globetrotter is in charge of all patient information. Get clearance from her, and I'll tell you. You'll find her in the south building.

*Reprinted with permission from Medical Economics, © 1962; 39(Jul 16):188–200, Medical Economics Company, Inc., Oradell, N.J. 07649.

DOCTOR: Thank you ever so much. Before I look for her, perhaps I ought to glance at the chart—if I may?

NURSE: The chart will be back from Miss Granite shortly. She's using it in a student nurses' class. Perhaps you'd care to sit and wait.

DOCTOR: Why, that's very nice of you, Miss Imperious. You don't find that kind of hospitality everywhere in this hospital! . . .

When it came to getting along with patients, the curmudgeon was in absolute command. Compared to the formidable old party of yesterday, we're pathetic weaklings. I can imaging this scene being played at the consulting room desk of the future:

PATIENT (barging in, unannounced): Sit down, Doctor. Dr. Zircon in Springfield suggested that when I moved to Bridgeport I should shop around for an obstetrician.

OBSTETRICIAN: How nice! I see you have a stenographer's pad with you, and I imagine you want to ask a few questions. But before we begin, let me give you this booklet. It tells all about me—my early childhood, my struggling years in—

PATIENT: No, no Doctor. My questions go deeper. I already know your medical background, basic experience, percentage of deliveries missed, and so forth. We *all* read Medical Consumer Reports.

OBSTETRICIAN: Yes, well, the reason Medical Consumer Reports gave me only an "Acceptable" rating last year was—

PATIENT: No need to apologize. I'm aware it was because the magazines in your waiting room were weeks old. Tell me, now: What do you think about when you deliver a baby at 4 o'clock in the morning?

OBSTETRICIAN: Often I think about George Muldoon, who sat next to me in high school and flunked out his second year, and who now makes $200,000 a year as a plumbing contractor.

PATIENT (writing furiously): I see. And how about your thoughts when you first hold in your hands the precious fruit of a mother's womb?

OBSTETRICIAN: Hold what?

PATIENT: The baby, the baby!

OBSTETRICIAN: Oh! Well—I think that if I can just get the episiotomy sewn up without sticking a vein, then maybe I can go home and get two hours' sleep before office hours.

PATIENT (sneeringly): Two hours' sleep! Doctor, you should be in some other line of work.

OBSTETRICIAN: Funny you should suggest that too. George Muldoon told me the same thing just the other day. . . .

But perhaps I'm being over-pessimistic. After a steady movement toward total docility, the medical pendulum could, I suppose, swing back again. For all I know, my colleagues have already started to lead the profession back toward wholesome curmudgeonism. Consider the following three conversations. Would you give Dr. A's responses or Dr. B's?

PATIENT (at 3 AM): I just thought I'd call and let you know I'm feeling much better, because I didn't want you to worry.

DR. A: You shouldn't have bothered. I like to worry.

DR. B: That's fine, but just to make sure you're OK. I'll give my answering service instructions to call you every hour on the hour for the next five nights.

FLOOR NURSE (at 9 AM): How did *I* know I wasn't supposed to wake the patient to give her the Seconal?

DR. A: That's perfectly all right. I should have been more explicit.

DR. B: And how did I know the hospital hired an imbecile?

Are you a Dr. A or a Dr. B? If you're a Dr. B, you're a curmudgeon, and there's hope for the rest of us.

CONSULTMANSHIP:

How to Stay One-up on Colleagues*
Anthony Shaw, M.D.

The art of consulting involves a good deal of medical one-upmanship. Such feats as feeling a spleen that's eluded all previous palpators or hearing a diastolic murmur that has previously gone undetected will score points for almost any consultant.

My first experience with the heady joys of consultmanship came when, as a senior surgical resident, I put on the consultant's hat. Often I'd be summoned by quaking medical residents to face down hemorrhage or to grapple with pus. Writing in a bold, steady hand, I'd speedily summarize a problem that had baffled another service for weeks, dismiss all the diagnostic possibilities studding the chart, and offer the correct diagnosis. Then in a spirit of noblesse oblige, I'd invite one and all to troop up to the O.R. and witness the cure. Now it's been some years since I was a surgical resident, and it may not have been exactly like that, but that's the way I prefer to remember it.

From my initial emergency consultation, though, I emerged not one-up, but definitely one-down. It started with an urgent call from the psychiatric wing of my medical center. The psychiatry resident, a young woman, had a patient—also a young woman—who'd suddenly started to hemorrhage from somewhere *down below*. She wanted a surgeon to come over and check it out. Not wanting to steal a case from GYN (especially at 4 AM), I asked which orifice the blood appeared to be coming from. There was a pause, during which I heard some whispering at the other end.

"She doesn't know," answered the psychiatrist.

"I see," said I. "Would you have a look and call me back?"

Her shock and dismay came through loud and clear: "Do you mean you want me to examine her perineum?"

"Well, yes," I said, falling back on my best 4 AM weapon, sarcasm. "I believe that even psychiatrists can tell which is which."

"Doctor," she said (you're in trouble when another doctor calls you Doctor), "I *never* examine my patients. It would ruin our rapport!"

I've told this story to a number of psychiatrists, and the first one has yet to laugh, which certainly must be an indication of something or other.

The techniques of consultmanship vary from specialty to specialty, but within each field of practice, certain consistencies may be recognized. Take the matter of consultation notes. The ophthalmologists', being in code, are comprehensible only to other ophthalmologists. Orthopedists' notes are brief. Typically, they say: "Chart read and patient seen. Will return after reviewing X-rays." Since the X-rays usually can't be located, this may be all there is to the note. One pediatrician got back at the orthopods. When he was called to see a young orthopedic patient with bilateral facial swelling, his entire succinct note read, "Mumps."

Neurologists' notes are paragons of organization, covering at least three sheets and ending with an offer to return and reevaluate the patient—if any change in condition should be observed. I don't think I've ever read a neurologist's note all the way through because I've always had to see another patient or have lunch or something. Nonetheless, as The New York Times ads say, "You don't have to read it all, but it's nice to know it's all there."

In many consultants' notes, various diagnoses are suggested not in order to establish them but to rule them out. Following a consultant's description of the physical findings of a patient howling with abdominal pain, one may read:

"Impression:

"1. Rule out peptic ulcer.

"2. Rule out acute pancreatitis.

*Reprinted with permission from Medical Economics, © 1970:47 (Aug 31):162–168, Medical Economics Company, Inc., Oradell, N.J. 07649.

"3. Rule out appendicitis.
"4. Rule out PID.
"5. Rule out twisted fallopian tube.
"6. Rule out splenic infarction."

"Rule out appendicitis" is a favorite pediatric note for a youngster with abdominal pain, McBurney's point tenderness, fever, vomiting, and elevated white blood cell count. I think this notation reduces the burden of guilt the pediatrician may feel when his little patient is carted off to be cut up by wicked surgeons. After all, he didn't say it *was* appendicitis, so he can't be blamed for what happens in that tiled chamber of horrors upstairs.

Every woman seen in the emergency room with abdominal pain and a little fever has pelvic inflammatory disease until the attending OBG man on call makes his appearance to rule it out. "Put her up in stirrups, and I'll be right over," comes the advance telephone warning. Most seasoned OBG's tend to affect a tremendously effective air of utter boredom that lends great authority to their consultative notes. Somehow they seem to be able to tell over the phone that young women awaiting them in the emergency room have pristine pelvic organs. While this clairvoyance rarely relieves them of the obligation to make the trip to the E.R., it does enable them to rouse themselves at 3 AM, amble over, in and out of the E.R., write "No GYN pathology" on the chart, and return home to slide back in the sack, having scarcely disturbed a good night's sleep.

Internists strain to outdo the neurologists in producing truly comprehensive consultative notes—a talent they acquired while surgeons were practicing square knots on bed posts. I remember one budding internist back in residency who would see a patient, and for two days no one could approach him nor would he discuss the case.

At the end of this time, an exquisitely typed "case report" would appear on the patient's chart. It not only would include the findings along with a diagnosis but also would provide a full review of the literature and bibliography on all diseases in any way related to the patient's. Sometimes his note would appear too late to help the patient, but it would be very useful in the subsequent CPC. That man is now solidly esconced on Park Avenue where he's able, in a busy week, to see five patients in consultation. His opinions are generally considered the last 10,000 words.

Surgeons on the other hand rarely write elaborate notes. As a matter of fact, surgeons are often much too busy to write notes at all. When the typical surgeon appears on the medical floor at 8 or 9 PM after his day in the O.R., he has in tow his resident or intern, whichever has a pen and legible handwriting. "Looks like perforated ulcer"—or hemorrhoids, or femoral thrombosis, or whatever— he barks. "Get him typed and cross-matched and we'll take him up!" After making sure the house officer is getting it straight on the chart, he rushes off to the coffee shop.

Occasionally a consultant feels that, while he doesn't know what a patient has, he could handle it better if the patient were in one of the consultant's own beds. Thus, a medical consultant's note may read in toto: "A fascinating case of vitiligo, nausea, and amnesia. I will be happy to accept this patient on my service." Surgical consultants are prone to a similar type of brevity: "Patient has gallstones. Will accept for transfer."

Sometimes the above formalities are dispensed with altogether. In that event, the consultant may substitute what I've heard some surgeons call "active" consultation—others call it case-stealing—for the more common "passive" kind. For example, a plastic surgeon I know of was once asked to evaluate a lump on the wrist of a medical patient. The next day, while making rounds, the primary physician noted a dressing on his patient's wrist and a sling on his arm. The complete "consultation" note on the chart included operative findings and a pathology report. One-up!

FOURTH AND GALL*

Leo A. Gordon, M.D., F.A.C.S.

"Good afternoon ladies and gentlemen and welcome to today's Southwestern conference matchup. We've got a dandy for you here. Dr. Floyd McKittrick, whom we've seen so many times before, will be going up against Lou Ronson—a big strapping hulk-of-a-guy with chronic biliary tract disease. We know you're gonna like this one. And doing the play-by-play is my good friend and colleague of so many American Surgical League broadcasts, the ol' Texan himself—Coach Dave Baker—David!"

"Good Morning Keith! And good morning everyone. It's a nippy November morning here in Houston. The room is in perfect condition and the participants are ready. You know, we've seen so many great match-ups on this very field. I believe you and I covered a GI bleeder here many years ago. McKittrick was just a student then, probably all wide-eyed watching the big boys. Now here he is himself—the main event. He is halfway through his eighth season in the American Surgical League. Most observers feel that he's just hitting his professional stride. He's got great hands and he's rugged. His greatest strength, though, is this innovative offense. He's not rigid, he adapts. That's been the key to his success in the league."

"Dave, how about this fellow Ronson?"

"Keith, Lou Ronson is a 52-year-old cost analyzer for an aeronautical research company. He has a long history of right upper-quadrant pain with two ER visits in the last month. Ultrasound shows stones in a contracted gallbladder with no other abnormalities. It's the general consensus of all players involved that cholecystectomy is indicated. He's a big man, 6 feet 2 inches, 195 pounds, and in good shape. He's eager and he's ready."

"How about the field conditions which you mentioned at the top of the broadcast?"

"The field is perfect, Keith. The lights are new. The table has recently been serviced. The floor is a bit slick, but otherwise playable. The suction is in peak condition. Temperature in the high sixties. Perfect biliary weather!"

"Thank you David. We'll be back with the starting line-ups after this commercial message."

Cut to commercial: Promo for "Greatest Surgical Legends" Special.

"Hello again, folks. The ol' Texan Dave Baker will go over the lineups. David!"

"Thanks, Keith. Floyd McKittrick will be working wiith his long-time first assistant, Dr. Calvin Duffey. They've been working together for years, although they are often viewed as unlikely teammates."

"How so?"

"Well, McKittrick is one of these Southwestern boys—good natured, low key, but not afraid to innovate in tight situations. Duffey is a product of that disciplined Northeast conference—very conservative on offense and unusually rigid on defense. Yet, when these two are on—when they really have it going—there is no finer duo in the league."

"How about anesthesia today?"

"Anesthesia controversy has dogged this conference for years. McKittrick has chosen his own for today's match. He's gone over his game plan repeatedly with the special teams and feels that they're ready."

"Thanks Dave. The patient is being induced. The prep is underway. The nursing staff is ready. We'll be back with the skin incision after these messages."

Cut to commercial: Promo for Network Investigative Report on "Medicine and Cognition—Fact and Fancy."

"Hello again everybody. Dave Baker and Keith Mattson bringing you a barnburner here from the rugged Southwestern Conference of the American Surgical League. McKittrick and company are going up against a tough rock-em sock-em bag of stones and we're going to stick with it all the way."

*Reprinted with permission from Surgical Rounds, © 1985;8 (11):80–87. Edited from the original.

"Here we go, ol' buddy. He's starting with a right subcostal."

"Yes. He's done this routinely for years. No reason to change with his record."

"Pesky bleeder at the midline."

"Nicely handled with the cautery."

"Okay, he's in. The abdomen is open."

"Now watch McKittrick on routine exploration, Cool, methodical, updating the team at every move."

"Great, no abnormalities on routine exam."

"Remember the unexpected pancreatic mass last season?"

"Yes indeed. The boys in programming really caught heat from our viewers when they elected to pull away from the broadcast after the cholangiogram."

"Here we go. He's begun dissection at the porta."

"Let's watch Duffey. He's short, but what strong hands! He can hold that position for a long t . . ."

"Fumbl-l-l-l-l-l-le!"

"The duodenum has slipped up and covered the field. Hold on a moment. Who recovered? It's Duffey. Somehow he replaced his hand on the duodenum. He definitely has possession. The porta is visible again."

"Okay folks. McKittrick has identified the cystic duct. He's looking for the artery. Hold on to your tickets. Wait a minute. Yes, I thought so. Bleeding during cystic duct dissection. This could result in a delay-of-case call."

"Watch Duffey with the suction, Keith. Very few players use it so well. Gentle, not abrasive. There's the vessel. He's quick clipping. Here it is on the replay. Vessel, bleeding freely. Duffey comes down, slight curving motion, he's around it, gently, firmly, clipped . . . stopped. What a player!"

"McKittrick has the cystic artery now. He'll doubly clip it, but not divide it, as is his usual move. He'll go up top."

"If our overhead camera can get a view of the fundus, we'll see him dissect out the gallbladder from the liver bed. But before that, a word from our sponsors."

Cut to commercial: Promo "The Halsted Chronicles."

"Welcome back folks. While we were away, McKittrick began his posterior dissection. What do you think Dave?"

"He's made his peritoneal incision. It's as thick as cow hide, buddy. Here he goes. Hold on . . . he's in the liver bed!"

"Not unusual in a match like this. Let's watch him work. Staying on the gallbladder as best he can. He's really in and out of it."

"Very dense inflammation."

"Yes, and you know how the men in the striped shirts can interpret that."

"Oh-oh! There's a lap on the play!"

"Watch McKittrick's face. He knows he must continue without arguing the call at this time. There he goes. The gallbladder is almost free. The vessel he clipped earlier is definitely the cystic artery."

"He's dividing it."

"What was the call?"

"Unnecessary roughness."

"Let's replay that on the monitor. There's the fundus. He dips behind. Well, the inflammation really obscured our angle. Let's just say it was close. Unnecessary roughness is subject to a lot of interpretation. This certainly wasn't the most obvious case."

"McKittrick kept his cool. He's fourth and gall. What do you think he'll call now?"

"No question in my mind."

"Cholangiogram?"

"Cholangiogram."

"Definitely. Cystic duct cholangiogram. The graphic shows McKittrick's record from last season. Thirty cholangiograms out of 39 cases for a cholangiogram rate of .769. Not bad."

"How about the positives?"

"Ten true positives last season."

"A great record."

"Here we go. Now watch Duffey duck out. He ducked out early, seeking the protection of the x-ray barrier. He's shown us just about his only fault as an assistant—leaving the field before the play is finished. That cost him last week."

"Okay. The gram is underway. No. He's hesitating. Oh-oh baby! Another flag."

"No question Keith—delay of case. No x-ray tech."

"Oh, that hurts."

"Here he is. The contrast is in . . . It's good!"

"Let's cut to the films for our viewers. There is the cystic duct entry. There's the distal duct with good emptying. There is the proximal duct. There's the right hepatic. There's . . . oh-oh Mama!"

"What?"

"Big stone in the left hepatic duct!"

"Great. We'll get a chance to see McKittrick shift from a one-one offense to a one-two with resident or nurse during the bile duct exploration."

"A real treat for our viewers—a common bile duct exploration. You're in for a thrill. We'll be back after these messages."

Cut to commercial: Promo for "Catgut Capers."

"Watch this folks, and watch it well. McKittrick routinely performs a Kocher during bile duct exploration."

"He Kochers as well as anyone in the league."

"There he goes. He'll get that distal duct and pancreatic head up lickety-split."

"Watch Duffey."

"Oh Sally-Jean! Duffey is out of bounds. He's over by the cava! O.K., he's recovering nicely."

"You think they'll call it."

"It's close. They'll let it go."

"McKittrick is opening the duct. He'll be using a biliary Fogarty. Here he goes. It's up. It's long enough. It's straight enough. Here it comes. It's GOOD! He's got the stone."

"How about a completion gram, Keith?"

"Floyd McKittrick is a wiley ol' fox of a player. He knows the value of a disciplined completion gram both for filling defects and, equally as important, for precise tube placement."

"O.K. Folks. In case you just joined us, we had a lulu of a hepatic stone extraction. Here's the replay of the stone extraction and completion gram. How about it Davey?"

"Here's the tape Keith. The catheter is up. It looked to me as if it veered to the right initially, but not so. Stone is out. The gram is perfect. Great placement and no other defects."

"Thanks, Dave. We're back live. Oh Nellie! Just hold on. The field is really unsteady. McKittrick feared this in a pregame interview."

"It's the anesthesia problem again, Keith. Another flag. He's getting a ten-minute major misconduct for improper abdominal relaxation. This could definitely shift the momentum."

"O-o-o-o he's hot! McKittrick is arguing. Very unusual for him to do this. He prides himself on good communication with the entire team. He's settled down now. The field is stable."

"He's using a round Silastic drain Keith. Any comments?"

"Well, Dave. What can you say about a league

that's spent the last 50 years arguing about a piece of rubber?"

"Right you are. He'll use it and use it well."

"Ronson is drained. Let's watch the closure. Oh-oh. Wait a minute. McKittrick is stopping. He's motioning for the room to quiet down. Crowd noise can be a problem late in the match. He's still motioning. There he goes. His assistant can rely on audibles now. Here's the closure. Remember last season when several players were deemed ineligible because of closure problems?"

"I sure do. The famous 'cheap bite' controversy in the Midwest Conference really cut into the credibility of a lot of the players."

"Can't fault McKittrick here—monofilament, running, locking, two layer. Skin clips. Great match."

"He's done. He's leaving the table quietly. Quite a change from last season."

"Yes. The ACS rule against postmatch celebrations within three feet of the playing field has really stopped a lot of the hoopla."

"Remember that anterior resection in the Big Eight we covered two years ago? Who was it, Slauson?"

"That's right. Big Daddy Slauson—had the lesion licked and lost it all on a high-five that contaminated his left glove. What a mistake!"

"Drama, controversy, success, failure, we've got it all in the American Surgical League broadcasts. Stay tuned folks, we'll be back with our postgame interviews and wrap-up after these messages."

Cut to commercial: Promo for the American Surgical League Playoffs.

"Welcome back, folks. We've been covering a real shoot-em-up for you here today. Things have gone well. We have Ahmal Ossard in the recovery area who'll be doing the postmatch interviews for us. Ahmal? Ahmal can you hear us?"

"Keith?"

"Ahmal?"

"Keith?"

"We seem to be having some tech . . ."

"Keith. I'm here in recovery with Lou Ronson who appears to be doing very well after the match. Vital signs are great, good respiratory effort. Clear bile in the bile bag. Lou, how do you feel?"

"Ahmal. I'm . . I . . . Where . . . The nurse. . . ."

"Well, Keith, Lou is a bit excited about the match. Perhaps we should come back to him."

"O.K., buddy. Maybe you could get over for a locker-room interview with McKittrick."

Cut to locker room.

"Floyd, you had problems early in the case. The bleeding around the porta, the poor relaxation, the unexpected hepatic duct stone. You came through. Things went well and the patient is fine. How do you feel?"

"Ahmal it was tough. I had a great team in there today. We all worked together to get the job done and emerged with a win."

"Your assistant, Cal Duffey. What can you say about him?"

"Cal was great. He protected me when he had to. He knew where I was during the entire match. His retraction was superb during the exploration of the duct."

"We have that on tape. Watch the monitor. Here he is positioning the duct."

"Yes. He had just the right amount of tension. Real steady. The fumble during the duodenal retraction had me concerned, but after Cal recovered, I knew we'd be all right. You know, Ahmal, everyone maligns the assistants, but they're key. Everyone in the league knows they can take a poor player and make him respectable, and take a mediocre player and make him a star."

"How about anesthesia?"

"We've had our problems with anesthesia all season. We shifted the line-up and brought up some rookies early in the year. Dr. Stanton came through today."

"What about the delay-of-case call during the cholangiogram?"

"Look, I know the refs have a tough job. I though it was unnecessary at that time. It's a judgment call. The x-ray tech was at lunch. You know how those things can happen."

"You looked real down after the unnecessary roughness call during the gall-bladder dissection."

"The patient had a lot of inflammation posteriorly. The gallbladder was partially intrahepatic. The line judge called it, I'm sure, because of the bleeding. You and the viewers realize that after years of inflammation, that plane can be hard to find and bleeding can result. I thought it was overcalling it, myself, particularly at the 150 cc line."

"What now Floyd? Where does Floyd McKittrick go now?"

"Ahmal, we did a great case today. I'll be stopping by recovery to review the orders and talk to Lou Ronson. Then I'll review everything with the family. After that, I'll go to the office to line up the rest of the schedule."

"We look forward to covering your cases in the future."

"Thanks, Ahmal. Can I say one thing?"

"Sure."

"Hi Mom!"

"Back to you Keith and Dave."

"Okay, friends—there you have it. A beautiful cholecystectomy with bile duct exploration and extraction of a left hepatic duct stone. A beautiful match with an early good result. Thanks for being with us. Please remember next week we'll be covering a big pancreatic tail lesion in the tough Western Conference. This is Keith Mattson and the ol' Texan, Dave Baker, saying good-bye for now."

She got her good looks from her father—he's a plastic surgeon.

Groucho Marx

THE ABDOMINAL SNOWMEN*

Anthony Shaw, M.D.

If public relations men had had their way, the first appendectomy would have been a different story.

Unfortunately for them, the citizens of the last century were denied the magnificent press coverage now given to surgical breakthroughs. One hundred years ago, surgeons gained recognition slowly— through the grueling process of publishing articles about their work in scientific journals and presenting the results at medical meetings. If they were lucky, their colleagues eventually recognized their achievements. For example, it took more than a century of contributions by many physicians, often working independently of one another in different countries, before appendicitis was acknowledged as a cause of abdominal distress. One of these physicians was Rudolph Krönlein of Zurich, Switzerland.

How different it would have been for Krönlein (and the rest of us) if modern communications had existed 100 years ago:

April 7, 1886—Radio Bulletin—

We interrupt this program to bring you a special report. CBS-Geneva has just learned that Switzerland's first human appendectomy is being performed at this moment in a Zurich hospital. Authorities at the hospital refuse to divulge the name of the patient, but the surgeon is said to be Dr. Rudolph Krönlein, head of the hospital's new division of abdominal surgery.

April 8, 1886—Zurich Straatszeitung (Reuters)—

A 3:42 PM Swiss time, the first human appendectomy in Switzerland was performed at Zurich's Allgemeinische Krankenhaus by Dr. Rudolf Krönlein and a team of six specialists. All that is known so far is that the patient is a 17-year-old female who is presently under the care of a special team of 23 nurses in the hospital's intensive care unit. In an effort to avoid accusations of publicity-seeking, Dr. Krönlein and his associates will not speak to reporters until tomorrow, when a ward in the Krankenhaus will be converted to a pressroom and Dr. Krönlein will hold a nationwide TV conference.

April 9, 1886—Zurich Zentralblatt (UPI)—Appendix Woman Passes Gas.

In the first release since yesterday's surgical breakthrough, spokesmen for Dr. Rudolf Krönlein have announced that Irmagaard Gluck, the 17-year-old woman who underwent Switzerland's first appendectomy, has, in scientific terms, broken wind. According to famed American surgeon Dr. Mondrian Kantor, this is a necessary first step in her recovery. Dr. Kantor, who has performed many appendectomies on dogs and rabbits, has been trying to find a suitable patient for the first American appendectomy. In a confidential report to UPI, Dr. Kantor predicted that in the future many appendectomies will be performed.

April 10, 1886—WCBS-TV (By Telstar)

MC: Welcome to "Face the World." Our guest today was, until two days ago, an obscure doctor known only to his medical colleagues. Today, he is an international celebrity. Ladies and gentlemen, it gives me great pleasure to introduce the Swiss surgeon Rudy Krönlein. Dr. Krönlein, how do you feel?

Dr. Krönlein: Humble and proud, of course.

*Reprinted with permission from MD, © 1986;30(12):112–117.

MC: Dr. Krönlein, can you now detail for us the events that led to this medical breakthrough?

Dr. Krönlein: I think there are many surgeons in the world today who are capable of removing the appendix from a living human being. The world is ready for this operation, and medical progress demands that it be done. We have done many appendix operations on mountain goats here in Switzerland, and when Ms. Gluck came into our laboratory—sorry, I meant hospital—we had our team ready to go.

MC: What was the most thrilling part of it all for you?

Dr. Krönlein: Toward the end—when I found myself looking into the right lower quadrant of a living human being and saw the big space where the appendix had been.

MC: Have you shown Miss Gluck her appendix?

Dr. Krönlein: Of course. Her comments will be published in her autobiography, which she has sold to an American publisher for an undisclosed sum.

MC: Dr. Krönlein, you have been accused of doing this operation as a publicity stunt in order to get your grant renewed. Is it possible that Miss Gluck did not need to have her appendix removed?

Dr. Krönlein: Why, my dear boy, our pathologists will tell you that I got it out just in time.

MC: Our reporter at the intensive care unit says that Miss Gluck has peritonitis and pneumonia, has become jaundiced, and is hemorrhaging.

Dr. Krönlein: These are things that can happen to any patient and have nothing to do with the success of the appendectomy.

MC: Are you planning to perform any other appendectomies?

Dr. Krönlein: I have six patients awaiting the operation at the Krankenhaus right now, and, as soon as I finish my world tour, I plan to perform it on them.

May 14, 1886—Zurich Zentralblatt (AP)—Commission Formed.

In the wake of proliferating appendectomies during the past month, a distinguished commission of army officers, clergymen, and lawyers has been appointed to study the deep moral and ethical issues raised by the operation. Expected to testify are Dr. Mondrian Kantor, who only this morning performed an appendectomy on a newborn anencephalic; Dr. Hector Gomez of Venezuela, who favors partial appendectomy; and Sir Osler Worthington, who feels that since the appendix is the seat of the soul it should not be tampered with under any circumstances.

Famous last words: Die! My dear doctor, that's the last thing I shall do!

Lord Palmerston

POSTMORTEM MEDICINE—
AN ESSENTIAL NEW SUBSPECIALTY*

Berril Yushomerski Yankelowitz, M.D.

With increasing technical knowledge, medical care has necessarily become more and more subspecialised.[1-14] Both the local community and the government have tried to approach the problem of delivering this care to as broad a segment of the population as possible. Especially notable are the heavily funded programmes in geriatrics research, as all segments of society have come to recognise the increasing proportion of old people in the population. The time has now come for us to focus on the medically most underserved population in the world today—the deceased. The urgency of this is quite apparent. There are more people who have already died than are alive today, and their number is increasing at an alarming rate. Physicians have not focused on the problems of the dead. Aside from anatomy, it is not a subject taught in most medical schools; as a result, early sensitivity of the medical student to the needs of the dead is never formally developed. Postmortem medicine is not a mere extension or subspecialty of geriatric medicine, but a major specific and unique problem in health-care delivery. We have therefore undertaken a pilot project to determine how the medical profession might better serve the dead patient, and this is the subject of the present paper.

The University of East Dakota Medical Center's pilot project on postmortem medicine is a broad-based multidisciplinary undergraduate and postgraduate study programme designed to investigate all aspects of diagnosis and care for the dead patient. Early in their training our medical students are given a one-semester course in psychosocial problems of the deceased human. In addition to didactic sessions, students are taken on field trips to cemeteries and funeral parlours, because we feel that classroom sessions alone depersonalise the dead patient in the student's mind. The members of our psychiatric faculty have responded enthusiastically and like this subject because they get to do most of the talking during patient interviews. Psychoanalysts are especially happy because of the long, meaningful silences they get when treating a dead patient. In the second year of medical school we provide courses in pharmacology and physiology in the dead patient. We have found that the pharmacokinetics of drugs in formalinised patients are quite different from those in the living. So far we provide only one clinical clerkship in cemetery medicine, but plan to offer a series of electives for interested students in funeral parlour physiology.

At this postgraduate level we have a pilot postmortem ward (separate from the morgue), which is staffed by two fellows who are supported by a National Institutes of Health (NIH) career development grant. The fellows are supervised by a senior attending physician, who is himself dead and therefore has an in-depth understanding of the specialty. The ward promotes active house-staff and nursing education and is a model for future programmes of similar type in the community. House staff who have just been on a ward with live patients have responded enthusiastically to the leisurely pace of the postmortem ward.

Research projects are going on, and we are fortunate to have received extensive Federal and local grant support for such studies as postmortem wound healing, the impact of embalming on social acceptability of the dead, management of the person who died before penicillin was available, and so on.

A series of new subspecialties is already appearing—postmortem endocrinology, postmortem podiatry, and postmortem neurosurgery to name a few. Some of our staff have developed a special in-

*Reprinted with permission from the British Medical Journal, © 1979;2:1639–1640.

terest in the long-dead patient, and we are considering a subsubspeciality of neanderthalogy.

In co-operation with the NIH and Rand Corporation, we have developed an extensive computerised programme of health-care services, delivery evaluation, assessment of the dead patient with peer review panels, and HMO (Heaven's Medical Offices). Our social-professional interface is progressing nicely. We already have a board certifying examination, and memberships are now open for our National College of Postmortem Medicine. The women's auxiliary of the American Dead Society has actively supported our many community efforts.

We have made substantial inroads in a neglected area and it is our hope that other universities will benefit from the billions that our government now wants to spend in this exciting new subspecialty.

References

1. Parlov SM: Death as a subspecialty. Sem Death 1979;1:6.

2. Parlov SM, Puttersberg RK: The mandate for internists to broaden their care for the dead. Sem Death 1979;1:100.

3. Puttersberg RK: Referral patterns in postmortem medicine. Sem Death 1979;1:120.

4. Puttersberg RK, Parlov SM: Health care delivery to the dead. Rand J Financial Medicine 1972;82:184.

5. Parlov SM, Yankelowitz BY: Management of the dead patient embalmed prior to 1842. Publications Unanimous 1648;2:15.

6. Yankelowitz BY: Outcome assessment and proven evaluation in postmortem care delivery. Rand J Grant Med 1987;8:43.

7. Yankelowitz BY: A randomised double-blind trial of formaldehyde versus placebo in third party olfactory detection of the dead patient. J Clin Invest Death 1979;49:862.

8. Yankelowitz BY: A longitudinal study of 357 dead patients. Ethiop J Anat 1257 AD; 27:4.

9. Puttersberg RK. The role of the physician's assistant in caring for the deceased—letter. Ann Int Death Med 2027 AD; 53:60.

10. Parlov SM: Federal regulation of rehabilitation of the patient embalmed with multiple chemical agents. Univ E Dak Newsletter 1979;(July 5):1.

RISKS OF CURB-SIDE CONSULTS*

To the Editor: Near dusk on a recent afternoon, I had just returned from a four-mile jog. One of my neighbors, a state trooper, was walking by with his medium-sized poodle on a leash. He beckoned me to the curb, "Hey, Doc, will you take a look at this?" He pointed to a small lesion on his nose. I walked over to him and leaned over with my steaming glasses in the fading sun to offer an opinion. I felt a sudden, piercing pain in my medial right thigh. The poodle had bitten through my sweat pants and punctured my leg in five places.

The lesson here is to be wary of giving advice at the curb side. Beside giving the wrong advice, you may get into more trouble than you bargained for, especially at dusk, with a state trooper and his poodle.

Hyannis, MA

William W. Stocker, M.D.

*Reprinted with permission from The New England Journal of Medicine, © 1980;302:1094.

Additional Readings

1. Barrett DS: Are orthopaedic surgeons gorillas? Br Med J 1988;297:1638–1639.

Extrapolating from the fact that hand size correlates with body size, this study shows that orthopedists are only slightly bigger than their colleagues in general surgery. The author concludes that "The image of the orthopaedic surgeon as a man of massive bulk and strength with a low hairline who communicates with his colleagues in a series of grunts while proceeding along the hospital corridor in a succession of ape like bounds is unfair."

2. Bornemeier WC: Sphincter protecting hemorrhoidectomy. Am J Proctol 1960;11:48–52.

This is a serious article with an amusing introduction: "It (the sphincter ani) is like the goalie in hockey—always alert . . . It apparently can tell whether its owner is alone or with someone, whether standing up or sitting down, whether its owner has his pants on or off . . . a muscle like that is worth protecting."

3. Bryant RD: An unusual obstetrical case history. Obstet Gynecol 1953;2:187–200.

This article is a tour de force. Using quotations taken directly from Shakespeare, the author pieced together a fascinating case report.

4. Burton JL: Skins are simpler than you think. Bristol Med Chir J 1986;101:15.

This article distills the practice of dermatology into a few easy to remember rules.

5. Cohen JHM: Pregnancy in elderly women. Lancet 1991;341:1668.

The title of this letter is a little misleading. A better one might be "A Report on the Methodologies Used in the Immaculate Conception."

6. Diamond EF: Why surgeons are real swingers. Med Economics 1977;54(Jan 10):200–207.

A nonsurgeon pokes fun at the two things that separate surgeons from the rest of us: a sense of style and a grasp of dramatic values.

7. Dias JJ, Brenkel IJ, et al: Orthopaedic surgery: a health hazard. Br Med J 1988;297:1637–1638.

The authors use a light touch to describe some of the dangers orthopedic surgeons face—both in and out of the operating room.

8. Gay SB, Selby B, et al: Autoradiology: patient heal thyself. AJR 1990;154:871–873.

In an effort to curb radiology costs, the authors studied the feasibility of patients performing radiology procedures on themselves. All necessary precautions were taken to prevent complications. For example, "When performing interventional procedures, we instruct patients to talk to themselves continuously and to notify the tech immediately if they get no response."

9. Goldberg JH: Would you swap a vasectomy for a new radiator? Med Economics for Surgeons 1984;3 (July):49–52.

The author presents some of the interesting solutions that patients have come up with to "pay" their doctors.

10. Gottschalk W: Dystocia on Mount Olympus. Obstet Gynecol 1959;13:381–382.

The author presents the obstetric histories of the Olympian Gods. For example, "Athene, Goddess of War, was delivered fully armed from her father's brow . . . The obstetrician in charge, far from being a physician (which is probably just as well) was Hephaestus, God of Fire." It's enough to make modern obstetricians quake in their booties.

11. Hoffman RS: Guidelines for equivocation in EEG reports. J Irreproducible Results 1993;38(6):20–22.

Since neurologists love qualified answers and the rest of us don't, the author presents his own solution to EEG equivocation. For example, "These findings are entirely nonspecific and consistent with a variety of medical conditions, most neurologic disorders, a state of excellent health, or electrode artifact."

12. Hulka JF: Multichannel automatic natality sensor with instantaneous computer-integrator and audiovisual recorder. Obstet Gynecol 1971;37:155–157.

Given all the high-tech equipment that's used in obstetrics, the author proposes "a new instrument" to monitor pregnant women: a physician's hands.

13. Merrel SW: Surgical aphorisms. West J Med 1991; 154:110–111.

This article contains two pages of witty sayings for surgeons. For example, "There's no such thing as bowel function at the VA," and "Never ask a surgeon whether you need an operation."

14. Novak DL, Bates BF: Digital radiology: uses and limitations of the method. AJR 1989;152:870–872.

Since rulers disappear from radiology departments as quickly as interns disappear on Friday nights, the authors advocate the use of fingers (digits) to quantify x-ray findings.

15. Pry P: Surgery in the future. Boston Med & Surg J 1892;127:395.

After observing that his cures by abdominal section had to be reopened at frequent intervals, a 19th century surgeon devised a technique whereby he could reinspect a patient's internal organs without the bother of parietal section: He simply closed the original incision with buttons and buttonholes. What is most interesting about this parody is that it anticipated by 90 years, the first implantation of a zipper into someone's abdominal wall (Leguit P: Zipper closure of the abdomen. Neth J Surg 1982;34:40).

16. Reid MH, Dublin AB: Simultaneous anthropomorphic projections. AJR 1985;144:861–862.

How to reduce radiology costs by overlapping body parts and x-raying them at the same time.

17. Rose I: Fellowshipmanship. Can Med Assoc J 1962;87:1232–1235.

This article is a satire on how to be a specialist. For example, "The specialist must always appear to be fond of the general practitioner, the same way a good citizen is fond of his dog or the Mountie of his horse."

18. Rose I: Counterfellowshipmanship. Can Med Assoc J 1964;90:1410–1413.

This article has some good lines for those of us who spend our time submitting consults rather than filling them out. It was published under the auspices of "The National Society for the Prevention of Cruelty to General Practitioners."

19. Ryall RL, Marshall VR: Point of view: laws of urodynamics. Urology 1982;20:106–107.

The authors bemoan all of the complicated formulas and biophysical jargon required to understand the idiosyncrasies of the urinary system. They present their own 7 laws of urodynamics. For example, "The patient with the best flow has the poorest aim."

20. Shaw A: Is there a surgeon in that quaking mass? Med Economics for Surgeons 1984;3(June):54.

The author reminisces about what it's like during a resident's first skin-to-skin operation. For example, when the attending says "Press a little more firmly on your scalpel," he really means, "This wimp's going to take three hours to get through the skin."

21. Shaw A: Today's most "in" specialty. Med Economics 1975;52(June 9):53.

This is a brief satire on the newest *specialty* in medicine—thanatology. Since all specialties need a board exam, the author has taken the liberty of writing one. Here's a sample question:

A Harvard ad hoc committee has made recommendations on how to determine when death has occurred. According to Harvard's criteria, a person is dead when:
  (a) His fingernails stop growing
  (b) He won't smile even when tickled
  (c) Blue Cross stops his payments
  (d) He graduates from Yale

MENTAL HEALTH HUMOR

Psychotherapy, like the rest of medicine, is serious business. It also has its own brand of inconsistencies and absurdities that make it a good target for one's sense of humor. Unfortunately, mental health journals have not opened their pages to much wit and humor. As a result, most of the barbs hurled in this direction have come from the entertainment industry which provides a rather two dimensional and stereotyped view of the field. The following articles provide a much needed dose of humor from the professional's point of view.

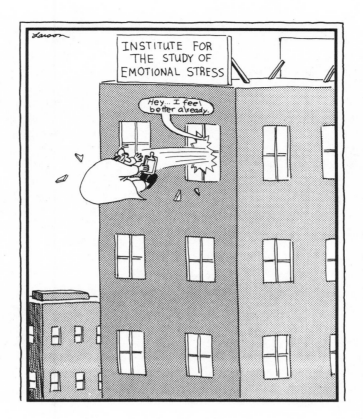

STREAMLINED TREATMENT IN THE ERA OF MANAGED CARE:

The Fast-Food-for-Thought Therapy Approach*
Jane P. Sheldon, Ph.D.

In our hectic, fast-paced world, clients cannot always afford the time it takes for traditional therapy. Additionally, managed care companies have shown a growing reluctance to pay for therapy services that require more than a few sessions of treatment. This has led to the development of a new, time- and cost-effective therapeutic approach, which takes its cue from the fast food industry. The following case study illustrates the effectiveness of this new approach.

THERAPIST: Hello, may I help you sir?

CLIENT: Umm, yes, I'm here because things aren't going well with my job and I just don't know what to do.

THERAPIST: What would you like?

CLIENT: To feel good and be happy in my life, that's what I'd like. That's why I'm here.

THERAPIST: Would you like a drink?

CLIENT: Oh, no! Just because my mother was an alcoholic doesn't mean I'll be! There's no way I'll ever become like her!

THERAPIST: Is there something else I can do for you?

CLIENT: Well, really the reason I'm here is because of my job. I'm just not satisfied at work and I'm constantly anxious.

THERAPIST: Chicken?

CLIENT: A little, I guess. I'm afraid to try things. I guess it's because I think I'll fail. And then work just piles up and I'm never on top of it. I guess you'd call me a procrastinator. I put things off, then they accumulate and suddenly I'm overwhelmed.

THERAPIST: Ketchup?

CLIENT: Exactly. I'm always behind and never seem to be able to catch up. Now and then I'll finally get a job done, but for some reason I still can't relax. I can never let up for a moment.

THERAPIST: Super fries, sir?

CLIENT: Oh, yeah! My supervisor fries my nerves. She's always breathing down my neck making sure I'm not slacking off. It's like having my mother around! Hey! I get it! She's just like my mom! No wonder I always feel so tense and incompetent at work! Wow, Doctor, you're great! I've only been here a few minutes, but I feel so satisfied!

THERAPIST: Anything else?

CLIENT: No, that's all. Thanks a lot, Doctor.

THERAPIST: Thank you, come again. Have a nice day.

After six months of therapy, a psychiatrist was making excellent progress with a patient who had a multiple personality disorder. Since things were going so well, he decided to submit a bill for his services. Two weeks after he submitted the bill, the following letter arrived in the mail:

Dear Dr. Pierce:

As you will undoubtedly recall, Myra was the one responsible for initiating these sessions. She also did most of the talking during the past few months. Since we don't know where she is any more than you do, we have no intention of paying this bill.

Sincerely,
Beth, Laura, Pat & John

DEVELOPING INSIGHT IN INTENSIVE-EXTENSIVE PSYCHODYNAMIC PSYCHOTHERAPY

A Case Study*

Don Yutzler, Ph.D.

Although a voluminous, if not tedious, literature exists on the theoretical construct of insight and its conceptual and dynamic underpinnings, as well as its cognitive and affective precursors and concomitants, little in the way of hard clinical data, drawn from actual real-life therapy cases, has been cited as a means of illustrating the dynamics of insight and "the working through process." The author presents, here, an annotated transcript of therapy sessions with one of his more successful therapy patients in order to vividly illustrate the development of therapeutic insight.

This is the case of a 34-year-old Caucasian male, who sought psychodynamic psychotherapy in order to gain insight into why he had left his ex-wife several years earlier. After a great deal of self-exploration, as well as another marriage and two children, the patient now wanted to embark on a formal journey of self-understanding.

The treatment began with 8 sessions of therapy, during which rapport and a strong "working alliance" were established. The following crucial interchange occurs in the 9th session:

THERAPIST: So, tell me about your ex-wife.
PATIENT: She was a short woman.

As is evident, this purely descriptive reply reflects no true insight. Note also the therapist's technique which, although highly directive, remains remarkably free of any countertransferential cathexes.

By the 14th visit, the therapist assessed that the patient was ready to tolerate more intensive, affectively charged material and so begins to probe more daringly:

THERAPIST: So, tell me about your ex-wife.
PATIENT: As I told you, she was a short woman.
THERAPIST: Um-hmmm. Tell me more.
PATIENT: Well, she weighted about 180 pounds.

In this lively interchange, we immediately note the gains in self-understanding. Although to the naive observer this patient seems rather superficial, the therapist begins to speculate that perhaps the patient is only superficial on the surface.

Again, to the casual listener, the juxtaposition of these descriptive concepts could immediately bring to mind an interpretative intervention; i.e., the woman was obese. But this patient clearly is not yet ready to draw such a conclusion himself and it would be a serious error if the therapist were to precipitously and wantonly blurt out such an anatomical observation. A premature insight could be extremely detrimental to the course of therapy, perhaps shortening it a great deal, perhaps even rendering any further sessions altogether unnecessary. Wisely, the therapist waits.

The next stage of therapy is focused on strengthening the patient's defenses to prepare him to handle the truth. Although the therapist thinks the patient is ready, he has erred, as the following dialogue in the 26th meeting reveals:

THERAPIST: 12 sessions ago, you described your ex-wife as a short woman weighing 180 pounds. Have you given any further thought to these two ideas?
PATIENT: No.
THERAPIST: Why not?

PATIENT: I don't know.

THERAPIST: Would you like to know?

PATIENT: I don't know. Do you think it's important?

THERAPIST: Important? I didn't say it was important. Do you think it is?

PATIENT: I asked you first.

Here, it is evident that the therapist has pushed too hard, and the patient is decompensating. The patient shows this by missing the next 2 appointments, thus requiring 4 more to explore resistance and billing issues.

A breakthrough occurs in the 33rd session when the patient refers to his ex-wife as a "tubster." The therapist, unfamiliar with this slang expression, asks for clarification:

THERAPIST: What?

PATIENT: Tubster.

THERAPIST: No, I mean what do you mean?

PATIENT: She was fat.

Here, the patient is obviously in touch with deeper levels of emotion, for he could have chosen a less pejorative term, e.g. "pleasingly plump," "rotund," or "the wide ride." In "fat," we have hit a nerve. But it was still too early to press for further insight. What remained, of course, was a fuller understanding of the many rolls of the ex-wife's fat in their marriage and its demise.

Finally, in the 40th session, the patient arrives at a marvelous insight:

THERAPIST: So, why did you leave your wife?

PATIENT: I just couldn't stand that short, stupid, fat woman any longer!

So this was it. He had left her because she lacked height and depth, while being overly wide. Notice the exclamation point at the end of the patient's statement, clearly signifying his angry yet liberated tone. Here, we have full simultaneous cognitive and affective insight.

The author is pleased to report that the treatment was successfully concluded in only 12 more sessions, as termination issues were worked through to satisfy the therapist's needs for closure and further income to cover malpractice insurance.

"Occasionally, I experience a complete loss of memory," Tracy said to her psychiatrist. "What do you recommend?"
"I recommend you pay me in advance."

A PROOF OF THE BENEFICIAL EFFECTS OF PSYCHOTHERAPY*

John Ellard, A.M., FRACP, FRCPsych, FRANZCP

There have been many attempts to estimate the positive effects of psychotherapy. Until now, these studies have been concerned with human therapists; none have addressed psychotherapy by members of other species. It's true that there is one report of monkeys as therapists,[1] but they were treating other monkeys, so it could be argued that the results do not apply to therapy with human beings.

The purpose of the study reported here is twofold:

1. To evaluate the effects of psychotherapy when the therapist is an animal other than *Homo sapiens*.

2. To compare the results achieved by two different psychotherapeutic techniques.

The first type of therapy is predominantly verbal, the therapist responding to the patient's communications with certain predetermined phrases, but nevertheless maintaining a neutral affective response to the patient's behavior.

The second type of therapy is non-verbal, comprising essentially non-possessively warm responses to the patient's behavior. The warmth is not endless and uncritical; should the patient behave negatively (for example, by kicking the therapist) then the therapist's response would be to discourage the repetition of such behavior.

The Population

On the premise that psychotherapy is good for everyone, patients were recruited from those seeking employment at the Employment Service agency nearest to the clinic. This was necessary because the available undergraduates have obtained a Supreme Court injunction which states that they cannot be compelled to be the subject of experiments in order to pass their examinations.

Patients were paid $15 for every day they remained in the study. Payment was by check.

Informed Consent

The patients were told that they would be paid to receive therapy which would certainly enrich their lives and make them live longer. Their personal attractiveness would increase dramatically, as would their capacity for experiencing sexual pleasure. It would be possible for the short in stature to gain as much as 2 cm in height. There were no known adverse effects of the projected treatment.

Thus informed, each patient signed the consent form.

Approval

The author thought it best to conduct the study during the summer so as not to add to the workload of the Ethics Committee. However, he has evidence in his possession that one member of the Committee is moonlighting in the armaments industry, another is being dried out in a private clinic under an assumed name, and that the third, widely believed to be studying elsewhere, is vacationing with his secretary. It is not anticipated that the Ethics Committee will offer public criticism of the project.

The Therapy

Verbal Therapy

The therapists were adult members of the species *Eolophus roseicapilla*, a pink and grey Australian

*Reprinted with permission of the Australian and New Zealand Journal of Psychiatry, © 1988;22:210–214. Edited from the original.

cockatoo, commonly known as the galah. Each was trained to repeat the following six phrases.

- "Tell me some more about that."
- "It must have been a difficult time for you."
- "Do you remember feeling like that when you were a child?"
- "You look sad, just now."
- "I guess people come and go all our lives."
- "It's important to be able to cry when you feel like it."

The patients lay on a couch, their feet pointing to the north, with the therapist on a perch 1.5 m high, and 1 m to the west of the patient's feet.

Each of the ten therapeutic sessions lasted twenty minutes, during which time the therapists uttered the therapeutic phrases randomly. The patients understood that if they did not listen attentively to the therapists' observations they would not be paid. The therapists maintained their affective distance by not changing their facial expressions, by becoming preoccupied with eating and drinking from time to time, and occasionally by defecating on the floor, while looking as if nothing had happened.

If was recognized that the therapists' neutral stance made them powerful transference figures, but analysis of this reaction was outside the present study.

Non-verbal Therapy

The therapists were Labrador retrievers, carefully selected from the author's collection of some three and a half thousand Labradors.

This part of the project drew heavily upon Bartz and Volger's magisterial study[2] on the use of hounds as therapists, for it was their realisation that hounds have "natural abilities of unconditional positive regard, warmth, compassion and the ability to openly express emotions" that inspired the present author in his development of the second part of this survey.

Bartz and Volger's reported experiences were very useful in devising the details of therapy. It may be observed that Labradors are very large dogs, with very short hair. This gives them an appearance of nakedness, introducing a variable into the study which is difficult to control. Anecdotes from patients who had encountered naked human

therapists persuaded the author that this was a situation to be avoided.

Accordingly, each Labrador was neatly dressed in a plain white T-shirt and jeans, the latter specially constructed so that their tails could protrude. This procedure removed some of the problems reported by Bartz and Volger; for example, the therapists were less inclined to urinate on the floor or to attempt to have intercourse with the patients' legs. They were also prevented from licking their genitals while in a reflective mood. As a measure of the success of this procedure, patients who had extensive therapy with human therapists reported that the human therapists were more inclined to do these things than were the Labradors in this study.

During therapy, the Labradors sat on a chair in the same spatial relationship to the patient as did the verbal therapists. They expressed their feelings for the patient by wagging their tails, by putting their heads to one side and looking wistful, and by whining and shifting about. Occasionally they jumped down and licked the patients' faces impulsively, and sometimes they offered to shake hands.

Measures of Outcome

Before the patients entered therapy they completed a number of psychological measures. They were also asked their favorite color, and to think of a number.

The same measures were completed on the day after the last psychotherapeutic session, permitting the benefits of therapy to be fully established before they were assessed. Those patients whose attention seemed to be flagging were reminded that they would not be paid until all protocols were completed.

Statistical Analysis

The large array of data collected was entered into a series of multiplexed Cray computers. After the usual Bayesian transformation they were confined within a region R enclosed by S, d being a volume element of R. The divergence theorem of Gauss states that under these conditions the following formula is true:

$$\iint_{S} \mathbf{f} \cdot \delta\sigma = \iiint_{R} (\mathbf{v} \cdot \mathbf{f}) \, \delta\tau$$

Results

Non-verbal affectively laden therapy was shown to be superior to verbal therapy provided by affectively neutral therapists.

The final score was: dogs 198 (31 goals, 12 assists), cockatoos 101 (14 goals, 17 assists)

Discussion

There is little to discuss. Whoever thought that a man's best friend was his cockatoo? The economic consequences of this study are important. The time spent in training the Labrador therapists (approximately seven hours) is significantly shorter than that required to become a Fellow of the Royal Australian and New Zealand College of Psychiatrists, or a fully accredited psychoanalyst. The author is seeking an item number for this form of therapy from Medicare.

References

1. Suomi SJ, Harlow HF. Social rehabilitation of isolate-reared monkeys. Developmental Psychology 1972;6:487.

2. Bartz WR, Volger RE. A proposal for eliminating the chronic shortage of mental health service providers: hounds as humanists. In: Ellenbogen GC, ed. Oral sadism and the vegetarian personality. New York: Brunner/Mazel, Inc. 1987:28–35.

A prescription for longevity: Swim a little, dance a little, go to Paris every August, and live within walking distance of two hospitals.

Horatio Luro (at 80)

THE ITEMIZED STATEMENT IN CLINICAL PSYCHIATRY*

A New Concept in Billing

Robert S. Hoffman, M.D.

Due to the rapidly escalating costs of health care delivery, there has been increasing pressure on physicians to document and justify their charges for professional services. This has created a number of serious problems, particularly in the field of psychiatry. Chief among these is the breach of confidentiality that arises when sensitive clinical information is provided to third-party insurance carriers, e.g. the patient's diagnosis or related details about his or her psychiatric disorder. Even when full disclosure of such information is made, insurance carriers frequently deny benefits because the description of the treatment appears imprecise or inadequate. There also has been some criticism of the standard hourly fee-for-service, the argument being that psychiatrists, like other medical specialists should be required to adjust their fees depending upon the particular treatment offered.

In view of these considerations, a method is required which will bring psychiatric billing in line with accepted medical practice. The procedure illustrated below, which we have successfully employed in our clinic for the past two years, achieves this goal. It requires only a modest investment in time and effort: the tape-recording of all psychotherapy sessions, transcription of tapes, tabulation of therapeutic interventions, and establishment of a relative value scale for the commonly used maneuvers. This can easily be managed by two full-time medical billing personnel per psychiatrist. The method, in our hands, has been found to increase collections from third-party carriers by 65% and to raise a typical psychiatrist's annual net income almost to the level of a municipal street sweeper or plumber's assistant.

Below is a specimen monthly statement illustrating these principles:

CALVIN L. SKOLNIK, M.D., Inc.
A Psychiatry Corporation

Jan. 5, 1978

Mr. Sheldon Rosenberg
492 West Maple Dr.
East Orange, N.J.

Dear Mr. Rosenberg:

In response to the request by your insurer, Great Lake Casualty and Surety Co., for more precise documentation of professional services rendered, I have prepared the enclosed itemization for the month of December. I trust that this will clarify the situation sufficiently for your benefit payments to be resumed.

Until next Tuesday at 11:00, 1 remain

Cordially,

Calvin L. Skolnik, M.D.

---

*Reprinted from the Journal of Irreproducible Results, © 1980; 26(3):7–8, with permission from Blackwell Scientific Publications.

FEE BREAKDOWN

Itemized Charges	No.		Charges ($)	Itemized Credits	No.		Credit
clarifications	140 @	.25	35.00	unusually interesting anecdotes	4 @	.45	1.80
restatements	157 @	.25	39.25	good jokes	3 @	.50	1.50
broad-focus questions	17 @	.35	5.95	item of gossip about another			
narrow-focus questions	42 @	.30	12.60	patient which was found			
reflections of dominant				useful in her therapy	1	3.50	3.50
emotional theme	86 @	.30	30.10	apology for sarcastic remark	1	1.00	1.00
resolutions of inconsistencies	38 @	.35	17.10	use of case history at American			
pointings out of nonverbal				Psychiatric Association convention	1		10.00
communications	22 @	.40	8.80	chicken salad sandwich on whole			
encouragements to say more	187 @	.15	28.05	wheat w/mayo	1/2 @	1.75	.86
sympathetic nods with				bummed cigarettes (1.00/pack)	7		.35
furrowed brow	371 @	.10	37.10	damaged Librium tablet returned	1		.10
acknowledgments of				unused			
information reception							
(Uh-huhs, Um-hmmm, etc.)	517 @	.08	41.36				
interpretations of unconscious							
defense configurations	24 @	.30	7.20				
absolution for evil deeds	16 @	.50	8.00				
pieces of advice	2 @	.75	1.50				
expressions of personal							
feelings	6 @	.50	3.00				
personal reminiscences	2 @	.65	1.30				
misc. responses (sighs, grunts,							
belches, etc.)	35 @	.20	6.00				
listening to remarks disparaging							
therapist's appearance, personal							
habits, or technique	7 @	1.75	12.25				
listening to sarcastic remarks							
about psychiatry	12 @	1.00	12.00				
listening to psychiatrist jokes	3 @	.80	2.40				
telephone calls to therapist	3 @	.15	.45				
telephone call to therapist at							
especially inopportune moment	1 @	10.50	10.50				
Kleenex tissues	22 @	.005	.11				
ashtray	1 @	3.50	3.50				
filling and repainting of ashtray-							
size dent in wall	1 @	27.50	27.50				
shampooing of soft drink stain							
on carpet	1 @	15.00	15.00				
letter of excuse from work	1 @	2.50	2.50				
surcharges for unusually boring							
or difficult sessions	2 @	35.00	70.00				

Subtotal: charges	$438.52	
	Subtotal: credits	$19.11
	Total: PLEASE REMIT—	$419.41

PRENATAL PSYCHOANALYSIS: A NEW APPROACH TO PRIMARY PREVENTION IN PSYCHIATRY*

Robert S. Hoffman, M.D.

Although it is widely appreciated that the emergence of psychoneurotic symptoms in adult life results from unconscious conflicts deriving from early childhood experiences, little effort has been directed toward primary prevention in this area. A possible approach to early intervention was evaluated by offering intensive psychoanalysis to third trimester fetuses during the two weeks prior to their delivery. Long-term followup was obtained on 46% of the sample (N=110) at age thirty, via interview and psychometric data. The primary criterion for adequate adult adjustment was an annual gross income exceeding $36,000.

Factor analysis of the data revealed that six therapeutic factors were correlated with good outcome:

1. Appropriate timing of interpretations, i.e. between contractions.

2. Analysis conducted with the fetus in the horizontal position. This can be achieved by first determining the alignment of the fetus in the uterus via sonography and then positioning the mother so that the fetus lies flat.

3. Thorough working-through of fetal feelings of anticipatory anxiety related to labor and imminent delivery.

4. Development of a full-blown transference neurosis wherein the fetus's behavior toward the analyst reflects earlier experiences with fellow germ cells in the prezygotic stage.

5. High forceps extraction, which appeared to enhance the effect of deep interpretations by pressing them into the fetal skull at the time of delivery.

6. The necessity that the fetus himself pay for the analytic sessions. Although this was impractical to arrange prior to delivery, it was found equally effective to inform the fetus that he would be billed at the age of 18.

In addition to the above therapeutic maneuvers, it was found that certain specific aspects of the fetal situation affected the subsequent course of personality development:

1. In several patients, inadequate materno-fetal circulation had a pronounced negative effect, a finding consistent with Melanie Klein's concept of "good and bad placenta."

2. Witnessing of the primal scene by the fetus was judged to be highly traumatic, no doubt due to close proximity to the action. This, of course, was predicted by Freud in his classic paper, "Kinderpeepinshtuppe" (1903), in which he noted that such experiences can eventuate in hysterical blindness, tunnel phobias, or plantar warts. Whether these effects are related to heightened Oedipal conflicts or to rhythmic compression of the fetal brain is still unclear.

3. Two sets of twins were followed in the study, and twinship was found to engender a certain degree of sibling rivalry. One twin garroted his brother with the umbilical cord. In the other pair, rivalry appeared to be less of a problem: since the mother had a bicornuate uterus, each twin had his own room.

These data suggest that psychoanalysis need not be delayed until neurotic symptoms emerge in adulthood, since efforts at early intervention *in utero* can be highly rewarding. Further research would be necessary to confirm these preliminary findings as well as to explore possible extensions of the technique. We are currently evaluating the effect of psychoanalytic therapy upon spermatogonia and primordial ovarian follicles prior to conception.

*Reprinted from the Journal of Irreproducible Results, © 1981; 27(1):5, with permission from Blackwell Scientific Publications. Originally appeared in Throwaway J Pyschoanal 46:4, Dec. 1978.

A PSYCHODIAGNOSTIC SYSTEM FOR MENTAL HEALTH CLINIC PATIENTS:

Diagnosis by Parking*

John B. Pittenger, Ph.D.

In a recent issue of the *Journal,* Schofield (1984) suggested that clients of mental health clinics park by diagnosis. Spaces in the parking lot would be marked with symbols indicating various diagnoses, thus allowing clients to park in a space appropriate to his/her problems as he/she perceives them. The author presents, here, a proposal to augment the diagnostic system through *observation of the parking behavior* of clients.

The therapist, or perhaps a full-time parking diagnostician, would observe the parking pattern of the client and note the problem indicated by the parking behavior. By inclusion of this aspect of adaptation to everyday life, we may be able to improve the accuracy of the diagnosis. Figure 1 illustrates a number of parking patterns and the diagnostic categories they indicate.

References

Shofield LJ Jr. A brief report of a psychodiagnostic system for mental health clinic patients: Parking by diagnosis. Journal of Polymorphous Perversity 1984;1(2):9.

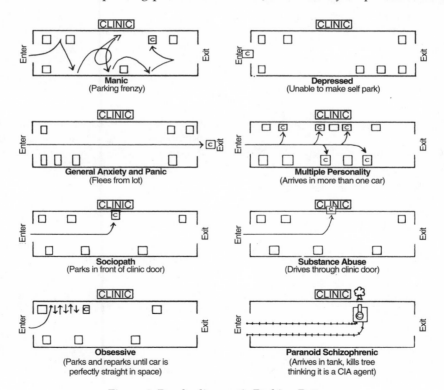

Figure 1. Psychodiagnostic Parking Patterns.

Additional Readings

1. Bentall RP: A proposal to classify happiness as a psychiatric disorder. J Med Ethics 1992;18:94–98.

This is a clever article that satirizes psychiatry's penchant for classifying and over-classifying human behavior. (For a review of this article, see Harris J. in the British Journal of Psychiatry 1993;162:539–542.)

2. Burns A, Howard R, et al: False teeth and Alzheimer's disease. Pyschiatric Bull 1992;16:227–228.

The authors of this research parody investigated the possible link between dentures and Alzheimer's disease. They found one.

3. Copans SA: Therapeutic effects of forceful goosing on major affective illness. J Irreproducible Results 1983;28(3):3–5.

This study compared the effects of antidepressants, electroshock therapy (ECT), and forceful goosing (FG) on four groups of patients. Goosing was superior to antidepressants and ECT in all parameters studied. The author recommends that FG be added to the armamentarium of all practicing psychiatrists.

4. Ellenbogen GC (ed): Oral Sadism and the Vegetarian Personality. New York: Brunner/Mazel, 1986.

A collection of readings from the first few years of the *Journal of Polymorphous Perversity.*

5. Ellebogen GC (ed): The Primal Whimper. New York: Guilford Press, 1989.

A second collection of amusing articles from *J.P.P.*

6. Ellenbogen GC (ed): Freudulent Encounters for the Jung at Heart. New York, W.W. Norton 1992.

This is the third collection of amusing articles from *J.P.P.*

7. Hillman J, Boer C (eds): Freud's Own Cookbook. New York: Brunner/Mazel, 1987.

This is a funny book that parodies the analytic theories of Freud and some of his contemporaries. Written in Freud's "own hand," the book contains analysis, commentary, and a number of delicious recipes: Birth Trauma Cake, Slips of the Tongue in Madeira Sauce, Erogenous Scones, and Fettucine Libido, to name just a few.

8. Holt RR: Researchmanship or how to write a dissertion in clinical psychology without really trying. Am Psychologist 1959;14(3):151.

In this brief satire, the author discusses eight techniques to help PhD candidates sail through their dissertations. It includes advice on how to survey the literature, how to be sure your dissertation will be publishable and how, in the name of science, to manipulate your subjects.

9. Karzin A, Durac J, et al: Meta-meta analysis: a new method for evaluating therapy outcome. Behav Res Therapy 1979;17:397–399.

As the name implies, meta-meta analysis involves doing a meta-analysis of other studies that used meta-analysis in their methodology. By using this innovative approach, the authors evaluated over 100,000 independent variables across 500,000 studies. Although clinical significance was not quite reached, the authors state unequivocally that, "Had there been a few more subjects, it is our firm conviction, we think, that the analysis might have shown a suggestive trend toward an almost significant effect."

10. Saretsky T: How to Make Your Analyst Love You: A Guide to Becoming a More Appealing Neurotic. New York: Citadel Press, 1993.

This book does for psychiatry what *That's Incurable* (p. 268) did for medicine. The author gives advice on everything from "How to Choose an Analyst Who Can Love You" to "Helping Your Analyst Work Out Separation Anxiety."

ODDS & ENDS

When I began my research, I had no preconceived ideas about the type of humor I would find. As the collection grew certain categories began to emerge, however, and the resulting chapters more or less fell into place. As you might expect, not all of the articles fit neatly into these chapters, so this one was created to handle the rest. Although the following selections defy organization into a single whole, they do add a dimension to the rest of the book. For example, the article by S. N. Gaño, "A Gloss Attributed to the Hippocratic School," is not only one of the funniest I found, but it was also published in a rather obscure journal: *The Leech* is the Journal of the Cardiff Medical Student's Club of the Welsh National School of Medicine.

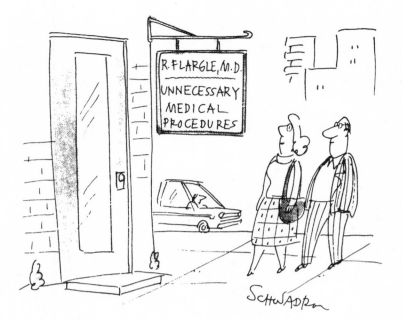

HOW TO SURVIVE YOUR NEXT VACATION*

Howard J. Bennett, M.D.

It's a well-known fact that doctors love vacations. Unfortunately, while it's nice to have a few weeks off, getting there is not always half the fun. Therefore, for all my tired and beleaguered colleagues, I offer the following guide to help smooth things over the next time you're planning a trip.

Try to get away in one piece. For most people, the week before vacation is pretty relaxing. Work slows to a crawl, and the biggest decision that needs to be made is where to go for lunch. For doctors, getting away is pure hell. The main problem, of course, is that it takes at least 2 weeks to dispose of all the clutter that's accumulated on your desk since your last vacation. There are patients to call, insurance forms to procrastinate over, and your "active"(ie, problem) patients to be signed out to your partners.

Why physicians feel the need to tie up loose ends before a vacation has never been formally studied, though I suspect it's due to a strong belief in one of Murphy's little-known laws: "If something can go wrong, it will probably happen while you're on vacation." What most physicians don't realize, however, is that Murphy was a malpractice lawyer before he went into the aphorism business, and this law is an obvious attempt to make the medical profession crazy. Therefore, unless you want to start preparing for vacations 6 months ahead of time, it would be better to heed a rule written by Hippocrates more than 2,000 years ago (before he left for a much-needed vacation in Crete): "The physician who goes on a journey with a cluttered desk may have fewer patients when he returns, but he will be happier for it."

Avoid trouble while you're away. When most people complain about vacations, they bring up such trivial matters as missing luggage, children who got sick the night before they were supposed

*Reprinted with permission from Postgraduate Medicine © 1992; 91(6):49–53. Edited from the original.

to leave, or unexpected hurricanes. The worst thing that can happen to a doctor on vacation is for someone else to discover that you're an MD. This not only encourages people to leave you the tab after dinner, but it's like wearing a sign around your neck that says FREE CLINIC: OPEN 24 HOURS A DAY.

I know of one doctor who took a chartered cruise in the Bahamas, only to discover that the two biggest hypochondriacs in his practice were on the same boat. After listening to 6 hours of symptoms and tales of past brushes with death, the doctor almost jumped overboard to have lunch with the sharks. The terribly irony of it all is that he was the one who suggested they take a vacation in the first place.

Then there was a doctor who inadvertently paid for room service with a credit card that had "MD" printed on it. For the rest of his vacation, instead of finding little chocolate mints on his pillow at night, there were notes from the maid with questions about her bursitis and the ailments of her 50-odd relatives.

So the next time you go on vacation, if you have a credit card that identifies you as an MD, make sure you leave home without it.

Be ready for your first week back. If the week before vacation was rough, the first week back is even rougher. To start with, turning patients over to your partners is like having house guests do the dishes—nothing is where you left it. Consequently, you know you'll have to check in with all your chronic patients to make sure everyone is okay. Also, because of some unknown force of nature, your desk is a bigger mess now than it was before you left: There are messages from patients you don't remember, results of lab work you'd swear you never ordered, and a new stack of charts to replace the ones you just tidied up. There is also a mountain of journals and promotional material from drug companies that must have taken a small forest to produce. The best way to handle this onslaught is to remember another wise saying from the father of medicine: "Life is short and vacations are shorter, but paperwork is eternal."

The final stumbling block you must overcome is that you invariably will be on call your first day back at work. This is a well-established ritual in medicine, whereby your colleagues punish you for having had a good time while they were left behind taking care of *your* patients. Although there are no foolproof ways to deal with this blow, the following strategies are worth considering: Offer someone a month's salary to take call for you. Don't come back in the first place. Go into the aphorism business.

A man is as old as his arteries.

Thomas Sydenham

JENNER AND THE AD-MAN*

What would have happened if Dr. Edward Jenner had called in a press agent to help him put across his smallpox vaccine discovery?

Well, Dr. Jenner, I'm Joe Blowhard—the XYZ agency has assigned me to work up something with you on this new discovery of yours . . . yes, yes, I know, we'll stick to the facts, but don't forget, we have to get people stuck on them, too—ha, ha. Now, let's see . . . you say this protects against smallpox . . . hmmm . . . maybe our best approach would be with the cosmetic angle . . . you know, "preserve your beautiful complexion, avoid disfiguring scars—get vaccinated the Jenner way"—how does that sound to you? . . . Oh, sure, I know people die from smallpox, but that sort of fright approach won't appeal like something that shows a woman how to be more beautiful. . . . We've got quotes from Helen of Troy on that. And if there had been any live wires in the Garden of Eden, I'll bet we could have worked up something from Eve on it, too.

Treatment or Application?

Now, Ed, just how do you go about this—er—treatment—or application, whatever you call it? . . . You *scratch the skin?* Isn't that a bit rough? We want people to get the idea you are helping them, not harming them. . . . Oh, sure, the help comes later, I know, but you have to allow for the shallow thinking of the average individual. Isn't there some other way . . . drinking the vaccine, say . . . or maybe just rubbing it in? . . . OK, Ed, if we have to do it that way, that's the way we'll do it . . . maybe we can hop it up a little—give it some schmalz—by calling it something like glorified scarification.

Next, Ed, just what is this vaccine? Something mysterious about it . . . comes from an isolated peak of the Andes . . . the tombs of the Pharoahs . . . a cauldron deep in the African jungle? . . . Ed, I guess I must have misunderstood you . . . I thought you said "cow" . . . oh, you did say cow . . . hmm . . . not very inspirational, is it? Well, a cow is a MOTHER, after all, so maybe we can work the angle of how

the young cows . . . it's calves? I'll make a note . . . how the Mother cow protects her young by producing this vaccine . . . oh, cows don't get smallpox? It's what? Cowpox? . . . Well, Ed, I guess you lost me on that last turn. Let's not get away from the central theme. Ed . . . none of this scatter-gun approach, you know . . . loses all its punch.

Let's try again . . . oh, it's the dairymaid? Well, that's better . . . chance for a lot of good buildup—got a couple of good models in mind already. Let's see . . . in her tender, loving care of her cow . . . yes, it fits right in, for who else would give a whoop for a cow, except perhaps a bull—ha, ha— the dairymaid is miraculously protected against this blight on fair womanhood by getting cowpox (whatever that is . . . we'll gloss it over), and now, as a result of your amazing break-through . . . conquest of another of Nature's mysteries . . . this boon is available to all! Sounds great, doesn't it?

Now, what about some color? Can't we get a cow in on this act . . . you know, all fluffed up, with a pink ribbon on her tail? We can put her up in a hotel . . . say the Savoy . . . and make with the idea she's really people . . . folks lap up that sort of whimsy, you know . . . Oh, I'll take care of the details . . . I'll find somebody to milk her, and all that sort of thing. . . . Yes, Ed, better start in production on the vaccine . . . no, better not bring a cow with the rash or whatever it . . . we could have a photogenic problem, and a cow's face isn't exactly . . . what's that? It's on the *udder?* Oh, oh . . . uh. . . . Well, Ed, that rocks the boat a little, you know . . . maybe a bit too sexy, I'm afraid.

Tell you what, Ed, let me dream over this stuff for a day or so . . . something will click, I know . . . but it takes some thinking-through right now. . . . OK, Ed, but don't release any of this info to anyone for the present—it's red-hot. . . . Sure, the scientists can wait just like everyone else.

Fine, Ed, and it's has been real great talking to you.

CONTRECOUP

*Reprinted from JAMA, © 1961;175(2):A234–236;with permission from the American Medical Association.

CD-ROMs I'D LIKE TO SEE*

Howard J. Bennett, M.D.

Every year, computer magazines publish review articles of the top CD-ROMs that were released in the previous twelve months. What would these articles look like if computer programs were written just for doctors? Here's a sample of what we might find.

Where in the World Are Carmen Sandiego's Veins?
Salmonella Software; $45 ★★★½

She may be a world traveler, but on her latest trip overseas, Ms. Sandiego got careless when she ate lunch at a seedy, out of the way restaurant. Now she's come down with a whopping case of diarrhea, and she shows up in your office with fever, abdominal pain, and 10% dehydration. What caused Carmen's illness? Is it contagious? Will you be able to save her so she can roam the globe again?

Doctors will love this interactive adventure. Not only do you have to find a vein in one of Carmen's vasoconstricted limbs, but most of her bodily fluids will need to be examined to come up with the correct diagnosis.

TurfWorks
Black Cloud Interactive; $38 ★★½

This program helps primary care docs turf unwanted patients to specialists. You answer a series of questions which include the diagnosis, insurance coverage, and whether or not the patient sends you candy or other gifts at Christmas. The program then generates a "dumping profile" and time honored methods to get the patient off your service and onto someone else's. On-line help offers clear examples and takes into account the day of the week, time of day, and other variables.

This program would have received a higher rating except that BCI also publishes *TurfWorks Pro*, which is designed for specialists who want state-of-the-art techniques to outmaneuver their primary care colleagues.

Cyst
Lipoma Productions; $59 ★★★★

The wonderful world of *Cyst* begins as you fall into the pages of a dermatology book and land in a strange island world. As you explore this world, you are presented with a series of challenging diagnoses. You discover patients with macules, papules, crusts, nodules, bullae, and papulosquamous eruptions—all beautifully rendered in 3-D. A haunting musical soundtrack enhances hours of game play. As an added bonus, Atarax samples are included to counteract the inevitable pruritus that comes from playing the game.

Vacation Doubler
Inspired Software; $79 ★★★★★

In the past, doctors had to work late, skip lunch, or die young to get managed care administrators off their backs. Now, however, by simply downloading *Vacation Doubler* onto your office computer, you can beat the bean counters at their own game. With the click of a button, *Vacation Doubler* inflates your productivity statistics so it will look as though you're Marcus Welby in overdrive. The administrators will be so pleased that you'll not only get more time off, but the CEO will probably give you the keys to his Swiss chalet.

Medicine's Greatest Hits
On-Call Entertainment; $55 ★★★½

This CD is filled with glorious moments from the pages of medical history. You can watch mold grow

*Reprinted from the Journal of Family Practice © 1996;42:88–90, with permission from Appleton & Lange, Inc.

in Alexander Fleming's kitchen, listen in on Harvey Cushing's first craniotomy, or see famous kings and queens as they are bled to death. The disc includes over 25 QuickTime movies starring today's most popular actors. Charlton Heston plays Hippocrates walking the streets of Cos. Tom Hanks does a deft turn as William Harvey. And Charles Bronson is perfect as Ignaz Semmelweis, pacing the floor of his asylum, muttering to himself about the importance of good hand washing. The CD also contains a trivia game and the 1996 edition of the *Guinness Book of Medical Records*.

Pathology Chess
Sarcoid Systems; $35 ★★½

The power of 3-D animation and fantasy meet in this medical version of an old classic. Players move pieces across a checkered battleground in an attempt to capture their opponent's king. When a piece is "captured," however, it doesn't just disappear off the board. In this chess game, the piece dies, and it's up to you to figure out what killed him. Animated orderlies carry the deceased to pathology where you review the history, perform an autopsy, and inform the grieving family why their little pawn (or knight, etc.) died. A special button transports you to the library where you can look up information about various diseases and other fatal conditions. Play is smooth and easy, and the program occasionally responds by voice. For example, after a clever diagnosis, you might hear, "Good job. Have you considered a career in pathology?"

SimCafeteria
Oat-Cell Productions; $32 ★★★

SimCafeteria is an animated game and planning simulator that lets doctors build a hospital cafeteria from the ground up. The program contains six modules which can be worked on in any order. You get to pick out the tacky decor. You get to hire the rude workers. You get to order the outdated equipment. And finally, if you select the executive privilege option, you get to overcook the food.

This program will keep doctors entertained for hours. It's a welcome addition to Oat-Cell's previous titles: *SimHMO*, *SimSurgeon*, and *SimNursing Home*.

ER—The CD
Central Line Publishers; $45 ★★★

Out-of-this-world graphics and a star-studded cast will keep you on the edge of your seat in this CD version of the hit TV series. In this interactive adventure, you get to play any character in the show. Then, as patients burst through the doors in various states of exsanguination, you get to bark out orders, fill out forms, or grill Carter to your heart's content. Your goal is to accumulate points by saving lives and keeping the ratings high. Extra points are made whenever you catch someone reading x-rays backwards or mispronouncing medical words.

Category 1 CME credit can be earned if you e-mail your scores to Michael Crichton or the publisher.

WHAT IF TELEVISION WAS JUST FOR US?*

Howard J. Bennett, M.D.

Although there are only a handful of medical programs currently on the air, it's only a matter of time before someone decides to exploit this market. In addition to MCN (Managed Care Network) and MNN (Malpractice News Network), here's what the listings might look like if television was just for us.

6 AM

- **Doctor's Call Hour**—*Discussion*
How to avoid getting up in the middle of the night to see patients.
- **CPC Festival**

7 AM

- **Captain Retractor**—*Cartoon*
- **Borborygmus**—*Talk Show*
The art of turfing.

8 AM

- **The Red Herring**—*Cartoon*
- **Stupid Advances in Medicine**
Topic: S.I. Units.

9 AM

- **Home CME**—*Instruction*
Neurosurgery for primary care physicians.
- **Koplick's Spot**—*Talk Show*
How to avoid drug reps in the office.

10 AM

- **Scoping for Dollars**—*Game Show*
- **I Dream of Tenure**—*Comedy*
Dr. Tony figures out a new way to pad his C.V.
- Movie—*Adventure*★★
"Abbott and Costello Go to Med School" (1952). Bud and Lou finally score well on their MCAT exams and head east for their freshman year at Harvard.

10:30 AM

- **Home Beeper Repair**—*Instruction*

11 AM

- **Where's That Chart?**—*Game Show*

- **QNS**—*Talk Show*
How to make really bad slides.

Noon

- **OOPS!**—*Game Show*
- **All My Interns**—*Serial*
- **Movie**—*Comedy*★★★
20,000 Lawyers Under the Sea" (1984). All the malpractice lawyers in the U.S. sign up for a conference in the Caribbean. The ship runs into high seas on the way back and sinks.

1 PM

- **The Joy of Cutting**—*Inspiration*
- **The Young and the Sleepless**—*Serial*

1:30 PM

- **Curbside**—*Discussion*
What to do when patients ask for free advice at the hardware store.

2 PM

- **Let's Make a Referral**—*Game Show*
- **One Life to Lose**—*Serial*
- **Wide World of Warts**
The 1994 World Cup Competition taped last March. Top dermatologists compete in the treatment of plantar warts.

3 PM

- **Stool Train**—*Music*
- **Movie**—*Adventure*★★
"A Fistula Full of Dollars" (1964). A savvy renal fellow (Clint Eastwood) figures out how to keep his dialysis unit in the black.
- **AMA Wrestling**

*Reprinted with permission from Resident & Staff Physician, © 1994; 40(9):43–44. Edited from the original.

4:30 PM
- **M*A*S*H**—*Comedy*
Trapper John does a hip replacement on himself.
- **Hemorrhoidectomy Awards**

5 PM
- **A Piece of My Behind**—*Essay*
- **Movie**—*Adventure*★★★
"Voyage to the Bottom of the Barrel" (1961). The Chief of Medicine (Richard Chamberlain) is faced with making his picks for the annual residency match.

6 PM
- **CYA News**
- **Billing the Rich and Famous**

7 PM
- **Wheel of Honors**—*Game Show*
- **Cisco & Ebert**
The hosts review articles from this week's *New England Kernel of Medicine*.

7:30 PM
- **Really Great Performances**
Dr. John Williams gets Medicaid to reimburse him in less than six months.

8 PM
- **Have Scut Will Travel**—*Drama*
Third-year medical students fight to see who can check the most lab results.
- **Supernova**
Remarkable footage of a 45-year-old surgeon burning out.

- **Movie**—*Drama*★★★
"Madam Ovary" (1989). Unhappy in her marriage to an attending, Emma (Julia Roberts) commits adultery with an ob/gyn resident. Unfortunately, he has too many debts, so she leaves him for an MBA.

9 PM
- **Guess Who's Pimping at Dinner?**—*Drama*
When Joanna brings a resident home for dinner, her father grills him on the differential diagnosis of splenomegaly.
- **Movie**—*Drama*★★★★
"The Answering Service Always Rings Twice" (1981). An internist (Jack Nicholson) tries to leave instructions with his service, but they always screw things up. He eventually goes insane and drives his car through their office building.
- **Movie**—*Adventure*★★
"The Towering Internal" (1991). Doogie Howser does his first pelvic exam.

10 PM
- **Stonewall & Bennetti**—*Drama*
Benetti tries to admit an adolescent with a lawn dart in his head, but Stonewall says to treat him at home.
- **House Calls**—*Science Fiction*

11 PM
- **On-Call Workout**—*Exercise*

11:30 PM
- **Sleeping Through the Night**—*Inspiration*

Concerned about your health? Of course you are!
That's why you need:

The BIG Book of Stuff Doctors Know But Just Won't Tell You*

DISCOVER:

☞ *Why colored toilet paper contributes to spontaneous human combustion!*

☞ *Why hysterectomies are completely unnecessary and only performed to put money into the pockets of greedy physicians!*

☞ *How to recognize and treat the symptoms of Alien Abduction!*

☞ *Why hanging upside down nude and eating oranges will prevent rickets!*
. . . and a wealth of other vital information!

Why remain a slave to the physician-promoted myth of maintaining health through tedious exercise, boring diet and giving up all the little pleasures of life like smoking, drinking and random, unprotected sex? This BIG Book has hundreds of nuggets of medical information that your doctor knows but won't tell you — so he can keep you under his fat, greedy thumb!

If you order now, we'll also send you, absolutely free of charge, this exciting companion volume:

Foods That Heal You Better Than Any Old Medicine

☞ *How to stop colon cancer dead in its tracks by eating an ordinary apple and a cup of oat bran!*

☞ *Foods that give you sexual prowess you never dreamed of! Including a special chapter on hundreds of aphrodisiacs your doctor knows about but won't admit to! (Ask him — you'll see!)*

☞ *How you can soothe almost any skin condition by smearing your entire body with salsa and used WD30 motor oil!*

- -

DON'T DELAY! ORDER TODAY! Can't you just imagine your doctor's face when you march into his office with this volume under your arm?

☐ YES, I need this BIG Book that will make those greedy doctors obsolete!

Bill my credit card	
17 monthly installments of	Name . . . .
ONLY $19.95	Address . . . .
Return to:	. . . .
Alarmist Press,	
Heartland, Ont.	Signature . . . .

Lisa Pardy

*Reprinted from Stiches (the Journal of Medical Humor) © 1994;
July/Aug:5, with permission from the author.

A MERCIFULLY BRIEF HISTORY OF MEDICINE*

Richard Armour, Ph.D.

Medicine began with the dawn of history. In fact it began shortly before dawn, at about 3 AM, when the first Stone Age doctor was roused from his bed by a patient who thought he was dying. Transportation being somewhat primitive (this being before the invention of the wheel), by the time the doctor arrived the patient was well.

Ancient

During the Stone Age the most common complaints were gallstones, kidney stones, and stumbling over stones. Surgery was in its infancy, largely because of the difficulty in making an incision with a sharpened stone. When a surgeon decided not to operate everyone breathed a sigh of relief, especially the surgeon and, if he was still alive, the patient.

Having no stethoscope, the Stone Age doctor had to place his ear directly against the patient's chest. This wasn't easy if the patient was male because the chest hair not only muffled sounds but in some cases pierced the doctor's eardrum. Small flat stones were used as tongue depressors. Only rarely were these stones swallowed by patients who mistook them for throat lozenges. The accidental swallowing of small stones, with dramatic improvement of sore throats, led to the invention of the placebo. It wasn't until the end of the Stone Age that chocolate-covered stones were available for children and others who had trouble getting the plain ones down.

The doctor's little black bag was at first a little brown bag, since it was made out of bark. A doctor with a friendly bedside manner often made a joke of this as he entered the sickroom. "My bark is worse than my bite," he would say, laughing so uproariously that it was hard to believe he used the same line at six previous calls that day.

Since everyone lived in caves during the Stone Age, the Stone Age hospital was also a cave. Attendants worked ceaselessly to keep the dirt off the dirt floors. Nurses hurried about, wearing sterilized bearskin and, in the interest of quiet, no shoes. In the operating room, the anesthesiologist stood by with a large club, ready to anesthetize the patient if he showed any signs of returning to consciousness.

Great strides in medicine were made in ancient Greece. The greatest strides were made by Hippocrates, who nervously walked up and down the halls. The reason he paced about was that he was the father of medicine and was pretty jumpy, especially when he was near the delivery room. Before Hippocrates, medicine was in the hands of priests. The priests thought diseases were caused by demons and angry gods, which still sounds pretty plausible. But Hippocrates thought sickness could be traced to natural causes such as bad diet, lack of fresh air, and falling off the top of the Parthenon.

It was in the time of Hippocrates that doctors learned to write prescriptions illegibly. Patients taking prescriptions to their apothecaries would try to read them but soon gave up saying, "That's Greek to me." They were Greek to everybody, but fortunately the Greek apothecary could read Greek, even when it was written by a physician.

Roman medicine made great contributions in the field of sanitary engineering and public health. The Romans drained swamps, built aqueducts, constructed sewers, and killed off enough people to keep cities from becoming overcrowded. The most famous doctor in Rome was Galen, who started his career by attending gladiators. Galen wrote many books about the four humors and was so obsessed with the idea that many thought him a better humorist than scientist.

Medieval

Medicine took an unexpected turn in the Middle Ages when it became affiliated with astrology. No

*Reprinted from JAMA, © 1965;192:129–131; with permission from the American Medical Association. Edited from the original.

one would swallow a pill without first checking to see if the stars were in a favorable position and, on a cloudy night, this could be difficult.

Blood letting was a popular cure in the Middle Ages. The idea was to get rid of impurities in the blood by opening a vein or (if in a hurry) an artery and letting the patient bleed to death. Much of the blood letting was accomplished by barbers, some of whom were very accomplished. There was also considerable therapeutic blood letting in tournaments, where knights with lances could lance a good deal more than a boil.

Knights in full armor were something of a problem when they came to the doctor's office for an examination. For one thing, they were noisy, clanking around the waiting room looking for an illuminated manuscript they hadn't already read. For another, it was hopeless to try to feel a pulse through a metal sleeve and rather silly to ask a grown man to stick out his tongue through a visor. But getting a knight to "disrobe" was no fun either, since he couldn't do it by himself and the nurse wasn't strong enough to lift some of the larger pieces of metal. This meant that the doctor had to lend a hand himself, when the waiting room was full and he had house calls to make.

Modern

Medicine developed rapidly in the Renaissance. The study of anatomy was advanced by an Italian, Vesalius, who is not to be confused with Vesuvius even though he occasionally blew his top. Vesalius was especially annoyed by the writings of Galen, which were full of errors about the human body. Galen, for example, believed that the pus which formed in wounds was good. Vesalius was less enthusiastic.

The greatest family in Italy during the Renaissance was the Medici family. The Medici were patrons of artists and writers rather than doctors, which may explain why they died out in 1743 surrounded by books and paintings but in bad shape physically.

During the Elizabethan period, an English physician by the name of Harvey (his last name, not his first) discovered the circulation of blood. Without the aid of a microscope, he found that blood goes around and around. This is very economical, since a little blood goes a long way, and people should be a lot more grateful than they are.

Probably the greatest development in the 18th century was Edward Jenner's discovery of a vaccine for smallpox. Jenner's description of his work, *Inquiry into the Causes and Effects of the Variolae Vaccinae* should have had a catchier title such as *A Pox on Pox,* but it was widely read in medical circles anyway.

During the modern era medical progress has been rapid. In England, Joseph Lister made operations safer by getting surgeons to wash their hands. In France, Louis Pasteur discovered how to keep food from spoiling and thereby made it necessary to eat leftovers. In Austria, Sigmund Freud discovered the id, ego, superego, and libido, all of which had been going unnoticed in the subconscious for years. Thanks to Freud, boys discovered it was normal to want to kill their fathers and marry their mothers. Also, people no longer had to listen to friends go on and on about their dreams now that there were psychiatrists who were paid to do it.

In recent years, there have been marvelous developments in medicine. Alexander Fleming, the discoverer of penicillin, proved that you should never throw something out just because it's moldy. Salk and Sabin have practically eliminated polio, at least in those patients who aren't too busy to drop in for the vaccine.

With x-rays, wonder drugs, and return envelopes for paying overdue accounts, medicine has come a long way since the Stone Age. Unlike the doctor awakened at the dawn of history by a patient suffering from a psychosomatic ailment, the modern doctor rouses himself only long enough to prescribe a couple of aspirin. He then goes back to bed and dreams of getting the Nobel Prize for curing the common cold. Or, better still, he leaves the whole thing to his answering service.

TOP TEN LISTS FOR DOCTORS*

Howard J. Bennett, M.D.

By now, most people are familiar with the Top Ten Lists that are featured on the *David Letterman Show*. For anyone who isn't, these nuggets of humor range from cutting political satire ("Top Ten Iraqi Nicknames for George Bush") to humorous commentary on modern culture ("Top Ten Rejected Names for Kentucky Fried Chicken"). Unfortunately, Letterman's writers don't realize how fond doctors are of lists, and they rarely come up with any medical topics. To remedy this situation, I've decided to concoct a few Top Ten Lists of my own.

Top Ten Journals Not Found at the National Library of Medicine

10. Journal of Really Rare Diseases
9. Annals of Insignificant Research
8. Hemorrhoid Clinics of North America
7. Journal of Anecdotal Medicine
6. Archives of the Frenulum
5. Journal of Unnecessary Procedures
4. UFO Medicine
3. Journal of Poorly Written Manuscripts
2. Annals of Unethical Research
1. Journal of Medical Misadventures

Top Ten Rejected Drug Names

10. Rectopen
9. Equivocort
8. Confusemol
7. Barfitol
6. Crockguard
5. Profitol
4. Ineffectin
3. Fraudusil
2. Placebobid
1. Terminol

Top Ten Medical Stories Buried in the Back Pages of the Newspaper

10. Nutrasweet Causes Kidneys to Grow Teeth
9. Infertility Linked to Not Having Babies
8. FDA Chief Addicted to Oxygen
7. Brain Stapling Cures Obesity
6. Renegrade Scientists Uses *Scrubbing Bubbles* to Unclog Fatty Deposits in Arteries
5. Sleep Causes Cancer
4. Kangaroo Brain Transplanted into Dan Quayle
3. Nitrite Levels Associated with High SAT Scores
2. Cholesterol is an Aphrodisiac
1. Flesh-Eating Bacteria Prefer Republicans

Top Ten Reasons to Stay in Medicine

10. McDonald's isn't hiring at the moment.
9. Avoiding lawsuits adds zest to life.
8. You get a lifetime supply of free pens from drug reps.
7. It will help with your insanity defense if you decide to "blow away" an HMO administrator.
6. To pimp medical students.
5. To provide excellent patient care, to advance the boundaries of medical science, and to take Wednesday afternoons off.
4. It beats selling Amway products.
3. So your mom won't be lying when she talks about you at weddings and Bar Mitzvahs.
2. In case Elvis shows up for a physical.
1. Somebody has to do it.

*Reprinted from the Journal of Family Practice © 1995;41:190–191, with permission from Appleton & Lange, Inc.

For additional Top Ten Lists, see pp. 91, 170, 191 and 258.—H.B.

MEDICAL HOROSCOPES*

Howard J. Bennett, M.D.

Aries *(March 21–April 20):* All endeavors of a creative nature will pay off this week, but first you must finish what you've started—like disimpacting the patient in room 419. Be on guard if a colleague asks you to switch call for the weekend. With Mars entering Venus, there's no telling how many STDs will walk through the door.

Taurus *(April 21–May 21):* This is a good time for pursuing your favorite hobby—filling out Medicare forms. Focus on your sickest patients and confuse things by using obscure CPT codes. With the moon in Pisces, hospital committee meetings will be even more boring than usual. Find a reason to stay late at the office.

Gemini *(May 22–June 21):* This is a favorable time for all Geminis. Expect no admissions after 3 PM, no calls after midnight, and no requests for free medical advice at dinner parties. The Sun in Aries makes this a good time to catch up on your journals. Don't worry if the articles are too long. Just read the abstracts.

Cancer *(June 22–July 23):* A managed care administrator figures prominently in your week. Attention revolves around fewer tests and early discharge. Be creative—turf the patient to surgery. Your lucky number is 14.

Leo *(July 24–Aug. 23):* Professionally you will be very much in demand this week and certain initials will play a prominent role in your work. Keep a watchful eye for I&D, QNS, CYA, and DNR. Be sure your beeper has a new battery.

Virgo *(Aug 24–Sept. 23):* Jupiter, the planet of good luck, crosses your solar chart on Monday making this a great week. You will pick up a physical finding that everyone else missed, an eager medical student will do all of your scut, and Mr. Smith's family won't be in his room when you stop by on rounds.

Libra *(Sept. 24–Oct. 23):* Attention to detail is the key to success this week. Don't forget to glove up for rectals, and be prepared to duck when culturing a 4-year-old with a sore throat and nausea. If you're suturing a routine laceration and the patient says he cut himself inside a UFO, call for backup.

Scorpio *(Oct. 24–Nov. 22):* A clash of ideas could lead to a food fight at your next staff meeting—Gemini, Virgo, and Scorpio are involved. The Capricorn moon emphasizes mystery and intrigue. Watch out for red herrings, lost specimens, and a lipoma the size of Nebraska.

Sagittarius *(Nov. 23–Dec. 21):* You may feel on top of the world, but nursing home requests are piling up like hotcakes. Placement is difficult, so bring lots of donuts to the nurse's station and stay on good terms with the social workers. A change in strategy is required if you plan on making it home by 9 PM. Don't forget flowers.

Capricorn *(Dec. 22–Jan. 20):* A dynamic aspect between the Sun and Mars signifies that you will ask some terrific questions at Grand Rounds. Take a moment to enjoy the accolades your colleagues bestow on you. Then get back to work and see a few hundred patients so your HMO doesn't fire you.

Aquarius *(Jan. 21—Feb. 19):* With Mars pulling in one direction and Pluto the other, expect to spend a lot of time in OB this week. Pitocin is good, but forceps are better. You will be told by someone you admire, "You have a way with foreskins."

Pisces *(Feb. 20–March 20):* An explosive aspect between the Sun and Mercury means there will be a lot of rota virus going around. Remember to wash your hands. Although your planetary influences are in a favorable position, no power in the universe can keep drug reps away from the office. Consider calling in sick.

*Reprinted from the Journal of Family Practice, © 1995;41:407, with permission from Appleton & Lange, Inc.

A GLOSS ATTRIBUTED TO THE HIPPOCRATIC SCHOOL*

S. N. Gaño

S.N. Gaño is the pen-name of a well-known New York M.D.—Editor

It's well known to students of ancient medicine that the Greek authors are incompletely represented in English translation. Similar neglect has befallen the Hippocratic writings. The text which follows has suffered the neglect of centuries. While thorough palaeographic and critical analysis must be reserved for the future, quite obviously the text is a gloss or series of notes on various familiar Hippocratic writings, and was probably prepared by a student or member of the Hippocratic group. The stylistic traits bear strong evidence of genuineness, and the reader cannot fail to be impressed by the conciseness, clarity, and sagacity which are displayed in every paragraph.

Prognostics

- Absence of respiration is a bad sign.
- It is unfavourable for the patient to be purple, especially if he is also cold. The physician should not promise a cure in such cases.
- Appetite is better without hellebore.[†]
- When bloodletting is followed repeatedly by sweating and convulsions, the patient will not have a crisis on the fortieth day.

Epidemics

- Plutocrates the moneylender, went to Potos during the Olympic Games. The itch appeared on the third day, followed by burning and discharge. Returned home to his wife—unfavorable crisis.

- On the island of Tenebros, in the spring of the year, several maidens were attacked by swelling of the abdomen and absence of the menstrual discharges. A voyage to Asia was recommended. Complete crisis at the end of the ninth month.

Aphorisms

- When the spleen is found on the right side, the patient should consider changing physicians.
- Patients who always wake up on the wrong side should be treated by purges.
- To have the mouth constantly open is common in persons entrusted with affairs of state. Usually nothing comes out.
- Fevers of eighty days where no cause is apparent produce alienation of mind in the physician.
- In cases of severe pain in the side of the chest, with profuse expectoration of blood and shortness of breath, it is best to observe carefully whether there is a knife between the ribs.
- Fevers, hemorrhages, and convulsions are bad; wine is good, in spring, summer or winter.
- Maidens, after the age of puberty, are subject to deep respiration at night, especially if the warm winds are blowing.
- When swarthy parents have a blonde child and a blonde serving-maid, the physician should suspect a displacement of humors.
- Logorrhea[‡] can be treated by placing a reed firmly beneath the tongue. In severe cases bandaging is helpful.

*Reprinted from the Leech, © 1958;4(8):17–19; with permission from the author. Edited from the original.
†poisonous herb
‡Excessive and often incoherent talkativeness.

Surgery

- The surgeon requires a steady hand and a calm disposition. It is also essential to have a patient.
- Great delay in resolution of the humors is more common among the rich than among the poor.
- Dislocation of the neck, which has been produced by a rope, cannot be treated with barley water.
- If the thumb is placed on the nose while the other fingers are alternately flexed and extended, fracture of the jaw may follow
- Those who have recently fractured both legs should not take part in the Olympic Games

Ancient Medicine

- In patients who are filled with nothing but crude humors, removal of all the blood relieves the symptoms.
- In those who hiccup and talk at random and cannot hold the head erect, the pneuma may have become mixed with undiluted wine. In such cases the crisis follows on the next day.
- Where symptoms are severe and protracted it is good (for the physician) if the patient's relatives are few, and best if they be absent altogether.
- The physician should not condemn ancient medicine merely because it was ineffective. The Art is eternal.

Answering Service Operators' Top Ten Pet Peeves*

10. Patients with multiple personalities who call in six times for the same complaint.
9. New digital headsets that keep picking up *Regis & Kathie Lee*.
8. Grouchy doctors who expect phone numbers to be accurate.
7. Choking patients who garble their phone number.
6. 911 operators who brag about the hunks they work with at the fire station.
5. Working the night shift, but not getting to wake anybody up.
4. People who like *Chicago Hope* more than *E.R.*
3. Tornadoes that knock out power but spare the phone lines.
2. No one has ever done a TV movie about answering service operators.
1. Prank calls from former co-workers who now have really good jobs that *don't* involve doctors.

*Reprinted from The Journal of Family Practice ©1996;43:110, with permission from Appleton & Lange, Inc.

Transcription errors and medical malapropisms are everyday occurrences in health care. Whether it's reading that a lesion was "two sontameters long" or that a patient was admitted with a "cerebral conclusion," it's amusing to see how medical reports can get turned on their ears. As much as doctors like to think that support staff and patients are the ones responsible for all of these goofs, the article by Dorothy Reid (p. 260) shows that this is not always the case.—H.B.

SERENDIPITOUS NEOLOGISMS*

Arlan L. Rosenbloom, M.D.

From time to time inadvertent witticisms shatter the repetitive jargon used in the communications between physicians. These nuggets of fortuitous humor arise either from erroneous translations of mumbled dictation or from conjectural interpretations of medical cryptography. Though blunders, they are welcome, since they often imply wildly improbable definitions. I have called them "serendipitous neologisms" (SN) because of their unpremeditated origin.

Notations

Over a two year period, I screened all my professional correspondence for errors, including letters, x-ray reports, medical records, and similar papers. Among several thousand misinterpretations encountered, a handful met the following criteria for SN:

1. The error *did not* result in a well-recognized word or phrase with an established meaning or connotation.

2. The error *did* result in the formation of a word or phrase not previously a part of the language (American).

3. The new word or phrase suggested a meaning whose only value was humorous.

Twenty-one discrete instances of SN are listed in the table.

Twenty-one Serendipitous Neologisms

What Was Intended	What Was Written	Connotation
1. ulcerative colitis	all-sorts-of-colitis	every bowel complaint possible
2. ultimate short stature	alternate short stature	every other patient is below the 3rd percentile
3. karyotype	carrier-type	mailman
4. chromosomal deletion	chromosomal delusion	inherited form of psychosis
5. consult	conslut	disreputable girl friend
6. double-blind study	double-lined study	insulated library
7. femoral vein	efemeral vein	one difficult to find
8. erythroblastosis fetalis	erythroblastosis vitalis	greasy kid stuff
9. phallic	fallic	sex-linked tendency to stumble
10. phospholipids	forceful lipids	the predominant fats
11. growth hormone	gross hormone	the one responsible for obesity
12. hirsute	hair suit	worn with a hair shirt
13. inborn error of metabolism	inborn era of metabolism	the current subspecialty fad
14. intersex	inner sex	mental masturbation
15. labia minora	lybia minor	prehistoric country in North Africa
16. myocardial infarct	myocardial infart	coronary air embolus
17. auto analyzer	otto analyzer	German psychiatrist
18. pregnanetriol	pregnant trial	pithy legal case
19. prepubertal	prepubital	sedative for children
20. siblings	siklings	unhealthy brothers and sisters
21. slightly ectatic ascending aorta	slightly ecstatic ascending aorta	a lukewarm affair of the heart

*Reprinted from Clinical Pediatrics, © 1972;11:496–497; with permission from J.B. Lippincott/Harper & Row. Edited from the original.

"THAT'S WHAT YOU DICTATED, DOCTOR!"*

Dorothy Reid

All the following gems are quotations from the dictation of staff physicians at Memorial Mission Hospital in Asheville, N.C., where I supervise the transcription unit. I don't intend this to be critical of our fine staff. It just shows how things sometimes come out no matter who happens to be doing the dictating.

The left leg became numb at times and she walked it off.

Patient has chest pain if she lies on her left side for over a year.

Father died in his 90s of female trouble in his prostate and kidneys.

Both the patient and the nurse herself reported passing flatus.

Skin: Somewhat pale but present.

On the second day the knee was better, and on the third day it had completely disappeared.

The pelvic examination will be done later on the floor.

Patient stated that if she would lie down, within two or three minutes something would come across her abdomen and knock her up.

By the time she was admitted to the hospital her rapid heart had stopped and she was feeling much better.

Patient has bilateral varicosities below the legs.

If he squeezes the back of his neck for 4 to 5 years it comes and goes.

Patient was seen in consultation by Dr. Blank who felt we should sit tight on the abdomen, and I agreed.

Speculum was inserted between the eyes.

Dr. Blank is watching his prostate.

Discharge status: Alive but without permission.

Coming from Detroit, Mich., this man has no children.

At the time of onset of pregnancy the mother was undergoing bronchoscopy.

She was treated with Mycostatin oral suppositories.

Healthy appearing decrepit 69 year old white female, mentally alert but forgetful.

When you pin him down, he has some slowing of the stream.

For another look into the world of medical malaprorisms, see p. 60 and the following.—H.B.

1. Dirckx JH: Doctor I'm (sic). Am J Dermatopath 1992;14:369–371.
2. Hale PN: Cheyanne strokes. N Engl J Med 1964;271:161.
3. Heath DS: [sic] Humor. Modesto, CA: American Association for Medical Transcription, 1995 (see the review on p. 268).
4. Kartman A: More malapropisms. J Fam Pract 1995;41:228.

*Reprinted with permission from Medical Economics, © 1973;50 (Oct 15):143; Medical Economics Company, Inc., Oradell, N.J. 07649.

Additional Readings

1. Armour, Richard: It All Started with Hippocrates.* New York, McGraw-Hill, 1966.

The author takes you on a hilarious romp through the history of medicine, from the Stone Age to the present (the present being 1966 of course). The book is an expansion of the article Dr. Armour has in this chapter.

2. Bennett HJ: My daughter is a Klingon. J Fam Pract 1994;39:295–296.

In this amusing essay, the author describes how his 15-month-old began to sound and act like a Klingon. The article generated a handful of letters which shows that medical folks definitely like *Star Trek*. (See *JFP* 1994;39:524–525 and 1995;40:408.)

3. Bennett HJ: The ins and outs of outies. JAMA 1993;270:1508.

After diagnosing an umbilical granuloma in his newborn daughter, the author muses on the origins of innies and outies.

4. Bluestone N: Alternative therapies. New Physician 1980;29(5):9–11.

The Chairman of Medicine at Farethewell Hospital is admitted to the Hospital for Alternative Therapies. The *chief* suffers from a severe case of role reversal as he's subjected to every oddball treatment in the book.

5. Burke BL, McGee DP: Sports deficit disorder. Pediatrics 1990;85:1118.

The authors describe a condition which is probably all too common among medical professionals. The major criterion for diagnosis is a history of always being the last one chosen for a team. A minor criterion is never having dated a cheerleader. While no definitive treatment exists, the authors suggest a combination of Ritalin and anabolic steroids. (A lively correspondence followed the publication of this article. See Pediatrics 1990;86:804–805 and 1991;87:126–127).

6. Danzl DF: Lunacy. J Emerg Med 1987;5:91–95.

This article examines whether the phase of the moon affects who rolls into emergency departments at night. The author makes a number of recommendations, including the development of the "Lunar Stress Syndrome" as a defense against malpractice litigation.

7. DePaolis M: The adventures of doctor TV. Postgrad Med 1990;88(6):22,23,26.

Can you make a difficult diagnosis on the first take? Can you stay cool when the chips are down, the music is building, and the last commercial is approaching? If not, check out this essay where the author compares TV medicine to the real thing.

8. Dooley MM: History of the condom. J Royal Soc Med 1994;87:58.

This letter, which is a response to an article on condoms, contains a priceless nugget of humor: "Rumor has it that Sir Winson Churchill was once asked by Stalin to help combat the Soviet condom shortage. He pursuaded a British manufacturer to have a special batch made twice as large as normal. These were shipped to the USSR marked 'Made in Britain—Medium'."

9. Escobar GJ: The genius of Friedrich Siegenthaler, M.D. Perspect Biol Med 1985;29:37–40.

This article contends that Dr. Siegenthaler is the real author of the works attributed to William Shakespeare. Dr. Escobar proves his point with some compelling analytic skills: "Macbeth, an allegory describing a chief resident's meteoric rise to the top, is replete with overt and symbolic references to the surgical world."

10. Galli-Resta L, Resta G: Not so humane care. Nature 1994;370:91.

This is an amusing letter about the inhumane way a primate is handled during labor and delivery. The "primate" in question is the first author.

11. Gaño SN: Computers and a paradox for librarians. Bull Med Libr Assoc 1963;51:499–500.

An essay satirizing the arrival of computers in the medical library. The main problem are the doctors who, according to the author, "Read less and less, but write more and more."

*This book is no longer in print, but should be available through interlibrary loan.

12. Hunter P: Developmental milestones for the TV generation. Pediatr Management 1992;June:38–39.

The author has created a new scale for developmental testing in the 1990s. For example, by 18 months of age, children should be able to put two words together: "Tastes great," "Less filling." "Buy now," "Pay later."

13. Karron R: Infectious diseases in bricks. J Irreproducible Results 1992;37(1):8–9.

The authors surveyed the brick population in and around Salt Lake City for evidence of infectious disease. Of the 120 million bricks studied, one was found to have syphilis. Their conclusion? Bricks may be prone to syphilis.

14. Newrick PG, Affie E, et al: Relationship between longevity and lifeline: a manual study of 100 patients. J Royal Soc Med 1990;83:499–501.

This is the first study to document a correlation between a person's lifeline and lifespan. The implications are far reaching—i.e., palmistry not only represents an inexpensive screening tool, but it may direct the allocation of medical resources in the future. It will also make a cushy elective for fourth year students.

15. Reyes MG, Teramura K: Ultrasound study of the faces of diseases. Mt Sinai J Med (NY) 1984;51:714–715.

Some interesting "faces" were found in the electronmicrographs of biopsy specimens. (For a similar effect, see Yokoo H: Smiling mitochondrion. N Engl J Med 1972;287:468–469; and Bainton DF: California bigfoot. N Engl J Med 1994;331:1693.)

16. Scanlon TJ, Nuben RN, Scanlon FL, Singleton N: Is Friday the 13th bad for your health? BMJ 1993;307: 1584–1586.

The authors did a retrospective analysis of the dangers associated with Friday the 13th. Their conclusions? "Friday the 13th is unlucky for some . . . staying at home is recommended."

17. Slay RD: the exploding toilet and other emergency room folklore. J Emer Med 1986;4:411–414.

The exploding toilet is one of many patient related stories that get told and retold in emergency rooms across the country. The author presents a few of these improbable case histories and discusses why they are so intriguing to emergency room personnel.

18. Terry JS: A proposal for new careers in health care. Perspect Biol Med 1984;28:35–39.

A satire which creates job descriptions for roles already operational (informally, that is) in many health care settings. Some examples are "Turf Monitor," "Nihilism Therapist," and "Liaison Jargonist and Director of Initials Management."

APPENDIX

Additional Journals of Interest

The Journal of Irreproducible Results (JIR): First published in 1955, JIR is the "Official Organ of the Society for Basic Irreproducible Research." It is published six times a year and features humor and satire from many disciplines: physics, mathematics, astronomy, medicine, education, and others. Blackwell Scientific Publications, Inc., Three Cambridge Center, Suite 208, Cambridge, MA 02142 (617) 225–0401.

Examples of medical articles include the following:

1. Eastern J, Drucker L, et al: The inheritance pattern of death. JIR 1982;28(1):22–23.

While attempting to stay awake during a boring departmental meeting, the authors accidently discovered "a classic Mendelian autosomal recessive pattern for the phenotype of death." The implications of this finding are discussed, including their recommendation to avoid marrying someone who has already shown evidence for expression of the gene.

2. Laerum OD: Rare diseases. JIR 1972;19(3): 61–63.

The author begins his article by reminding us that rare diseases are uncommon in medical practice. He then goes on to categorize them according to their various subgroups. For example, "Diseases which have not yet occurred, but will be discovered some time in the future—sooner or later," and "Diseases which have not yet occurred and will never occur in the future either." It is not necessary for the clinician to know anything about this latter group.

Note: In 1994, there was a falling out between the publisher and the editorial staff at JIR. Consequently, the editors jumped ship and created the Annals of Improbable Research.

The Annals of Improbable Research (AIR): First published in 1994, AIR is the "Journal of Record for Inflated Research and Personalities." It is published six times a year and features humor and satire similar to JIR. The MIT Museum, 265 Massachusetts Ave., Cambridge, MA 02139 (617) 253–4462.

The Journal of Polymorphous Perversity (JPP): First published in 1984, JPP features humor and satire in the fields of psychology, psychiatry, social sciences, education, and related disciplines. It is published twice a year. Wry-Bred Press, Inc. P.O. Box 1454, Madison Square Station, New York, N.Y. 10159 (212) 689-5473.

Examples of articles include the following:

1. Smoller JW: The etiology and treatment of childhood. JPP 1985;2(2):3–7.

The author describes the causes of this highly prevalent disorder and its clinical features (congenital onset, emotional lability, legume anorexia, etc.). Despite wide-spread treatment facilities (public schools) and its 95% remission rate, childhood remains one of the most costly disorders facing health care professionals today.

2. Polloway EA: The influence of tenure on the productivity of faculty in higher education. JPP 1986;3(2):7.

This article is similar to one I heard about on writer's block a few years ago: It's a blank page!

The Journal of Nursing Jocularity (JNJ): First published in 1991, JNJ features humor and satire in the fields of nursing, medicine, and related disciplines. They also publish serious articles on the importance of humor in health care. It is published four times a year. JNJ Publishing, Box 40416, Mesa, AZ 85274 (602) 835-6165.

Examples of articles include the following:

1. The editors: Ninja school of nursing. JNJ 1991;1(2):26–27.

This article is presented as an advertisement for the Ninja School of Nursing. It consists of testimonials like this one: "We had to get this patient to surgery, and the hypo wasn't knocking him out. But one swoop with my Ninja Nurse Numchucks against his temple put him out faster than lightning."

2. Gish S: Romancing the CVP. JNJ 1994;4(3): 14–15.

This article begins with the following introduction: Assisting a doctor for the first time with a CVP line is a little like making love for the first time (but without the dim lights and soothing music). It's awkward, time consuming and after it's over, neither of you is quite satisfied—but at least you got the job done.

Lite Medicine: First published in 1996, Lite Medicine is a newsletter of "Insight, Humor and Information for Healthcare Professionals." It is published monthly and features cartoons, jokes, anecdotes, short essays, and other interesting material. P.O. Box 4444, Vancouver, WA 98662 (888) 548–3633.

Stitches (The Journal of Medical Humour): Stitches was first published in 1990 as Punch Digest for Canadian Doctors. The name changed in 1992 and, for a brief period, a separate edition was published in the U.S. The magazine features stories, anecdotes, cartoons, and satire. It is published ten times a year. Stitches Publishing, Inc. 16787 Warden Ave., R.R. #3, Newmarket, Ontario L3Y 4W1, Canada (905) 853-1884.

Examples of articles include the following:

1. Scott M: The canteen audit. Stitches 1992; Oct:34–37.

Since hospital food is notoriously bad, the author satirizes what would happen if he submitted some cafeteria food to a pathologist. Here's one of the "reports." Specimen #4: Lunch meat. Gross: A 2.0 × 2.0 × 0.1 cm, square of pale tan tissue. Microscopic: An almost acellular stroma, consisting of sheets of intertwined degenerating collagen fibers. Numerous vacuoles are present, and some of the cells that can be identified are retinal, intestinal, pulmonary and testicular tissue of porcine origin. The differential diagnosis would be between a hamoma and a spaminoma; the absence of teeth and hair favors the latter. Diagnosis: Spaminoma (malignant).

2. Wood RP, Clark J: The autopsy waiting room. Stitches 1994;Nov/Dec:23–24.

Two family members are waiting anxiously for an autopsy to be completed on their recently deceased grandfather. When the pathologist finally emerges, the dialogue goes something like this: **Dr. Clark:** Well, you'll be glad to know there was no evidence of cancer. **Brother:** Wonderful! **Sister:** Thank God! **Brother:** What did Grandad die of? **Dr. Clark:** I'm not 100% sure—but I can tell you it was nothing serious.

Additional Books of Interest

1. Abrahams, Marc (ed): Sex as a Heap of Malfunctioning Rubble. New York: Workman Publishing, 1993.

This is the fourth collection of the best articles from *The Journal of Irreproducible Results*.

2. Bosker, Gideon: Medicine is the Best Laughter. St. Louis: Mosby-Yearbook, 1995.

This is a marvelous collection of cartoons and anecdotes taken from a variety of magazines and newspapers. The material is not only funny but many of the cartoons would make great slides to spice up your lectures.

3. Brallier, Jess M: Medical Wit & Wisdom. Philadelphia: Running Press, 1993.

This is a compilation of amusing medical quips from Hippocrates to Groucho Marx. A number of quotations from the collection appear as filler throughout the book.

4. Buxman, Karen and LeMoine, Ann (eds): Nursing Perspectives on Humor. Staten Island, NY: Power Publications, 1995.

This book is similar in scope to Vera Robinson's but is multiauthored. It includes a wealth of practical information on how to use humor with patients.

5. Cocker, John: Stitches: Off-the-Wall Tales from the Doctor's Office, Hospital, and Operating Room. Toronto: Stoddart Publishing, 1993.

This is a funny collection of anecdotes and cartoons from the first few years of *Stitches: The Journal of Medical Humour.*

6. Cowan, Lore and Cowan, Maurice (eds): The Wit of Medicine.* England: Leslie Frewin Pub Ltd, 1972.

This is an interesting collection of witty sayings by famous doctors from Hippocrates to Osler. The editors have thrown in some amusing poetry as well.

7. Dirckx, John: Roundsmanship: An Introductory Manual. Modesto, CA: Prima Vera Publications, 1987.

If you liked The Art of Pimping (p. 47), you'll love this book. Dr. Dirckx has written a complete guide for the serious roundsman (or roundswoman). Study it at night instead of Harrison's and you'll be a full professor in no time.

8. Ellenbogen, Glenn C (ed): The Directory of Humor Magazines & Humor Organizations in America (and Canada). New York: Wry-Bred Press, 1992.

This reference book provides information on humor magazines and organizations, including those that study humor as well as publish it. The book is broad in scope and contains material on both trade and professional organizations. The publications are cross referenced under 43 subject headings, including medicine, nursing, psychiatry, psychology, and the social sciences.

9. Fishbein, Morris: Tonics & Sedatives.* Philadelphia: J.B. Lippincott, 1949.

A collection of anecdotes, jokes, poems, and other humorous items from *JAMA*'s Tonics & Sedatives column, selected by one of the journal's former editors.

10. Gordon, Leo A: Gordon's Guide to the Surgical Morbidity and Mortality Conference. Philadelphia: Hanley & Belfus, 1994.

This is a serious book on the M&M conference that deftly incorporates humor into the text. The author does a great job analyzing and humanizing this important aspect of surgical training.

11. Hawkins, Clifford (ed): Alimentary, My Dear Doctor: Medical Anecdotes and Humour. Oxford: Radcliffe Medical Press, 1988; New York: Scovill Paterson.

This is an amusing collection of anecdotes and poetry that has an interesting story behind it. The book is the result of a competition on humor sponsored by the publisher. All of the contributors are members of The General Practitioner Writers Association (GPWA) which is based in Great Britain. As the title suggests, each of the pieces lands on some niche within the GI tract. For example, "The general practitioner's association with the bowels begins with the digestion of large amounts of information at medical school. Quite often the intellectual nutri-

---

*These books are no longer in print, but should be available through interlibrary loan.

tion is in a high fibre form; much of it is unabsorbed and goes straight through."

Since the publication of Hawkins' book, Radcliffe Press has come out with two similar collections: Gray, Ian: Myocardial Medley, 1990 and Sandler, Merton: Nervous Laughter, 1991. Sandler's book contains material in the areas of psychiatry and neurology.

12. Heath, Diane S (ed): [sic] Humor: A collection of bloopers, malaprops, and other humorous material from the world of medical transcription. Modesto, CA: American Association of Medical Transcription, 1995.

This is a marvelous collection that contains just about every malapropism and transcription blunder you could imagine. Most of the entries are amusing and some are hilarious.

13. Mould, Richard F. Mould's Medical Anecdotes.* Bristol, England: Adam Hilger; Philadelphia: Taylor & Francis, 1984.

The items collected in this book range from brief notations to short articles. Although some of the material is funny, most of it can be described as amusing curiosities of medicine. For example, "Head Shrinking," "Foreign Bodies," and "Internal Combustion," to name a few.

14. Mould, Richard F: More of Mould's Medical Anecdotes.* Bristol, England: Adam Hilger, 1989.

This is Dr. Mould's second collection of anecdotes. If you liked his first book, you'll enjoy the sequel as well.

15. Ricks, Anne E: The Official M.D. Handbook.* New York: New American Library, 1983.

A ribald look at medicine that begins with getting into medical school, winds its way through internship and residency, and ends up with a chapter on "Doctor-speak." Along the way, the book also lampoons specialists, all types of medical practice, and much more.

16. Robinson, Vera M: Humor and the Health Professions. Thorofare, NJ: Slack, Inc., 1991.

This is a great book for anyone who wants a serious look at humor in medicine. The author examines the topic from many viewpoints: the nature of humor, humor in health and illness, and cultivating the use of humor.

17. Scherr, George H (ed): The Best of the Journal of Irreproducible Results. New York: Workman Publisher, 1983.

This is the third collection of the best articles from the *Journal of Irreproducible Results.*

18. Spence, Wayman R: Perez on Medicine—The Whimsical Art of Joses S. Perez. Waco, TX: WRS Publishing, 1993.

This is a collection of marvelous paintings that poke fun at medicine and its various specialties. The originals were exhibited at the National Library of Medicine in the summer of 1994.

19. Thomas, George and Schreiner, Lee: That's Incurable: The Doctor's Guide to Common Complaints, Rare Diseases, and The Meaning of Life.* New York: Penguin Books, 1984.

This is one of the funniest medical books to ever hit the stands. The authors counsel the reader on everything from "Ten Diseases You Were Better Off Not Knowing About" to "How to Get into the Hospital." (For a small taste of what the book is like, see the excerpt, "A Hypochondriac's Handbook" which was published in Esquire, March 1984, pp 81–88.)

*These books are no longer in print, but should be available through interlibrary loan.

Getting Humor Published in Medical Journals

Most of the humor that appears in the medical literature turns up sporadically as letters to the editor, anecdotes, essays, and parodies.[1] Although some journals publish humor more than others, getting something funny into a medical journal is always a little iffy. The person who determines the type of material a journal publishes is the editor. Not surprisingly, then, a journal's emphasis may change over time. For example, in the past *JAMA* published a number of columns that featured cartoons, anecdotes, poetry, humor, and satire (see p. xviii). At the present time, however, the only journal that features a column devoted to all types of medical humor is the *Journal of Family Practice* (Table). Nevertheless, a journal does not have to publish a regular column to accept humor. A brief look through the collection will show how many journals have published humor over the years.

How to Write Medical Humor

Although no one can teach you how to be funny, there are a number of steps you can follow to help turn an amusing idea into a finished product. With that in mind, here's a list of things to consider the next time your Muse drops in for a visit.

- Keep your eyes open for amusing anecdotes and stories you run into at work. Comedians extract humor from their daily lives and the newspapers. The same thing can be done in medicine.
- Write down your ideas for later use. William Carlos Williams, the famous doctor-poet, was known for jotting down ideas in between patients. While this might be difficult given today's medical demands, consider stealing a few moments during the day to record your thoughts and observations.
- If you were involved in follies during medical school, you might be able to recycle or update some of this material for current use.
- Anecdotes, letters, and verse are easier to write than full length articles. Therefore, consider starting out with one of these shorter forms. It's also easier to get this material accepted for publication.

Journals with Columns that Feature Humor & Satire*

Journal	Column	Comments
Annals of Internal Medicine	Ad Libitum	occasional humor
JAMA	A Piece of My Mind	occasional humor
Journal of Emergency Medicine	Humanities and Medicine	occasional humor
Journal of Family Practice	Humor in Medicine	monthly column
Lancet	Diverticulum	occasional humor
Obstetrics & Gynecology	After Office Hours	occasional humor
Postgraduate Medicine	Physician at Large	occasional humor
Survey of Ophthalmology	Time Oph	poetry

*Note: Some journals publish humor at specific times of the year as AJR does with its April issue (see p. 154) and the British Medical Journal does with its Christmas issue (see p. 149).

- Read (and study) the humor you find in this book and the journals you get on a regular basis. Reading is one of the best ways to get ideas for your own work.
- Read (and study) nonmedical humorists. People like Dave Barry, Garrison Keillor, Art Buchwald, etc. can both teach and inspire you to write. However, don't be intimidated by these folks—they are professionals and you're not. You don't have to write as well as they do to be funny or to get published.
- Determine which journals you would like to publish in.
- Review the type of humor they have published in the past.
- Don't forget to read the Instructions for Authors page. It doesn't help if you submit papers that contain stylistic errors.
- Write up your comic morsel and tailor it, if possible, for the intended audience. Some humor is too unique to conform to a journal's standard forms, and this should not inhibit you from writing the piece. It may make it a little harder to get accepted, however.

- Rewrite it 5–10 times.
- Rewrite it some more.
- Ask a colleague or two to read your article to get some feedback on what works and what doesn't. Keep in mind that what's funny to one person, may not be to another.
- Submit the article.
- Keep your fingers crossed.
- If rejected, take a deep breath and submit it to the next journal on your list. It's unsettling to have your work rejected, but there's no way around this if you're infected with the writer's bug. Just remember that being rejected does not mean a piece isn't good. The editor may have a different sense of humor than you do, or a piece like yours may not fit the editorial needs of the journal. The first edition of this book was rejected by fifteen publishers before it was accepted by Hanley & Belfus.
- If have trouble getting your work accepted by a national publication, try a state medical journal, a medical newspaper, or one of the non-medical journals listed in the section Additional Journals of Interest.
- Keep writing.

References

1. Bennett HJ: Humor in the medical literature. J Fam Pract 1995;40:334–336.

Humor in Serious Medical Articles

Hilarity and good humor . . . help enormously both in the study and in the practice of medicine.—William Osler[1]

For the most part, doctors write humor as a break from the serious side of medicine. Although humor is commonly used during lectures and other presentations, physicians rarely incorporate humor into their serious publications. Given the purpose of the medical literature, this is not surprising. When authors do rely on humor, it is usually to catch the reader's attention or to emphasize a specific point in the paper.[2] Since humor has the potential to facilitate teaching,[3-5] one could argue that it has a role, albeit a limited one, in serious medical publications. Because this is the least common expression of medical humor, I wanted to give readers a taste of how this is done. If anyone is aware of additional examples, please send them my way.

- William Bennett Bean had a penchant for incorporating light verse into his serious work (see p. 100).
- Henry Schneiderman wrote an article that addressed how we evaluate medical students during their clinical clerkships. Although his essay was serious, he included some humor to help make his point (see p. 46).
- Many physicians enjoy writing brief case reports about the *hazards* of daily living. These reports are frequently humorous (see p. 130).
- William Bornemeier wrote an article on hemorrhoidectomies many years ago that began with a humorous introduction (see p. 227).
- In some cases, authors use a light touch throughout an entire article as in a 1988 report about a patient who got her tongue stuck in a bottle.[6] When referring to a literature search on the topic, the authors quote the following fictitious study—"Quickknife IM: Surgical management of the tongue in bottle syndrome. J Medical Misadventures 1980;1:1 (first and last volume issued)."
- Some authors approach a serious topic with

an idea that is so clever you cannot help but smile. For example, in an effort to address society's changing attitudes toward a woman's ideal weight, the body types of mannequins were compared over a 70 year period.[7] This article appeared in the *British Medical Journal's* Christmas issue, which is known for publishing lighter medical articles (see p. 149).

- In some situations, authors use figures instead of text to make their point. For example, I have seen two articles that used the same humorous device. In both cases the authors covered the eyes of an illustration with a black bar to "conceal" its identity—one was a chimpanzee[8] and the other was a cat.[9] Although this is a simple device, it immediately catches the reader's eye and beckons you to read the article.
- Sydney Gellis, the editor of *Pediatric Notes*, is well known for including amusing quips that highlight his commentary on the pediatric literature. A few years ago, he reviewed an article where a husband and wife did some research on their son when he had chickenpox (they clothed him in specially made garments to test the theory that skin temperature affected the number of skin lesions). After he abstracted the article, Dr. Gellis added the following remark:

"This is a beautiful example of clinical research in the home. I keep wondering if the couple obtained informed consent."[10]

- In 1988, a plastic surgeon described a method for determining facial growth following the repair of unilateral cleft palates.[11] While his intent was serious, the author included a "rating scale" that was clearly tongue-in-cheek.
- Humor occasionally finds its way into books as well as journals. In *Nutrition During In-*

fancy, the authors replaced the traditional introduction with a series of illustrations that were amusing and informative.[12] Leo Gordon recently published a book on morbidity and mortality conferences which is a brilliant mix of humor and serious discourse.[13] When discussing the etiology of hepatitis, the following comment appeared in a textbook of pathology:

"It has been estimated that the chance of acquiring the infection from oysters is about 1 in 10,000; therefore, no more than 9,999 of these delicacies should be consumed in one sitting."[14]

- For additional examples culled from the medical literature, see the article by Richard Reece.[2]
- The final area to consider is satire. Although the line between humor and satire can blur at times, the author's intent with satire is more serious. Medical satire commonly appears in essays and editorials where the author uses irony or wit to make his point. Frederick Brancati writes brilliant medical satire (see pp. 26, 28, 47, 159). Other examples include articles that have lampooned medicare,[15] medicine's preoccupation with disease,[16] and the reporting of medical news.[17]

Although most medical humor turns up as essays, verse, and parodies, it occasionally works its way into serious publications. This material can surprise and delight. It also has the potential to make weighty information more palatable and might aid in our ability to retain what we read. However, like all types of humor, one must be careful about how and when it is used.

References

1. Bean WB: Sir William Osler's Aphorisms: From His Bedside Teachings and Writings. New York: Henry Schuman, Inc., 1950, p. 81.

2. Reece RL: Humor in scientific medical writing. Minn Med 1968;51:563–566.

3. Felson B: Humor and medicine. Semin Roentgen 1987;22:141–143.

4. White LA, Lewis DJ: Humor: a teaching strategy to promote learning. J Nurse Staff Devel 1990;6(2):60–64.

5. Leidy K: Enjoyable learning experiences—an aid to retention. J Contin Educ Nurs 1992;23:206–208.

6. Mills JC, Simon JE: Tongue in cheek? Or in bottle? Pediatr Emer Care 1988;4:119–120.

7. Rintala M, Mustajoki P: Could mannequins menstruate? BMJ 1992;305:1575–1576.

8. Simkin PA: Simian stance: a sign of spinal stenosis. Lancet 1982;2:652–653.

9. Montague LR: Cross species applicability of psychiatric diagnosis and treatment. BMJ 1989;299:1569.

10. Gellis SS: Modifying chickenpox. Pediatr Notes 1992;16:1.

11. Ross RB: Testing surgical success. Plast Reconst Surg 1988;82:921–922.

12. Tsang RC, Nichols BC: Nutrition During Infancy. Philadelphia: Hanley & Belfus, 1988.

13. Gordon LA: Gordon's Guide to the Surgical Morbidity and Mortality Conference. Philadelphia: Hanley & Belfus, 1994.

14. Robbins SL, Cotran RS, Kumar V: Pathologic Basis of Disease. Philadelphia: W.B. Saunders, 1984, p. 900.

15. Vosk A: New stratagems for dealing with Medicare's prospective payment system and other cost-containment measures. JAMA 1991;266:121–122.

16. Meador CK: The last well person. N Engl J Med 1994;330:440–441.

17. Reemtsma K, Maloney JV: The economics of instant medical news. N Engl J Med 1974;290:439–442.

Selected References on Humor & Medicine

1. Ackerman MH, Henry MB, Graham KM, et al: Humor won, humor too: a model to incorporate humor into the healthcare setting. Nurs Forum 1993;28(4):9–16.

2. Aring CD: A sense of humor. JAMA 1971;215: 2099.

3. Bean WB: Some notes of parodies. Arch Intern Med 1962;110:819–822.

4. Bennett HJ: Humor in the medical literature. J Fam Pract 1995;40:334–336.

4a. Bennett HJ: Using humor in the office setting: a pediatric perspective. J Fam Pract 1996;42:462–464.

5. Berk LS, Tan SA, Fry WF, et al: Neuroendocrine and stress hormone changes during mirthful laughter. Am J Med Sci 1989;298:390–6.

6. BeSaw L: Sick jokes—doctor, it hurts when I do this. Texas Med 1995;91(9):28–34.

7. Black DW: Laughter. JAMA 1984;252:2995–2998.

8. Blair W: What's funny about doctors. Perspect Biol Med 1977;21:89–98.

9. Burson-Tolpin A: A travesty tonight: satiric skits in medicine. Lit Med 1993;12(1):81–110.

10. Carlyon W, Carlyon P: Humor as a health education tool. In Lazes PM, Kaplan LH, and Gordon KA (eds): The Handbook of Health Education,* Rockville, MD, Aspen, 1987, pp 111–121.

11. Coombs RH, Chopra S, et al: Medical slang and its functions. Soc Sci Med 1993;36:987–998.

12. Coser RL: Some social functions of laughter: a study of humor in a hospital setting. Human Relations 1959;12(2):171–182.

12a. Coser RL: Laughter among colleagues: a study of the social functions of humor among the staff of a mental hospital. Psychiatry 1960;23:81–95.

13. Cousins N: Anatomy of An Illness (As Perceived by the Patient). New York: W.W. Norton, 1979.

14. Cushner FD, Friedman RJ: Humor and the physician. South Med J 1989;82:51–52.

15. D'Antonio IJ: The use of humor with children in hospital settings. In: McGhee P (ed): Humor and Children's Development: A Guide to Practical Applications.* New York: Haworth, 1989, pp. 157–171.

16. Editorial: The "sense" of humor—art and science. JAMA 1970;212:1697–1698.

17. Elliot-Binns CP: Laughter and medicine. J Royal Coll Gen Pract 1985;35:364–365.

18. Felson B: Humor and medicine. Semin Roentgen 1987;22:141–143.

19. Fishbein M: Medical hoaxes. Med World News 1972;13(13):52.

20. Fry WF: The physiologic effects of humor, mirth, and laughter. JAMA 1992;267:1857–8.

21. Garfield E: Humor in scientific journals and journals of scientific humor. Curr Contents 1976;(Dec 20):5–11.

22. Gilbert SF: Bacchus in the laboratory: in defense of scientific puns. Perspect Biol Med 1985;29:148–152.

23. Hunt AH: Humor as a nursing intervention. Cancer Nurs 1993;16:34–9.

24. Hunter KM: An N of 1: syndrome letters in The New England Journal of Medicine. Perspect Biol Med 1990;33:237–251.

25. Jarcho S: Some hoaxes in the medical literature. Bull Hist Med 1959;33:342–347.

Note: Dr. Jarcho also wrote under the psuedonym, S. N. Gaño. He has an article in the chapter "Odds & Ends" and a couple of "Additional Readings" in the book.

25a. Keeler ML: Memo. J Emer Med 1996;14:105–106. (This is an essay about humor in the E.R.—H.B.)

26. Kimmel PL: Francois Rabelais: satire as therapy for the body politic. The Pharos 1992;55(3):7–12.

27. King LS: New movie monsters from the medical world. JAMA 1972;220:90–91.

28. Klass P: Sick jokes. Discover 1987;Nov:30–35.

29. Klatz IM: Munchausen's syndrome: hoaxes, parodies, and tall tales in science and medicine. Perspect Biol Med 1992;36:139–154.

30. Klawans HL: Vaginismus and other medical satires. In The Medicine of History from Paracelsus to Freud.* New York, Raven Press, 1982, pp 167–180.

31. Lefcourt, Herbert M, and Martin, Rod A: Humor and Life Stress: Antidote to Adversity.* New York, Springer-Verlag, 1986.

32. Leiber DB: Laughter and humor in critical care. Dimens Crit Care Nurs 1986;5(3):162–170.

33. Leidy K: Enjoyable learning experiences—an aid to retention? J Continuing Educ Nursing 1992;23: 206–208.

34. Liechty RD. Humor and the surgeon. Arch Surg 1987;122:519–522.

*These books are no longer in print, but should be available through interlibrary loan.

35. Lindsey D, Benjamin J: Humor in the emergency room. In Mindess H, and Turek J (eds): The Study of Humor.* Los Angeles, Antioch College, 1979, pp 73–76.

36. Linn LS, DiMatteo MR: Humor and other communication preferences in physician—patient encounters. Medical Care 1983;21:1223–1231.

37. London SJ: The whimsy syndromes: the fine art of literary nosology. Arch Intern Med 1968;122:448–452.

38. Louros NC: Molière and medicine. International Surg 1978;63:71–74.

39. Madden T: Joking relationships. J Royal Coll Gen Pract 1986;36:197.

40. Mandell HN: Frivolity in medicine: Is there a place for it? Postgrad Med 1988;83(8):24–28.

41. Millar TP: Humor: the triumph of reason. Perspect Biol Med 1986;29:545–559.

42. Nelson DS: Humor in the pediatric emergency department: a 20-year perspective. Pediatrics 1992;89:1089–1090. (This article inspired a handful of letters that questioned the appropriateness of humor in medical settings. See Pediatrics 1993;91:680–681.)

43. Nezu AM, Nezu CM, et al: Sense of humor as a moderator of the relation between stressful events and psychological distress: a prospective analysis. J Pers Soc Psychol 1988;54(3):520–525.

44. Nilson DL: Medicine and physiology. In Humor Scholarship—A Research Bibliography. Westport, CT, Greenwood Press, 1993, pp 15–20.

45. Papper EM: Satire of medicine: the 18th century and beyond. J Royal Soc Med 1990;83:524–528.

46. Powell BS: Laughter and healing: the use of humor in hospitals treating children. J Assoc Care Child Hosp 1974;3(2):10–16.

47. Price PB, Lewis EG, et al: Attributes of a good practicing physician. J Med Educ 1971;46:229–237.

48. Rakel RE: Humor and humanism. Houston Med 1989;5(1):7–9.

49. Reece RL: Humor in scientific medical writing. Minn Med 1968;51:563–566.

50. Robinson VM: Humor is serious business. Dimens Crit Care Nurs 1986;5(3):132–133.

51. Robinson, Vera M: Humor and the Health Professions. Thorofare, NJ: Charles B. Slack Co., 1991.

52. Robinson VM: Humor and health. In McGhee, PE and Goldstein JH (eds): Handbook of Humor Research, Vol. 2.* New York, Springer-Verlag, 1983, pp 109–128.

53. Rodning CB: Humor and healing: a creative process. Pharos 1988;51(3):38–40.

54. Rohtbart M: Therapeutic humor: an interplay of physiology and people. Resid Staff Physician 1991;37(10):39–42.

55. Roland CG: Thoughts about medical writing: can it be funny and medical? Anesth Analg 1971;50:229–230.

56. Rosenberg L: A qualitative investigation of the use of humor by emergency personnel as a strategy for coping with stress. J Emer Nurse 1991;17:197–203.

57. Scarlett EP: Some hoaxes in medical history and literature. Arch Intern Med 1964;113:291–296.

58. Schwartz AJ, Black ER, et al: Levels and causes of stress among residents. J Med Educ 1987;62:744–753.

59. Segal D: Playing doctor seriously: graduation follies at an American medical school. Int J Health Serv 1984;14:379–396.

60. Silberman IN: Humor and health: an epidemiological study. Amer Behav Scientist 1987;30(3):100–112.

61. Silverstein S: Mixing humor with medicine. California Physician 1991;8(6):44–47.

62. Smith DP: Using humor to help children with pain. Child Health Care 1986;14:187–8.

63. Stevens H: Humor plus humility equals humaneness. JAMA 1964;190:88–91.

64. Thomas P: The anatomy of coping: medicine's funny bone. Med World News 1986;27(13):42–66.

65. Thorson JA, Powell FC: Sense of humor and dimensions of personality. J Clin Psychol 1993;49:799–809.

66. White LA, Lewis DJ: Humor: a teaching strategy to promote learning. J Nurse Staff Devel 1990;6(2):60–64.

67. Williams H: Humor and healing: therapeutic effects in geriatrics. Gerontion 1986;1(3):14–17.

68. Woodhouse DK: The aspects of humor in dealing with stress. Nurs Admin Q 1993;18:80–89.

INDEX

Note: Numbers in parentheses refer to citations in the Appendix or in one of the Additional Readings sections in the book. For example, reference 7 on page 155 will be listed as 155(7).

Wellness—*continued*
  humorous quotations, 37, 237
  last well patient, 174(15)
  NEJM spoof and, 179
Western Journal of Medicine,
    228(13)
Western Journal of Surgery, Obstetrics,
    *& Gynecology,** 119
*World Medicine,** 76
Writing and Publishing, 71–91. *See*

also Case Reports, Curriculum
    Vitae
  advice for authors, 90(1)
  book collecting, 66(4)
  book reviews in verse, 104
  case reports, 119–135
  editing a journal, 90(7)
  how to write medical humor, 269
  journal names, parody of, 7, 147,
    226, 255

  letters to the editor, spoof of, 79
  medico-literary tenesmus, 69
  multiple authorship, 73, 99, 113
  poem on, 114(10)
  poor writing, 88, 90(9,11), 98
  publication game, 76, 81, 90(5),
    156(13)
  rejected manuscripts, 90(2), 155(3)
  titles, spoof of, 71
  visual aids, 91(12)

*These journals are no longer being published.